Substance Abuse in the Mentally and Physically Disabled

Substance Abuse in the Mentally and Physically Disabled

edited by
John R. Hubbard and Peter R. Martin
Vanderbilt University Medical Center
Nashville, Tennessee

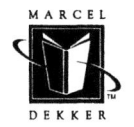

MARCEL DEKKER, INC. NEW YORK · BASEL

Library of Congress Cataloging-in-Publication Data

Substance abuse in the mentally and physically disabled / edited by John R. Hubbard, Peter R. Martin.
   p. cm.
   Includes index.
   ISBN 0-8247-0587-4 (alk. paper)
   1. Dual diagnosis. 2. Chronically ill—Substance use. I. Hubbard, J. R. (John R.) II. Martin, Peter R.

   RC564.68 .S83 2001
   616.86—dc21
                                                                    2001032419

This book is printed on acid-free paper.

Headquarters
Marcel Dekker, Inc.
270 Madison Avenue, New York, NY 10016
tel: 212-696-9000; fax: 212-685-4540

Eastern Hemisphere Distribution
Marcel Dekker AG
Hutgasse 4, Postfach 812, CH-4001 Basel, Switzerland
tel: 41-61-261-8482; fax: 41-61-261-8896

World Wide Web
http://www.dekker.com

The publisher offers discounts on this book when ordered in bulk quantities. For more information, write to Special Sales/Professional Marketing at the headquarters address above.

Copyright © 2001 by Marcel Dekker, Inc. All Rights Reserved.

Neither this book nor any part may be reproduced or transmitted in any form or by any means, electronic or mechanical, including photocopying, microfilming, and recording, or by any information storage and retrieval system, without permission in writing from the publisher.

Current printing (last digit):
10 9 8 7 6 5 4 3 2 1

PRINTED IN THE UNITED STATES OF AMERICA

In Memoriam

This book is dedicated to Pietro Castelnuovo-Tedesco, M.D., a dear friend who passed away on January 16, 1998. His contribution to this volume—retrieved from his briefcase by his wife, Lisbeth—represents the last contribution to psychiatry from this compassionate and fertile mind. He brings to us an erudite essay on how psychoanalytical theory may inform our approach to treatment of individuals who suffer from drug and alcohol dependence. He draws on a long career devoted to explorations in psychotherapy, psychoanalysis, and psychosomatic medicine. His contribution is all the more valuable as he addresses the issues of the alcohol- and drug-dependent patient, at our request, in what was for him a new area, elucidated by his extensive experience in delivering the highest quality of psychiatric care throughout a lifetime.

Before his death, Pietro Castelnuovo-Tedesco was the James D. Blackmore Professor of Psychiatry at Vanderbilt University School of Medicine and a supervising analyst in the St. Louis Psychoanalytic Institute. Prior to his arrival at Vanderbilt in 1975, he was Chairman of Psychiatry at Harbor General Hospital in Los Angeles and Professor of Psychiatry at UCLA School of Medicine. In addition to his leadership role in American psychoanalysis, he is perhaps best known for two seminal books: *The Twenty Minute Hour: A Guide to Brief Psychotherapy for the Physician* and *Psychiatric Aspects of Organ Transplantation*.

Preface

The important interrelationship between substance abuse and psychiatric or general medical illness has become increasingly clear from both clinical and scientific sources. Growing attention to this issue is evidenced by the establishment of subspecialties in addiction psychiatry and addiction medicine. This book provides current clinical, scientific and epidemiological information on the etiology, detection, pathology, and treatment of substance abuse patients who have a comorbid psychiatric or general medical disorder.

Substance Abuse in the Mentally and Physically Disabled is divided into there parts. Part 1 provides an overview. Assessment instruments, laboratory data, and major comorbidity epidemiological studies are discussed, in addition to general information on comorbidity. Part 2 is composed of six chapters on specific psychiatric illnesses (including anxiety, depression, bipolar disorder, schizophrenia, personality disorders, and mental disorders of childhood.) It also includes a chapter by Dr. Castelnuovo-Tedesco (now deceased) on psychoanalytically informed treatment of alcoholism. Part 3 comprises four chapters on substance abuse in special subpopulations of general medicine (including cardiovascular disease, HIV-related illnesses, chronic pain, and neurological disorders). In addition, a chapter on substance abuse in the elderly has been provided in light of the ever-increasing age of our population and in recognition of their special problems.

We wish to thank the many excellent chapter authors who contributed to this book. Distinguished scientists were recruited from numerous leading universities in the United States. It is our hope that the information and analysis contained in this text will be helpful to substance abuse clinicians, general medical doctors, medical specialists, clinical researchers, and basic scientists who are interested in this exciting and rapidly expanding field.

In addition, we are very grateful to the many administrative assistants who have helped make this book possible. Our deepest appreciation is also extended to our families, including Suzanne Hubbard, Tara Hubbard and Erin Hubbard, Barbara Martin, and Alec Martin for their inspiration, love, and support.

John R. Hubbard
Peter R. Martin

Contents

In Memoriam   *iii*
Preface   *v*
Contributors   *ix*

INTRODUCTION

1. Substance Abuse in the Mentally and Physically Disabled: An Overview   1
   John R. Hubbard and Peter R. Martin

SUBSTANCE ABUSE AND MENTAL HEALTH

2. Comorbidity of Anxiety Disorders in Substance Abuse   11
   Robert R. Swift and Timothy Mueller

3. Substance Abuse and Depression   33
   Lauren P. Lehmann, John R. Hubbard, and Peter R. Martin

4. Bipolar Disorder and Comorbid Substance Use Disorders   59
   Carlos A. Zarate, Jr., and Mauricio F. Tohen

5. Substance Abuse in Schizophrenia: Biological Factors Mediating Comorbidity and the Potential Role of Atypical Antipsychotic Drugs 77
Myung A. Lee and Herbert Y. Meltzer

6. Substance Abuse and Personality Disorders: The Impact of Three Personality Clusters on Prevalence, Course, and Treatment 103
Lisa A. Ottomanelli and Bryon Adinoff

7. Comorbid Mental Disorders in Adolescents with Substance Use Disorders 133
Duncan B. Clark and Jeanette Scheid

8. Comments on the Psychoanalytically Informed Treatment of Alcoholism 169
Pietro Castelnuovo-Tedesco

SUBSTANCE ABUSE AND PHYSICAL DISABILITIES

9. Cardiovascular Disease and Substance Use Disorders 179
Robert P. Albanese, Jr., W. Blake Haren, and John R. Hubbard

10. The Relationship of Substance Abuse to the Human Immunodeficiency Virus: Background and Management 203
Stephen A. Wyatt and Richard S. Schottenfeld

11. Chronic Pain and Substance-Related Disorders 241
John R. Hubbard and Edward A. Workman

12. Substance Dependence in the Elderly 265
Richard R. Irons and Donald E. Rosen

13. Neurological Disorders and Head Injuries 277
David D. Weinstein and Peter R. Martin

Index 307

Contributors

Bryon Adinoff, M.D. Department of Psychiatry, University of Texas Southwestern Medical Center, and VA North Texas Health Care System, Dallas, Texas

Robert P. Albanese, Jr., M.D. Departments of Psychiatry and Internal Medicine, Medical University of South Carolina, and Ralph H. Johnson VA Medical Center, Charleston, South Carolina

Pietro Castelnuovo-Tedesco, M.D.[†] Department of Psychiatry, Vanderbilt University School of Medicine, Nashville, Tennessee

Duncan B. Clark, M.D., Ph.D. Department of Psychiatry, Pittsburgh Adolescent Alcohol Research Center, and University of Pittsburgh, Pittsburgh, Pennsylvania

W. Blake Haren, M.D. Departments of Psychiatry and Internal Medicine, Medical University of South Carolina, and Ralph H. Johnson VA Medical Center, Charleston, South Carolina

---

[†]Deceased.

John R. Hubbard, M.D., Ph. D.* Division of Addiction Medicine, Department of Psychiatry, Vanderbilt University Medical Center, and Nashville VA Medical Center, Nashville, Tennessee

Richard R. Irons, M.D. Professional Renewal Center, Lawrence, Kansas

Myung A. Lee, M.D. Department of Psychiatry, Vanderbilt University Medical Center, Nashville, Tennessee

Lauren P. Lehmann, M.D. Department of Psychiatric Medicine, University of Virginia Health Sciences Center, and Salem VA Medical Center, Salem, Virginia

Peter R. Martin, M.D. Division of Addiction Medicine, Department of Psychiatry, Vanderbilt University Medical Center, Nashville, Tennessee

Herbert Y. Meltzer, M.D. Department of Psychiatry, Vanderbilt University Medical Center, Nashville, Tennessee

Timothy Mueller, M.D. Department of Psychiatry, Brown University Medical School, Providence, Rhode Island

Lisa A. Ottomanelli, Ph.D. Department of Psychiatry, University of Texas Southwestern Medical Center, and VA North Texas Health Care System, Dallas, Texas

Donald E. Rosen, M.D. Department of Psychiatry, Oregon Health Sciences University, Portland, Oregon

Jeanette Scheid, M.D., Ph.D. Department of Psychiatry, Pittsburgh Adolescent Alcohol Research Center, and University of Pittsburgh, Pittsburgh, Pennsylvania

Richard S. Schottenfeld, M.D. Department of Psychiatry, Yale University, New Haven, Connecticut

Robert Swift, M.D., Ph.D. Department of Psychiatry, Brown University Medical School, and ACOS for Research and Education, Providence VA Medical Center, Providence, Rhode Island

Mauricio F. Tohen, M.D., Dr.P.H. Eli Lilly Laboratories, Indianapolis, Indiana, and Consolidated Department of Psychiatry, Harvard Medical School, Boston, Massachusetts

---

*Currently in private practice.

Contributors

David D. Weinstein, M.D. Division of Addiction Medicine, Department of Psychiatry, Vanderbilt University Medicinal Center, Nashville, Tennessee

Edward A. Workman, M.D., Ed.D., F.A.A.P.M. Pain Medicine & Neuropsychiatry Associates of Tennessee, and Lakeshore Mental Health Institute, Knoxville, Tennessee

Stephen A. Wyatt, D.O.[*] Department of Psychiatry, Yale University, New Haven, Connecticut

Carlos A. Zarate, Jr., M.D. Mood and Anxiety Disorders Program, National Institute of Mental Health, National Institutes of Health, Bethesda, Maryland

---

[*]*Current affiliation*: Stonington Institute, North Stonington, Connecticut

1
Substance Abuse in the Mentally and Physically Disabled: An Overview

John R. Hubbard*
*Vanderbilt University Medical Center
and Nashville VA Medical Center
Nashville, Tennessee*

Peter R. Martin
*Vanderbilt University Medical Center
Nashville, Tennessee*

INTRODUCTION

Drug and alcohol abuse is an enormous societal problem due to individual suffering as well as associated disruption of families and communities through criminality and violence, lost productivity, and healthcare costs. The relationship between substance-related disorders and other psychiatric disorders or general medical illnesses is accordingly of significant interest. The medical profession readily recognizes the causal relationship between alcohol/drug abuse and certain devastating medical problems such as cirrhosis of the liver, HIV, stroke, and dementia. However, the importance of comorbid substance abuse and psychiatric disorders and the contribution of alcohol/drug abuse to

---

*Currently in private practice.

the management and outcome of chronic medical illnesses is only now starting to gain significant attention.

Until recently, substance abuse and comorbid psychiatric/medical problems were typically treated independently of each other. In recognition of how co-occurring illnesses can directly and indirectly have an impact on each other, current trends promote coordinated treatment of comorbid substance abuse, psychiatric, and general medical problems in order to optimize patient care and reduce cost. The recent establishment of "addiction psychiatry" as a subspecialty of psychiatry attests to the importance of simultaneously treating comorbid psychiatric and substance abuse problems.

In this chapter, we begin the discussion of comorbidity of substance abuse and psychiatric and/or medical problems by providing background information on substance abuse assessment tools and laboratory tests and reviewing some of the major epidemiological studies that are discussed in greater detail in the remainder of the book. The word "abuse" is used interchangeably in this chapter (and in other chapters in this volume) with "dependence" or "addiction" simply for the sake of convenience and in accordance with common usage. The reader is directed to the DSM-IV, in which a clear distinction between the terms "abuse" and "dependence" are made, but "addiction" is not defined (1).

ASSESSMENT INSTRUMENTS FOR SUBSTANCE ABUSE SCREENING

Patient questionnaires and laboratory tests are commonly used to screen for possible substance abuse problems. Several common questionnaire screening instruments include:

1. CAGE
2. Michigan Alcoholism Screening Test (MAST) or the Brief MAST
3. Drug Abuse Screening Test (DAST)
4. Alcohol Use Disorders Identification Test (AUDIT)
5. Alcohol Urge Questionnaire (AUQ)

Other questionnaires have also been developed to screen for substance abuse. In addition, many screening psychiatric and general medical questionnaires are available. It is important that screening tools detect any possible signs of substance abuse (high sensitivity, low specificity), but in so doing some patients may be inaccurately identified (false positives) who actually do not have a substance use disorder. Tests with greater specificity and a clinical evaluation should follow in management of those patients who are identified by screening tests.

The CAGE is a simple four-question verbal or written screen. C, A, G, and E represent symptoms of an alcohol problem (2): C = difficulty Cutting back alcohol consumption; A = others are Annoyed at your alcohol use; G = Guilt over alcohol use, and E = need for an alcohol Eye-opener in the morning. A score of two or more "yes" answers is considered a positive screen for probable alcoholism. This screen is well known, easy to use, and can be routinely used in both psychiatric and general medical settings.

The AUQ consists of eight questions concerning the current desire to drink alcohol (3). Each question is scored on a six-point scale, from "strongly disagree" to "strongly agree." The MAST is a more comprehensive self-administered questionnaire for diagnosing alcoholism (4,5). It consists of 25 simple yes or no questions. A score of 5–7 or more is indicative of alcoholism. The brief MAST, which consists of 10 questions and takes less time to use, is highly correlated with the complete 25-question MAST (6). The DAST is similar to the MAST, except that it is used to screen for drug abuse (4). It consists of 28 simple true or false questions. Internal reliability of the DAST has been reported to be about 0.92 or better (4). The AUDIT consists of 10 items associated with drinking behaviors, alcohol intake, and alcohol-related problems (7,8).

The more comprehensive instruments that have been developed are generally used for research purposes only. Two commonly used tools are the Structured Clinical Interview for DSM-IV Disorders (SCID) and the Psychiatric Research Interview for Substance and Mental Disorders (PRISM) (9). Their primary drawback is the extensive time and training needed to use these tools. The advantage of these validated diagnostic instruments is that the detailed substance abuse information obtained is combined with historical data related to comorbid psychiatric disorders, allowing for a more meaningful diagnostic formulation.

LABORATORY TESTS

Several laboratory tests are particularly useful for substance abuse assessment. Common markers for heavy drinking include gamma-glutamyl-transpeptidase (GGT), the liver function tests aspartate amino transferase and alanine aminotransferase, and carbohydrate-deficient transferrin (CDT) (10–12). GGT is a glycoprotein located in the membrane fraction of numerous tissues such as the liver, brain, kidney, and heart. Increases in serum GGT may be due to heptobiliary and pancreatic disease but can also result from heavy drinking with minimal hepatic cell injury. CDT is an abnormal form of serum transferin (12). Increased CDT is caused by a transferrin molecular deficiency in a terminal triglysaccharide associated with active alcohol abuse and resolves with abstinence (12). Since CDT is not typically elevated in hepatic disease alone, it is also a good measure of noncompliance with alcoholism treatment.

Urine drug screens (UDSs) provide important objective information about recent alcohol and drug use, but many drugs of abuse are not automatically detected and the clinician must be aware of the limitations of the particular laboratory he or she uses. In addition, drugs have very different elimination rates from the body, which can also influence interpretation of a positive UDS. For example, chronic use of cannabinoids can lead to cannabinoids being detected in a UDS weeks to even months after the last use of marijuana. Detection of urine dilution may suggest that a patient is trying to "beat" a UDS by diluting the urine with water or another liquid.

MAJOR COMORBIDITY EPIDEMIOLOGICAL STUDIES

Throughout this book references are made to several large population studies documenting the significant comorbidity of psychiatric disorders and substance use disorders. We describe here some background information on three of the most often quoted epidemiological studies on psychiatric comorbidity (9,13–15).

1. Epidemiological Catchment Area Survey (ECA) of 1984 (13)
2. National Comorbidity Survey (NCS) of 1994 (14)
3. National Longitudinal Alcohol Epidemiological Survey (NLAES) of 1996 (15)

The ECA gathered data from catchment areas in Baltimore, Los Angeles, St. Louis, Durham, and New Haven (9,13). The sample size was over 20,000, with a response rate of about 78%. Diagnoses were based on DSM-III criteria utilizing an instrument called the Diagnostic Interview Schedule (DIS) (9,16). "Current" (referring to a 6-month period prior to actual interview) and lifetime prevalence rates and the "co-occurrence" of multiple diagnoses were determined (9,13). The NCS provided data based on DSM-III-R diagnostic criteria. The sample size was over 8000, with a response rate of about 83% from a full national sample population (9,16). Interviews were conducted using the Michigan Modification of the Composite Intervention Diagnostic Interview (UM-CIDI). The NLAES focused largely on depression and alcohol and drug disorders (9,15). The over 40,000 people surveyed were from the general U.S. population; the response rate was approximately 89% (9,15). An interview tool called the Alcohol Use Disorder and Associated Disability Interview Schedule (AUDADIS) was used for eliciting the diagnostic criteria (9,17). These epidemiological studies have served as stimuli for more specific and detailed clinical and family studies of the relationship between substance abuse and other psychiatric disorders, and ultimately as the foundation for investigations of shared psychobiological features of these disorders.

OVERVIEW OF SUBSTANCE ABUSE AND PSYCHIATRIC/MEDICAL DISORDERS

The term "dual diagnosis" is often used to describe patients who meet diagnostic criteria for a substance use disorder and another axis I psychiatric disorder. It is in the diagnosis and treatment of the dually diagnosed patients that psychiatrists can make a special contribution by virtue of their knowledge and ability to treat relevant psychiatric disorders, substance abuse issues, and associated medical problems.

Substance-related disorders are the most common form of psychiatric illness, with a lifetime prevalence of about 17% to 27% (14). In addition, many other psychiatric disorders are very common in the general population. For example, the lifetime prevalence of depression and various anxiety disorders is about 5–17% and 25%, respectively (14,18). The lifetime prevalence for any psychiatric disorder (other than a substance-related disorder) is approximately 23–48% (14,18). Accordingly, even if no causal relationship existed between substance abuse and another psychiatric disorder, many patients may have comorbid conditions based on chance associations alone, and these could affect the treatment of these patient and their prognosis.

Data presented in this text (as well as anecdotal clinical experience) support the contention that the co-occurrence of substance abuse and other psychiatric problems extends beyond chance in many instances. Alcohol and illicit drugs have been shown in many studies to cause disturbances of mood, thought, and cognitive functions and affect interpersonal relationships. Thus, substance-related disorders can sometimes mimic other psychiatric illnesses. In addition, emotional and serious physical disabilities often appear to promote alcohol or illicit drug abuse/dependence as a form of inappropriate "self-medication."

The significant statistical association between substance-related and other psychiatric disorders in the general and several clinical populations (indicated by an odds ratio [OR] above 1) suggest that these disorders may be causally associated with one another. Some of the most powerful associations among substance use and other psychiatric disorders are shown below with lifetime odds ratios (9):

Alcohol use disorder and a drug use disorder; OR ≈ 6–13
Bipolar disorder, type I, and alcohol use disorder; OR ≈ 6
Bipolar disorder, type I, and a drug use disorder; OR ≈ 11
Bipolar disorder, type I, and any substance use disorder; OR ≈ 8
Bipolar disorder, type I, and an alcohol use disorder; OR ≈ 6
Schizophrenia and an alcohol use disorder; OR ≈ 4
Schizophrenia and a drug use disorder; OR ≈ 6
Affective disorder and any substance use disorder; OR ≈ 3
Major depressive disorder and a cannaboid use disorder; OR ≈ 5
Major depressive disorder and an alcohol use disorder; OR ≈ 3–4
Major depressive disorder and a cocaine use disorder; OR ≈ 5
Substance use disorder and schizophrenia; OR ≈ 4
Nonaffective psychosis and an alcohol use disorder; OR ≈ 2
Nonaffective psychosis and a drug use disorder; OR ≈ 3
Posttraumatic stress disorder and a substance use disorder; OR ≈ 3
Phobias and substance use disorder; OR ≈ 2

These strong statistical associations underline our contention that substance abuse patients require evaluation and treatment for psychiatric comorbidity and that general psychiatric patients should be comprehensively evaluated for substance abuse problems and receive treatment, as indicated. In addition, in order to gain a better understanding of psychiatric disorders in general, it is important not to overlook dually diagnosed patients as an important clinical research population. Detailed discussions about the existence and implications of associations between individual psychiatric disorders and substance abuse are provided in specific chapters of this book.

Physical disability causes adverse effects on a patient's daily routine, self-image, and ability to work and to interact socially (19). Such consequences of physical disability can greatly enhance the risk of alcohol/drug abuse and dependence. In addition, although the cause of a patient's clinical morbidity or mortality may be documented as traumatic injury, AIDS, cirrhosis, heart failure, or other medical problems, closer investigation will often show that the given illness or injury was actually caused or greatly exacerbated by substance abuse. For example, it has been reported that nearly 80% of rehabilitation patients have alcohol-related injuries (20). In addition, about 50% of motor vehicle deaths, 35% of motor vehicle injuries, 30% of noncommercial airplane crashes, and 40% of drownings are associated with alcohol use (20). Emergency room data indicate positive blood alcohol levels in about 30–60% of head injury patients (19,21–23). In a 1989 investigation of over 100 spinal cord injury patients, nearly 40% were intoxicated with alcohol when they were injured (24). Other studies on spinal cord injury patients reported intoxication levels ranging from 17 to 79% (19,25). Injury due to hypothermia is also frequently alcohol-related. In one study of over 1000 patients with frostbite, 405 had associated alcohol intoxication (26). Much less data exist on drug (nonalcohol) associated injuries. Studies suggest that about 9–18% of injuries are related to intoxication with drugs other than alcohol (19,27).

It has been recognized for many years that many general medical problems are caused by chronic abuse of alcohol and/or other drugs. However, coordinated treatment of the medical and the substance abuse disorders has frequently been overlooked. Treatment of acute medical/surgical problems without treating the underlying substance abuse (and perhaps comorbid psychiatric disorder) will often lead to repeated cycles of hospitalization and progressive worsening of the patient's medical condition. An example of recent coordinated efforts in substance abuse and medical management has been the mandatory treatment of alcoholism or drug dependence in appropriate surgical patients awaiting a liver transplant.

A recent study by Moore and Li (28) evaluated illicit drug use in over 1800 people with physical disabilities. They found high rates of illicit drug use in this population, including 16% marijuana abuse in the past year and 9% in the past month, 3% cocaine abuse in the past year and 19% lifetime, 7% lifetime heroin abuse, 16% lifetime hallucinogen abuse, and 10% lifetime inhalant abuse. As in the general population, illicit drug use was often associated with male gender, younger age, and low income (29). Use of illicit drugs by a "best friend" increased risk of drug use, with a represented odds ratio (OR) of about 8.

Substance abuse problems may interfere with physical recovery and rehabilitation (19). For example, the lack of knowledge about alcohol or drug dependence can result in unexplained agitation, drug craving, and even withdrawal symptoms (19). Several studies confirm increased medical complications during recovery of alcoholics (25,28–30). Emotional healing may also be delayed in alcohol and drug abusers, especially if drug-related acts contributed to the psychic or physical trauma (19,31). Patients with a history of alcohol abuse were found to participate less actively in vocational, rehabilitation, and educational activities and programs than otherwise similar patients in a study of over 100 spinal cord injury subjects (24).

The remaining chapters in this book discuss some of the important medical/surgical illnesses (such as chronic pain, AIDS, neurological illness, and heart disease) that may be most closely associated with alcohol and drug abuse. A chapter on substance abuse and aging has also been included since aging has an increasingly greater impact on the physical health and behavior of these patients. Fittingly, the book ends with a discussion by Pietro Castelnuovo-Tedesco, M.D. (to whom this book is dedicated), of the psychodynamic principles that should guide the treatment of the *individual patient* with substance use disorder whether or not this co-occurs with medical/surgical or other psychiatric problems.

REFERENCES

1. American Psychiatric Association. Diagnostic and Statistical Manual of Mental Disorders. 4th ed. Washington, DC: American Psychiatric Press, 1994.
2. JA Ewing. Detecting alcoholism: the CAGE questionnaire. JAMA 252:1905–1907, 1984.
3. MT Boher, DD Krahn, BA Staehler. Development and initial validation of a measurement of drinking urges in abstinent alcoholics. Alcoholism: Clin Exp Res 19:600–606, 1995.
4. LC Morey, PR Martin. In: Measuring Mental Illness: Psychometric Assessment for Clinicians. S Wetzler, ed. Washington, DC: American Psychiatric Press, pp 163–181, 1989.
5. ML Selzer. The Michigan Alcoholism Screening Test: the quest for a new diagnostic instrument. Am J Psychiatry 127:89–94, 1971.
6. AD Pokerny, BA Miller, HB Kaplan. The brief MAST: a shortened version of its Michigan Alcoholism Screening Test. Am J Psychiatry 129:118–121, 1972.
7. TF Babor, JR De La Fuente, JB Saunders, M Grant. AUDIT: The Alcohol Use. Disorders Identification Test, Guidelines for Use in Primary Healthcare. Geneva: World Health Organization, 1989.
8. JB Saunders, OG Aasland, TF Babor, JR De La Fuente, M Grant. Development of the Alcohol Use Disorders Identification Test (AUDIT): WHO collaborative project on early detection of partners with harmful alcohol consumption. II. Addiction 88:791–804, 1993.
9. DS Hasin, EV Nunes. Comorbidity of alcohol, drug, and psychiatric disorders: epidemiology. In Dual Diagnoses in Treatment. HR Kranzler, BJ Rounsaville, eds. New York: Marcel Dekker, pp 1–30, 1998.
10. RZ Litten, JP Allen, JB Fertig. Gamma-glutamyl transpeptidose and carbohydrate deficient transferrin: alternative measure of excessive alcohol consumption. Alcoholism Clin Exp Res 19:1541–1547, 1995.
11. AA Mihas, M Tavassoli. Laboratory markers of ethanol intake and abuse: a critical appraisal. Am J Med Sci 303:415–428, 1992.

12. RF Anton, DH Moak, P Latham. Carbohydrate-deficient transferrin or an indicator of drinking status during a treatment outcome study. Alcoholism: Clin Exp Res 20:841–847, 1996.
13. D Regier, J Myers, M Kramer, L Robins, D Blazer, R Uhough, et al. The NIMH Epidemiologic Catchment Area program. Arch Gen Psychiatry 41:934–941, 1984.
14. R Kessler, K McGonagle, S Zhav, et al. Lifetime and 12 month prevalence of DSM-III R psychiatric disorders in the United States: results from the National Comorbidity Survey. Arch Gen Psychiatry 51:8–19, 1994.
15. B Grant, M Pickering. Comorbidity between DSM-IV alcohol and drug use disorders: results from the National Longitudinal Alcohol Epidemiologic survey. Rockville, MD: National Institute on Alcohol Abuse and Alcoholism, 1994.
16. L Robins, J Helzer, K Ratcliff, W Seyfired. Validity of the Diagnostic Interview Schedule, version II DSM-III diagnosis. Psychology Med 12:855–870, 1982.
17. B Grant, D Hasin. The Alcohol Use Disorders and Associated Disabilities Interview Schedule, Rockville, MD: Watson Institute in Alcohol Abuse and Alcoholism, 1992.
18. HR Kranzler, B Mason, V Modesto-Lowe. Prevalence, diagnosis, and treatment of comorbid mood disorders and alcoholism. In: Dual Diagnosis and Treatment. HR Kranzler, BJ Rounsaville, eds. New York: Marcel Dekker, pp 107–136, 1998.
19. JR Hubbard, AS Everett, MA Khan. Alcohol and drug abuse in patients with physical disabilities. Am J Surg Alcohol Abuse 22:215–231, 1996.
20. SN Applegate, WP Arnold, RJ Canterbury III, JH Duffee, WL Fang, GF Grossman, SJ Grossman, JL Krag, JL Lohr, JA Morse, JH Pryor, DE Smith, University of Virginia Health Sciences Center PROJECT SAGE. In: Substance Abuse Curriculum for Medical Students, Housestaff and Physicians in Primary Care. JA Lohr, RJ Canterbury III, WL Fang, eds. Charlottesville, VA: University of Virginia, pp IV-14–15, 1990.
21. FR Sparadeo, D Strauss, JT Barth. The incidence, impact, and treatment of substance in head trauma rehabilitation. J Head Trauma Rehabil 5(2):1–8, 1990.
22. B Brismar, A Engstrom, U Rydberg. Head injury and intoxication: a diagnostic and therapeutic dilemma. Acta Chirung Scand, 149:11–14, 1982.
23. F Sparadeo, D Gill. Effects of prior alcohol use on head injury recovery. J Head Trauma Rehabil 4(1):75–82, 1989.
24. AW Heinemann, N Goranson, K Ginsburg, S Schnoll. Alcohol use and activity patterns following spinal cord injury. Rehabil Psychol, 34(3):191–205, 1989.
25. JJ O'Donnell, JE Cooper, JE Gessner, I Shehan, J Ashley. Alcohol drugs and spinal cord injury. Alcohol Health Res World 82:27–29, 1981.
26. BJ Miller, LR Chasmar. Frostbite in Saskatoon: a review of 10 winters. Can J Surg, 23(5):423–426, 1980.

27. JB Parkerson, Z Taylor, JP Flynn. Brain injured patients: comorbidities and ancillary medical requirements. MMJ 39(3):259–262, 1990.
28. D Moore, L Li. Prevalence and risk factors of illicit drug use by people with disabilities. Am J Addiction 7:93–102, 1998.
29. SW Glenn, OA Parsons, L Stevens. Effects of alcohol abuse and familial alcoholism in physical health in men and women. Health Psychol 8(3):325–341, 1989.
30. GJ Jurkovich, FP Rivara, JG Gurney, C Fligner, R Ries, BA Mueller, M Copass. The effect of acute alcohol intoxication and chronic alcohol abuse on outcome of trauma. JAMA 270(1):51–56, 1993.
31. JJ O'Donnell, JE Cooper, JE Gessner, I Shehan, J Ashley. Alcohol, drugs and spinal cord injury. Alcohol Health Res World 82:27–29, 1981.

2
Comorbidity of Anxiety Disorders in Substance Abuse

Robert Swift
*Brown University Medical School
and Providence VA Medical Center
Providence, Rhode Island*

Timothy Mueller
*Brown University Medical School
Providence, Rhode Island*

INTRODUCTION

Anxiety disorders and addictive disorders are common problems and therefore are encountered regularly by health care practitioners of all disciplines. The anxiety and addictive disorders coexist at a rate greater than chance, suggesting that the etiology of the two types of disorders may be linked. Patients with both disorders provide a particular challenge for clinicians. In these patients, treatment interventions must be integrated to consider both disorders. This chapter provides information on the assessment and treatment of patients with anxiety and substance use disorders.

DEFINITIONS AND DIAGNOSES
Anxiety Disorders

Anxiety is a universal human experience. Loosely defined, anxiety is a sensation of uneasiness, worry, or apprehension about future events, actions, or uncertainties. In spite of its universality, for some individuals, the anxiety can occur in situations not usually considered anxiety-provoking or the intensity of anxiety becomes debilitating. Such individuals are considered to have an "anxiety disorder." Several types of anxiety disorders are described in the fourth edition of the American Psychiatric Association's *Diagnostic and Statistical Manual of Mental Disorders* (DSM-IV) (1). The most common of these anxiety disorders are described in Table 1. Anxiety disorders are extremely common in the population, with an overall lifetime prevalence rate of 24.9%.

Table 1. DSM-IV Anxiety Disorders

Generalized anxiety disorder
 Characterized by persistent, excessive worrisome thoughts and tension about everyday routine life events and activities, lasting at least 6 months. Almost always anticipating the worst even though there is little reason to expect it; accompanied by physical symptoms, such as fatigue, trembling, muscle tension, headache, or nausea.
Phobias (simple, social, agoraphobia)
 Characterized by persistently recurring, irrational, severe anxiety of specific objects, activities, and situations, with avoidance of the phobic stimulus. Two major types of phobias are specific phobia and social phobia. People with *specific phobia* experience extreme, disabling, and irrational fear of something that poses little or no actual danger, such as certain animals, the dark, heights; the fear leads to avoidance of objects or situations and can cause people to limit their lives unnecessarily. People with *social phobia* have an overwhelming and disabling fear of scrutiny, embarrassment, or humiliation in social situations, which leads to avoidance of many potentially pleasurable and meaningful activities.
Panic disorder (with and without agoraphobia)
 Sudden overwhelming feeling of terror and apprehension with marked physiological responses produced by a benign situation. Panic disorder may occur with and without agoraphobia, a term that literally means, "fear of the marketplace" and refers to the fact that crowded places may precipitate panic attacks for some persons and leads to avoidance of public places and social withdrawal.
Obsessive-compulsive disorder
 Obsessional thoughts that are impossible to stop or to control associated with severe anxiety. The individual engages in idiosyncratic compulsive behaviors and rituals that are necessary to reduce the anxiety.
Posttraumatic stress disorders (acute, delayed, and chronic)
 A state of anxiety and distress secondary to a catastrophic emotional event, outside of the realm of normal human experience, such as a physical or sexual assault or natural disaster. Nightmares, flashbacks, numbing of emotions, depression; feeling angry, irritable, and distracted; and being easily startled are common.

Source: Adapted from Ref. 1.

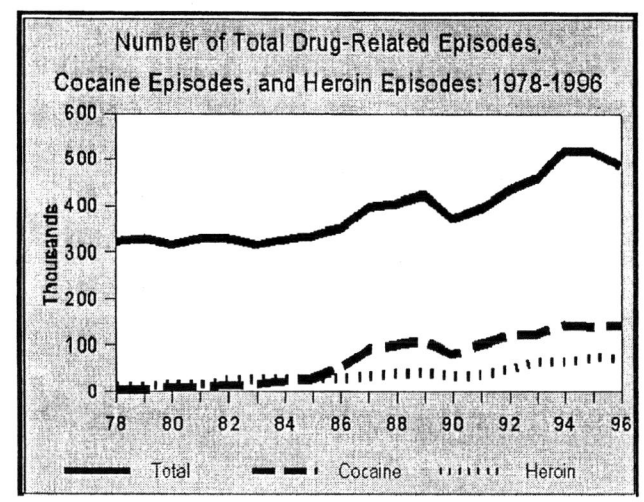

Figure 1 Estimated prevalence of any illicit drug use in the past month (1974–1995)

Source: Substance Abuse and Mental Health Services Administration. Office of Applied Studies. National Household Survey.
Note: Estimates with low precision or years with no estimates reported are excluded.

In addition to its occurrence as a distinct disorder, anxiety may occur *secondary* to other mental or physical disorders. For example, anxiety symptoms are common in psychotic disorders, such as schizophrenia, and in affective disorders, such as major depression and bipolar disorder. Several medical illnesses may engender or mimic anxiety disorders as well. Mitral valve prolapse can produce mental and physical symptoms that may be indistinguishable from a panic attack. Endocrine disorders, including hyperthyroidism, Cushing's disease, pheochromocytoma, and hypoglycemia, sometimes present with anxiety symptoms. Anemia, migraine, epilepsy, and organic brain syndromes can also be associated with significant anxiety signs and symptoms.

Substance Use Disorders

The use of psychoactive substances is also common. However, when drug or alcohol use becomes excessive, is uncontrolled, and continues to be used in spite of adverse social, psychological, or medical consequences, the users are considered to have a "substance use disorder." In DSM-IV, the acute effects of psychoactive substances are classified under two major categories: substance use disorders and substance-induced disorders. Substance-induced disorders include the behavioral and neurological effects of acute and chronic drug use. These are "substance intoxication," "substance withdrawal," "substance-induced psychotic disorder," "substance-induced mood disorder," "substance-induced anxiety," "substance-induced sleep disorder," "substance-induced persisting dementia (and amnestic) disorders," and "substance-induced sexual dysfunction."

The two substance use disorders are "substance dependence" and "substance abuse." These describe behavioral symptoms and maladaptive behaviors resulting from the acute or chronic effects of the drug (see Table 2). DSM-IV describes 11 distinct classes of psychoactive substances associated

Table 2. Characteristics of Substance Dependence and Substance Abuse

Psychoactive *substance dependence* is defined by the presence of at least three of the following, persisting over a 12-month period:

1. Tolerance occurs; that is, there is a need for increasing amounts of the substance in order to achieve intoxication or other desired effect.
2. Characteristic withdrawal symptoms (may not apply to cannabis, hallucinogens, or PCP), or the use of the substance (or a closely related substitute) to relieve or avoid withdrawal.
3. The substance is taken in larger amounts or over a longer period of time than the person intended.
4. There is a persistent desire or one or more unsuccessful attempts to cut down or to control substance use.
5. A great deal of time is spent in activities necessary to get the substance (e.g., theft), taking the substance (e.g., chain-smoking), or recovering from its effects.
6. Social, occupational, or recreational activities are given up or reduced because of substance use.
7. There is continued use despite knowledge of having a persistent or recurrent social, psychological, or physical problem that is caused by or exacerbated by use of the substance.

The term *substance abuse* is a residual category that describes patterns of drug use that do not meet the criteria for "dependence." Substance abuse is a pattern of substance use of at least 1 month's duration that causes clinically significant impairment. This may include impairments in social, family, or occupational functioning, use in the presence of a psychological or physical problem, or use in situations in which use of the substance is physically hazardous, such as driving while intoxicated or using alcohol in spite of knowledge of cirrhosis.

Source: Adapted from Ref. 1.

Anxiety Disorders

with abuse and dependence: alcohol; amphetamine and related substances; caffeine; cannabis; cocaine; hallucinogens; inhalants; opioids; nicotine; phencyclidine and related substances; and sedatives, hypnotics, and anxiolytics. Ten of these classes (all but nicotine) are associated with abuse and dependence; dependence only is defined for nicotine. "Polysubstance dependence" is defined as using three or more categories of substances. The category "Other Substance Use Disorders" includes use of anabolic steroids, nitrate inhalants, anticholinergic agents, and other psychoactive substances. Substance use disorders are the most prevalent psychiatric disorders, with a 26.6% lifetime prevalence rate according to population surveys. Table 3 compares the overall lifetime prevalence rate of substance use disorders to those of other psychiatric disorders.

The Comorbidity of Anxiety Disorders and Substance Use Disorders

Strictly speaking, the term comorbidity signifies the co-occurrence of any two diagnoses. In psychiatry, comorbidity usually refers to the co-occurrence of a major psychiatric disorder, such as schizophrenia or major depression, and any

Table 3. Lifetime Prevalence Rates for Substance Use Disorder Comorbidity with Selected Mental Health Disorders

	Lifetime prevalence (%)	Lifetime prevalence with comorbid substance use disorder (%)	Odds ratio[a]
Any substance use disorder	16.7	—	—
No mental disorder	77.5	13.2	1.0
Any mental health disorder other than a substance use disorder	22.5	28.9	2.7
Schizophrenia	1.4	47.0	4.6
Major depression	5.9	27.2	1.9
Any anxiety disorder	14.6	23.7	1.7
Panic disorder	1.6	35.8	2.9

[a]Odds ratios are calculated for comorbid risk compared to a nonaffected population, i.e., a population without the diagnosis in the row.
Source: Adapted from Ref. 6.

other major psychiatric disorder, such as a substance use disorder, also coded on Axis I of the DSM-IV multiaxial diagnostic system. The term "dual diagnosis" is a popular designation also used to indicate the co-occurrence of major psychiatric disorders and substance use disorders. The anxiety disorders in general, and panic disorder in particular, co-occur with substance use disorders at rates that exceed their association by chance.

Surveys of patients in substance abuse treatment show increased rates of anxiety disorders (2,3) and surveys of psychiatric patients with anxiety disorders show increased rates of substance use disorders (4,5). However, these samples could be biased, because data derived from treatment samples may represent more severely ill patients who enter treatment. However, two national surveys of psychiatric disorders in the general population also showed increased comorbidities between anxiety disorders and substance use disorders. The National Institute of Mental Health Epidemiologic Catchment Area Program (ECA) survey estimated the rates of psychiatric disorders in the U.S. population through its structured interviews of 20,291 people in five areas of the country. The ECA findings detail the comorbidity of mental disorders with substance use disorders (6). Overall, those with any anxiety disorder had a 70% greater likelihood of also having a substance use disorder (odds ratio = 1.7). Those with obsessive-compulsive disorder and panic disorder were most likely to also have a substance use disorder, with odds rations ranging from 2.5 to 4.4, depending on the specific substance. Table 3 summarizes the findings with special attention to panic disorder.

The U.S. National Comorbidity Survey (NCS), a household survey of 5877 respondents aged 15–54 years conducted between September 1990 and February 1992, also found similar increases in risks for alcohol and drug dependence in the presence of anxiety disorders (7)—19.4% of individuals with alcohol abuse or dependence and 28.3% of individuals with drug abuse or dependence had comorbid anxiety disorders.

Theories for the Comorbidity of Anxiety Disorders and Substance Use Disorders

There are several theories to explain the relationship between anxiety disorders and substance use disorders. The self-medication hypothesis of addiction holds that persons with psychiatric disorders preferentially use psychoactive substances to treat their dysphoric states (8). In the case of anxiety disorders, the experience of intense anxiety can be so unpleasant that persons so afflicted tend to avoid situations that trigger the anxiety and do whatever they can to reduce it when it does occur. Some self-administer drugs and/or alcohol to reduce their acute anxiety and distress. Although these substances may initially provide relief, their addictive nature ultimately leads to comorbid abuse and dependence and greater stress in their lives.

It has been proposed that comorbid anxiety disorders and substance use disorders may derive from a common, shared factor (9). Because both anxiety and substance use disorders cluster within families, it has been suggested that the disorders have a common genetic predisposition (10). For example, in families having members with panic disorder and agoraphobia, first-degree relatives are at three times greater risk for alcoholism, compared to families not having these disorders. However, family studies in this area also suggest specificity in the association between anxiety disorders and substance use disorders; there is only a slightly greater than average risk of alcoholism in the relatives of family members with panic disorder without agoraphobia.

The similarity between the symptoms of anxiety disorders and drug intoxication or withdrawal has suggested that common neurobiological mechanisms may lead to relationships between these groups of disorders (11). Central noradrenergic systems become activated during both panic and withdrawal. Many substance withdrawal syndromes (e.g., alcohol withdrawal, sedative withdrawal, and opioid withdrawal) are associated with intense anxiety and are often treated clinically with anxiolytic medications, including adrenergic blockers. Individuals who develop primary substance use disorders commonly develop anxiety and panic symptoms secondary to their drug or alcohol use (12). Intoxication with cocaine, stimulants, or caffeine frequently produces significant anxiety. Drug craving, defined as a strong urge to use the drug, is commonly associated with significant anxiety (13).

The Primary-Versus-Secondary Distinction

Historically, comorbid anxiety and substance use disorders were categorized as being primary or secondary disorders, based on the age of onset of one disorder in relation to the other. Thus, if an individual's substance dependence began at age 16 and his anxiety disorder at age 21, he could be considered as having a primary substance dependence disorder and a secondary panic disorder. In DSM-IV nomenclature, such a patient is considered as having substance dependence and a "substance-induced" anxiety disorder. Conversely, a patient with an anxiety disorder that preceded the onset of comorbid substance dependence would be considered to have a primary anxiety disorder. By this logic, the order of onset offers a suggestive causal relationship. If primary panic disorder is seen in patients with comorbid substance dependence, it would suggest that the psychoactive substance is used to treat panic symptoms. Alternatively, the drug would appear to be the cause of panic disorder if only secondary panic is seen. Primary and secondary distinctions may also be useful in predicting long-term outcomes and determining optimal treatment. There is some evidence that anxiety symptoms may abate over time in patients with primary alcohol dependence and secondary anxiety. However, in practice, determining the temporal relationship between the disorders is often difficult, particularly if the course of both disorders is chronic and long-standing and the patient is a poor historian.

In the case of alcohol, there exist empirical data to suggest that consistent temporal relationships between substance use disorders and anxiety disorders exist for some disorders or for certain individuals. A recent review on the comorbidity of alcohol abuse and anxiety disorders notes that simple panic disorder has no consistent relationship to the onset of alcohol abuse, whereas panic with agoraphobia usually precedes the onset of alcoholism (7). This temporal relationship suggests that alcohol abuse may not have a causal relationship to uncomplicated panic, whereas patients with panic and agoraphobia may use alcohol to self-medicate.

However, other studies find no definite temporal relationships between the disorders. The Harvard Anxiety Research Project (HARP) recruited 711 patients into a longitudinal outcomes study and identified 181 patients with anxiety disorder who also had a history of a substance use disorder. Subjects whose anxiety disorder had an onset before their substance use disorder (primary anxiety), compared with those whose substance use preceded onset of an anxiety disorder (secondary anxiety), did not have different ages of onset for substance use disorder, nor was there greater likelihood for choosing alcohol for any of the anxiety disorders (14). It was noted that there is a lower risk of alcohol use in the small group of generalized anxiety subjects and a greater risk of opioid use in the small group of posttraumatic stress disorder subjects.

TREATMENT

Treatment Outcomes for Anxiety and Substance Use Disorders

Anxiety disorders and substance use disorders both result in considerable morbidity, mortality, social problems, and high healthcare costs. Anxiety disorders, especially panic disorder, are associated with high utilization of health services and high costs to society (15,16). It has been estimated that the annual costs to the U.S. economy from anxiety disorders approaches $63 billion and from drug and alcohol abuse and dependence $98 billion. Of the latter, almost $10 billion is attributed to direct healthcare costs.

In general, the presence of comorbid anxiety and substance use leads to worse clinical outcomes for dual diagnosis patients than for patients with single disorders (17). It is generally held that it is the overall degree of psychopathology rather than the specific diagnosis that foretells more unfavorable treatment and psychosocial outcomes for these patients (18,19). One major clinical outcome of concern that is more likely in patients with panic disorder and alcohol or drug abuse is suicide (20). The ECA data convincingly corroborated earlier evidence that suicide attempts are more common in subjects with panic disorder than in subjects with any other psychiatric diagnosis and no psychiatric diagnosis, with odds ratios of 2.62 and 12.18, respectively. This risk was even greater in panic patients who were comorbid for alcohol or drug abuse, with odds ratios of 3.28 and 4.03, respectively, compared to panic patients without the comorbidity.

While some of the poorer clinical outcomes in dual diagnosis patients may result from greater psychopathology, at least part of the outcome must be blamed on the existing treatment system. In many situations, treatment facilities focus primarily on treating mental disorders or substance use disorders and have difficulty accommodating and treating patients with dual disorders. Third-party insurers that manage care and pay for treatment frequently have different treatment-necessity criteria for the various classes of disorders. Thus, dual diagnosis patients can easily "fall through the cracks" and receive suboptimal treatment. A recent Treatment Improvement Protocol (TIP) for dual disorders identifies these issues and suggests solutions (21).

Overview of Treatment

The most effective way to reduce the medical, social, and psychological impact of mental disorders, including addictive disorders, is through effective treatment. Clinical treatment outcome studies with anxiety disorders and addictive disorders have demonstrated that treatment can be effective. The optimal goal of treatment should be remission of anxiety symptoms and abstinence from psychoactive substances with addictive potential. Patients benefit from effective treatment by having the quality of their lives improved, their morbidity minimized, and their lives prolonged. Research studies have demonstrated that effective treatment of anxiety disorders and addictive disorders is also cost-effective. In the CALDATA Study of addiction treatment, approximately $7 was saved for every dollar invested in treatment (22). Likewise, reviews of published studies on the treatment of anxiety disorders find significant savings in total healthcare costs when effective anxiety disorder treatments are available. However, since these conditions are chronic, relapsing disorders, treatment may not be completely effective or may require multiple treatment episodes before a successful outcome is achieved.

Clinicians treating patients with comorbid anxiety and substance use disorders should possess knowledge about both disorders and interactions between the disorders and potential treatments. From the anxiety disorders perspective, this includes behavioral and pharmacological therapies for the management of anxiety. From the addictive disorders perspective, this requires knowledge of therapies for the acute management of intoxication and withdrawal, as well as knowledge regarding long-term treatment and rehabilitation. An overall biopsychosocial approach to treatment is preferred. A treatment plan should be based on scientific evidence of treatment efficacy but individualized as necessary, to match the patient to the best modality of treatment for the type and severity of the problems. The ability of the clinician to work with professionals from other disciplines is important, as treatment often involves other family members, legal and forensic systems, public assistance services, schools, and child-protection agencies. Although treatment of dual diagnosis patients can present challenging issues for the clinician, a flexible combination of psychotherapeutic/behavioral, social, and judicious pharmacological therapies can be successful in most patients.

Components of Treatment

While specific treatment options for patients with comorbid psychiatric and addictive disorders may depend on whether they present to a medically oriented, substance abuse–oriented, or mental health–oriented treatment system, there are commonalties among all the treatment systems. Treatment usually consists of the following components, listed in the Table 4.

Table 4. Phases of Treatment According to Mental Health and Substance Abuse Treatment Models

Phase of treatment	Mental health model	Substance abuse model
Assessment	Diagnosis	Initiation of treatment
Initial intervention	Stabilization, symptom reduction	Detoxification
Consolidation	Induction of remission	Rehabilitation
Long-term	Maintenance	Aftercare

Assessment and Diagnosis: Diagnosis, Initiation of Treatment, and/or Referral

For all patients, a supportive, therapeutic relationship is the best way to elicit accurate information. In the context of this relationship, the clinician should conduct a detailed psychiatric examination, including an alcohol and drug history, conduct a physical and mental status examination, order and interpret necessary laboratory tests, and meet with family or significant others to obtain additional information.

The assessment of anxiety should follow the algorithms for diagnostic criteria, as presented in DSM-IV. Of particular interest are the type and pattern of anxiety symptoms (frequency, duration, intensity), whether there are specific triggers or precipitants, age at onset, family history, and effect on the patient's life.

Information about a patient's alcohol and drug use is best obtained in the context of asking about such habits as caffeine and nicotine consumption. Quantity and frequency questions about psychoactive substances, such as "how much" and "how often" are useful in low to moderate users, but are unreliable for detecting substance abuse or dependence, especially when such use is illegal. A useful method to assess dependence explores whether the patient has experienced deleterious social or behavioral consequences from psychoactive substances, or has poor control of use. In assessing alcohol dependence, formalized interviews have been developed using these criteria.

The CAGE questionnaire is a simple four-item test that uses the letters C, A, G, and E as a mnemonic for questions about alcohol use. The questions are listed in Table 5. A positive answer on more than two questions is considered suspicious for alcohol abuse. The CAGE may be a better predictor of alcoholism in medical patients than laboratory tests (23). The CAGE is often adapted to drug use, as well.

The Michigan Alcohol Screening Test (MAST) is a widely used screening instrument to assess for alcohol and drug use and a presumptive diagnosis of alcoholism. It is a 25-item scale that identifies abnormal drinking through its social and behavioral consequences (24). A shortened, 10-item test, the

Table 5. The CAGE Interview

Have you ever felt the need to Cut down on drinking (or drugs)?
Have you ever felt Annoyed by criticisms of drinking (or drugs)?
Have you ever had Guilty feelings about drinking (or using drugs)?
Have you ever taken a morning Eye opener (or used drugs to get going in the a.m.)?

Brief MAST, has similar efficacy in the diagnosis of alcoholism. Another instrument, which is quite useful for screening for alcohol use, is the AUDIT, developed by WHO for a multinational project; it is effective in screening both patients and nonpatients for problem drinking (25). Two interviews that effectively address the behavioral consequences of drug abuse are the Drug Abuse Screening Test (DAST) (26) and the Addiction Severity Index (ASI) (27). These instruments have been utilized primarily in clinical research and have not been widely used in clinical practice.

Other items in the medical history that should increase suspicion about substance use include: divorce, problems at work (job loss, tardiness, absenteeism, work-related injuries), injuries (falls, auto accidents, fights), arrests, driving while intoxicated, leisure activities involving drugs or alcohol, and financial problems. Having an alcohol- or drug-abusing biological parent or spouse also increases the risk for substance use.

Serum and urine toxicological screens can have an important role in the assessment and treatment of patients with substance use disorders. However, it is important for clinicians to know how to properly conduct such testing and how to interpret the results. Optimally, informed consent should be obtained for all drug and alcohol testing unless the patient is unable to give consent or laws require testing. Most toxicological analyses are conducted on urine, although analyses are sometimes conducted on blood, amniotic fluid, saliva, or hair. To minimize adulteration and collection errors, all samples should be obtained under direct observation. Positive test results should always be confirmed with a second test using a different analytical method, because chemically similar compounds in foods or medications can give false positive results. Although a positive test suggests use of a psychoactive substance, it does not indicate whether use was acute or chronic, how much was used, when it occurred, or whether there was behavioral impairment because of the use.

Initial Intervention: Stabilization and Detoxification

Patients with comorbid anxiety disorders who have substance dependence should undergo treatment that addresses both disorders, as residual symptoms from one disorder may interfere with treatment of the other. For example, agoraphobia and other anxiety symptoms can impair the ability of patients to participate in treatment activities such as therapy groups or self-help groups. Since withdrawal can exacerbate anxiety symptoms, all patients with should undergo a supervised detoxification and any emergent withdrawal symptoms should be treated. Detoxification may be accomplished in an outpatient, inpatient, or residential setting depending on the drug used, the level of dependence, the severity of psychiatric problems, and the presence of coexisting medical problems. More severe and disabling problems are more likely to require inpatient treatment.

Withdrawal is a distinct physiological and/or behavioral state that follows cessation or reduction in the amount of drug used. In general, the signs and symptoms of withdrawal are the opposite of those that the drug produces (e.g., withdrawal from depressants produces excitation). Patients with anxiety disorders and substance dependence are more likely to use sedatives (alcohol, barbiturates, benzodiazepines, opiates) rather than stimulants (amphetamines, cocaine), since sedatives are anxiolytic and stimulants are usually anxiogenic.

The proposed neurobiological mechanism for withdrawal is a change in the number of postsynaptic neurotransmitter receptors or in receptor sensitivity that occurs with chronic drug use. It should be emphasized that withdrawal is not specific to addictive substances; chronic use of medications such as beta-adrenergic blockers, antihistamines, cardiac antiarrhythmics, and antidepressants may be associated with a withdrawal syndrome following discontinuation of drug. General methods for the therapeutic detoxification from drugs and alcohol are presented in Table 6. The use of such methodology minimizes withdrawal signs and symptoms.

The patient with an anxiety disorder usually comes into treatment distressed and wishing relief from the distress. Unfortunately, for the patient with combined anxiety disorders and substance dependence, removal of the psychoactive substance and probable withdrawal signs and symptoms will generally exacerbate the anxiety disorder and increase distress, leading to the patient's leaving treatment. For this reason, it is particularly important to attempt to aggressively minimize anxiety through slow tapering of medications, judicious use of other anxiolytic medications, and use of nonpharmacological anxiety-reduction techniques, including relaxation and other

Table 6. Methods of Detoxification from Drugs and Alcohol

1. Controlled administration of the drug, with a slow taper in the daily drug dose (example: tapering sedatives over days in patients with sedative dependence)
2. Administration of a cross-tolerant agent that is slowly tapered over time (example: chlordiazepoxide in alcohol withdrawal, methadone in opioid withdrawal)
3. Administration of an alternative agent to suppress signs and symptoms of withdrawal (example: clonidine in opioid withdrawal, anticonvulsants in sedative withdrawal)
4. Nonpharmacological detoxification, with supportive care (example: social-setting detox in alcohol dependence)

behavioral therapies. Providing education about anxiety disorders and its relationship to substance use for the patient is important. Finally, it is important to engender hope, in that both disorders are potentially treatable; although symptoms may worsen in the short run, they will improve over time.

Consolidation/Rehabilitation Treatment

Consolidation therapies for anxiety disorders include psychosocial therapies consisting of various psychotherapies and pharmacotherapies. These are described below.

Psychosocial Treatments for Anxiety Disorders and Substance Use Disorders. The two most effective forms of psychotherapy used to treat anxiety disorders are behavioral therapy and cognitive-behavioral therapy (28). Behavioral therapy tries to change actions through techniques that replace anxiety-related behaviors with other behaviors. Commonly used behavioral techniques include progressive muscular relaxation, diaphragmatic breathing, guided imagery, and gradual and controlled exposure to the frightening thoughts or situations. Progressive muscular relaxation is a technique for reducing muscular tension and anxiety. During a relaxation session, the therapist instructs patients to become aware of specific muscle groups and learn to tense and relax them, leaving them in a relaxed state. Usually, the session begins by relaxing the lower extremities and then, moving rostrally, the arms, shoulders, neck, and head. Diaphragmatic breathing teaches patients to take voluntary control of their breathing by using the diaphragm to breath, rather than the accessory chest muscles. Focusing on and controlling breathing in this manner reduces hyperventilation and anxiety symptoms. Guided imagery has the patient imagine a pleasant, peaceful situation, such as relaxing on the beach or floating in water. Focusing on this pleasant situation displaces anxiety and tension.

Exposure techniques present the patient with real or imagined situations that routinely provoke or worsen his or her anxiety. However, the therapist controls the exposure to the provocative stimulus so that the magnitude of the anxiety is tolerable. Gradually, the anxiety diminishes. Exposure techniques are particularly useful in phobias and posttraumatic stress disorder.

Cognitive-behavioral therapy teaches patients to understand their thinking patterns so they can react differently to the situations that cause them anxiety. They learn how their thinking patterns contribute to their symptoms and how to change their thoughts so that symptoms are less likely to occur. In coping-skills therapy, a variant of cognitive-behavioral therapy, patients learn

Anxiety Disorders

behavioral skills and techniques to avoid anxiety-provoking situations and to better contend with anxiety when it occurs.

Addiction rehabilitation treatments consist of medical, psychological, and social measures to help avoid the use of psychoactive substances in the future. Psychosocial rehabilitation treatments consist of individual and group therapies, residential treatment in alcohol-free settings, or self-help groups such as Alcoholics Anonymous (AA), Narcotics Anonymous (NA), ALANON, and Rational Recovery. Almost all advocate the total avoidance of alcohol and addictive drugs. Individual and group psychotherapy can be useful for understanding the role of the drug in the individual's life, improving self-esteem and relieving psychological distress. Cognitive-behavioral therapy and its variant, coping-skills therapy, have been widely utilized to assist patients in remaining abstinent from alcohol and drugs (29). Changes in living situation, work situation, or friendships may be necessary to decrease availability of drugs and to reduce social pressure to use drugs. While most treatment can be provided in an outpatient setting, halfway houses, therapeutic communities, and other residential treatment situations may be necessary to ensure a drug-free environment.

In any treatment situation, the adequate treatment of underlying psychiatric symptoms, medical illness, and pain is important, as this may reduce the need for self-medication. Psychotherapies and social interventions should incorporate integrated anxiety treatment and substance abuse treatment into the treatment plan.

Pharmacotherapies for Anxiety and Substance Use Disorders. Although there are many anxiolytic medications that can be used to treat anxiety disorder patients, some of these can be abused or cause dependence in patients with comorbid substance use disorders. Thus, anxiolytic medications that have little or no potential for abuse or harmful overdose are preferred. These include antidepressants, especially the selective serotonin-reuptake blockers (SSRIs) the anxiolytic drug buspirone, antihistamines, and beta-adrenergic blockers (30). For generalized anxiety disorder (GAD), buspirone or antidepressants are usual first-line treatments; for panic disorder, obsessive-compulsive disorder (OCD), posttraumatic stress disorder (PTSD), and social phobia, antidepressants are the preferred first-line therapy (Table 7). Benzodiazepines and other dependence-producing sedative medications are sometimes used during detoxification and acute treatment; however, their use in long-term anxiolytic treatment must be carefully considered, because of the potential for abuse (31,32). The use of benzodiazepines often becomes an issue for clinicians who have a strong negative position on the use of potentially abusable or addictive medications in patients with substance use disorders.

Table 7. Drug with Anxiolytic Effects

Drug class	Examples	Potential for abuse and dependence
Adrenergic blockers	Clonidine, propranolol	Minimal
Alcohol	Ethyl alcohol	Yes
Antihistamines	Diphenhydramine, hydroxizine	Minimal
Barbiturates	Butabarbital, phenobarbital	Yes
Benzodiazepines	Alprazolam, diazepam	Yes
Buspirone	Buspirone	None
Neuroleptics	Chlorpromazine, olanzepine	None
Opiates	Codeine, morphine, oxycodone	Yes
Sedative hypnotics	Meprobamate	Yes
SSRIs	Fluoxetine, sertraline, paroxetine, trazodone	None
Tricyclic antidepressants	Imipramine, desipramine	None

In spite of the risk of dependence in patients with a history of a substance use disorder, benzodiazepines are the most effective medications for treating the acute symptoms of panic. In general, long-acting benzodiazepines with slow onset of action, e.g., clonazepam, are preferable to short-acting, rapid-onset agents, e.g., lorazepam, alprazolam. However, slower-onset agents are much better for preventing an attack than treating the acute symptoms. In the future, newer benzodiazepines may be developed with less potential for producing dependence. A new class of medications, benzodiazepine partial agonists, may have anxiolytic effects without producing dependence.

If patients require pharmacological sedation, antihistamines such as diphenhydramine and hydroxazine can be used for short-term anxiolytic effects and sedation, without producing dependence. Sedative antidepressants, including trazodone, nefazodone, and doxepin, are also effective for sedation and hypnotic effects.

Buspirone is a nonbenzodiazepine anxiolytic medication that has partial agonist activity at the serotonin-1a receptor and serotonin-2 receptor, as well as having dopamine-2 receptor antagonist activity. It has been demonstrated to be an effective anxiolytic in anxiety disorders, particularly GAD. One study with anxious alcoholics found improved treatment retention in patients receiving buspirone (33). However, a double-blind study of buspirone in 67 anxious alcoholics found the medication to have no effect compared to placebo (34). The anxiolytic effects of buspirone may take several weeks to be manifest, and substance-abusing patients, who are used to experiencing an immediate effect of drugs, require education about its delayed therapeutic effect. The usual dose of buspirone ranges from 15 to 60 mg per day.

All antidepressants appear to have anxiolytic as well as antidepressant properties, and all appear to act by increasing the amounts of norepinephrine, serotonin, and dopamine neurotransmitters in synapses. This is thought to lead to receptor down-regulation and other adaptive changes in neurons. Antidepressants have been shown to be effective in the treatment of GAD, panic, OCD, and PTSD (35,36). Three classes of antidepressants are used for the treatment of anxiety disorders: SSRIs (e.g., fluoxetine, sertraline, paroxetine, citalopram, trazodone), tricyclic antidepressants (e.g., imipramine, desipramine, doxepine, nortriptyline), and MAOIs (phenelzine, tranylcypromine). In general, the selection of specific antidepressants should depend on evidence-based practice, the clinical state of the patient, and drug pharmacokinetics. Patients should be started on low doses of antidepressant medications, with the dose gradually increased.

The antidepressant effect of these medications is helpful for patients with significant depressive as well as anxiety symptoms. For patients with suicidal potential, SSRIs are preferred over tricyclic antidepressants because of the relative lack of toxicity in overdose. MAOIs should be used with great care and only in patients who can adhere to the dietary guidelines (avoiding foods containing tyramine) and who do not use stimulants or narcotics. These medications can also cause significant weight gain and hypotension. Because of the induction of hepatic enzymes in alcohol and drug users, higher doses of antidepressants may be required to achieve therapeutic levels of medication (37). All antidepressants lower the seizure threshold and may present some risk in substance-abusing patients with a history of seizures. In an anxious elderly patient, consideration should be given to using lower doses of medication, owing to slower hepatic metabolism, increased sensitivity to side effects, and a greater chance of interaction with other medications.

Adrenergic blocking agents reduce the peripheral manifestations of anxiety and may have central anxiolytic effects as well. Beta-blockers appear to be effective for the short-term treatment of mild to moderate situational anxiety, such as anxiety associated with performances and examinations. For patients with addictive disorders, beta-blockers may have an advantage over benzodiazepines, as they cause minimal effects on cognition and have little potential for abuse. Alpha$_2$-agonists, such as clonidine, reduce central and peripheral adrenergic activity and have anxiolytic effects. Side effects of beta-blockers and alpha$_2$-agonists include bradycardia and hypotension. Also, chronic use of adrenergic medications can produce up-regulation of receptors and rebound adrenergic hyperactivity if the medication is abruptly stopped; adrenergic medications should therefore be tapered over time when discontinued.

Neuroleptics have anxiolytic effects and are used to treat anxiety associated with psychosis or delirium and PTSD. They are also effective in reducing severe anxiety and agitation associated with situational distress, panic attacks, and OCD. Since they have significant side effects, including weight gain, sedation, akathesia, parkinsonism, and tardive dyskinesia, consideration needs to be given to the relative risks and benefits.

A number of pharmacological therapies have been shown to be effective in the treatment of substance use disorders when used as a component of a comprehensive treatment program (38). Pharmacotherapies can treat alcohol and drug dependence through several mechanisms that reduce the impetus for drug use. Since drugs and alcohol produce pleasure, and this may maintain use, pharmacological agents that reduce the pleasurable effects or increase the aversive effects of drugs can reduce use. Medications that suppress the punishing effects of withdrawal by substituting for the drug or by blocking withdrawal signs and symptoms could reduce drug use. Finally, drug and alcohol dependence are characterized by craving or an overwhelming urge to use the substance. Medications that block craving can reduce drug use.

In the case of alcohol, three medications have been approved for the treatment of dependence in Europe or the United States (39). Disulfiram is a medication that increases the aversive effects of alcohol. Naltrexone blocks the pleasurable effects of alcohol and also blocks craving. Acamprosate is a medication approved in Europe that blocks alcohol withdrawal distress and craving. For opioid dependence, substitution therapies such as methadone, buprenorphine, and l-alpha-acetylmethodol (LAAM) reduce withdrawal signs and symptoms and reduce craving for opioids.

Aftercare/Maintenance Treatment

Following completion of briefer treatments, patients should be engaged in longer-term maintenance treatments that address both anxiety and substance use. The objectives for longer-term treatment or rehabilitation include: 1) maintenance of the alcohol- or drug-free state, 2) maintenance of a remission in anxiety symptoms, and 3) psychological, family, and vocational interventions to ensure compliance. Dramatic changes in living situation, work situation, or friendships may be necessary to decrease drug availability and reduce peer pressure to use drugs. Halfway houses, therapeutic communities, and other residential treatment situations are useful in this regard. Ongoing individual and group psychotherapy can be useful for understanding the role

Anxiety Disorders

of the drug in the individual's life, to stabilize the family system, to improve self-esteem, to provide alternative methods of relieving psychosocial distress, and to reinforce the need for abstinence. Treatment of underlying psychiatric or medical illnesses should be coordinated with the substance abuse treatment. Continued involvement in self-help groups such as AA or NA can be helpful to maintain sobriety and provide social support.

Medications that are effective in reducing anxiety symptoms or substance use should be continued into the maintenance phase of treatment. Since the course of both anxiety disorders and substance use disorders is chronic and characterized by exacerbations and remissions, dosage adjustment and medication adjustments may be required over time.

The treatment plan developed for patients with anxiety and substance abuse should be formulated into a written contract signed by both the clinician and the patient. A copy should be given to the patient—and family members, if appropriate—and placed in the patient's medical record. Although treatment plans should be individualized according to the patient's clinical situation, there are several elements that should be a part of any plan. These include: only one physician to prescribe psychotropic medications and one pharmacy where prescriptions are filled, avoidance of alcohol and medications that produce dependence, procedures for drug and alcohol screening, and a policy on changes in medication and medication dosage and required treatment, such as addiction counseling and/or participation in self-help programs. For patients who receive benzodiazepines, pain medications, or other potential substances of abuse, the contract should include a policy for prescription refills and for dealing with lost prescriptions. The consequences of noncompliance with the contract, for example, required inpatient treatment or termination with the clinician, should be clearly stated.

Certain habits that contribute to anxiety should also be addressed. Caffeine, and the related methylxanthines theophylline and theobromine, are found in coffee, tea, cola, and other carbonated drinks, in chocolate, and in many prescribed and over-the-counter medications. Even low to moderate doses of caffeine (one or two cups of coffee per day) may significantly increase anxiety and panic symptoms and worsen sleep disturbances. Limiting the patient's use of caffeine and other methylxanthines is important in the overall treatment of the anxiety disorder patient. Smoking is also prevalent among substance users and should be addressed. Nicotine is a psychomotor stimulant and may exacerbate anxiety. Moreover, the use of nicotine products is associated with cardiovascular and respiratory disease and cancers of the lung and oropharynx. In fact, alcoholics who smoke are more likely to die from tobacco-related illness than from alcoholism. Thus, all patients who smoke or use tobacco products should receive education and be offered treatment for nicotine dependence.

CONCLUSIONS

There is a greater than average likelihood that patients with anxiety disorders will have coexisting substance use disorders. Alhough treatment presents challenging issues in this group, a flexible combination of psychotherapeutic/ behavioral and judicious pharmacological therapies can lead to successful treatment outcomes in most patients.

REFERENCES

1. American Psychiatric Association. Diagnostic and Statistical Manual of Mental Disorders. 4th ed. Washington, DC: American Psychiatric Press, 1994.
2. Schuckit MA, Hesselbrock V. Alcohol dependence and anxiety disorders: what is the relationship? Am J Psychiatry 151:1723–1734, 1994.
3. Kranzler HR, Liebowitz NR. Anxiety and depression in substance abuse. Med Clin North Am 72:867–885, 1988.
4. Galanter M, Castaneda R, Ferman J. Substance abuse among general psychiatric patients: place of presentation, diagnosis and treatment. Am J Drug Alcohol Abuse 14:211–235, 1988.
5. Brady KT, Lydiard RB. The association of alcoholism and anxiety. Psychiatric Q 64:135–149, 1993.
6. Regier DA, Farmer ME, Rae DS. Comorbidity of mental disorders with alcohol and other drug abuse. JAMA 264:2511–2518, 1990.
7. Kessler RC, Crum RM, Warner LA, et al. Lifetime co-occurrence of DSM-III-R alcohol abuse and dependence with other psychiatric disorders in the National Comorbidity Survey. Arch Gen Psychiatry. 54:313–321, 1997.
8. Khantzian EJ. The self-medication hypothesis of addictive disorders: focus on heroin and cocaine dependence. Am J Psychiatry 142:1259–1264, 1985.
9. Kushner MG, Sher KJ, Beitman BD. The relation between alcohol problems and the anxiety disorders. Am J Psychiatry 147:685–695, 1990.
10. Merikangas KA, Stevens D, Fenton B. Comorbidity of alcoholism and anxiety disorders. Alcohol Health Res World 20:100–105, 1996.
11. George DT, Nutt DJ, Dwyer BA, Linnoila M. Alcoholism and panic disorder. Is the comorbidity more than coincidence? Acta Psychiatria Scandinavia 81:97–107, 1990.
12. Brown SA, Irwin M, Schuckit MA. Changes in anxiety among abstinent male alcoholics. J Stud Alcohol 52:55–61, 1991.

Anxiety Disorders

13. Swift RM, Stout RL. Relationship between craving and anxiety in opioid withdrawal. J Substance Abuse 4:19–26, 1992.
14. Goldenberg IM, Mueller T, Fierman EJ, et al. Specificity of substance use in anxiety-disordered subjects. Compr Psychiatry 36:319–328, 1995.
15. Rees CS, Richards JC, Smith LM. Medical utilisation and costs in panic disorder: a comparison with social phobia. J Anxiety Disord 12(5):421–435, 1998.
16. Katon W. Panic disorder: relationship to high medical utilization, unexplained physical symptoms, and medical costs. J Clin Psychiatry 10:11–22, 1996.
17. Ries R. Clinical treatment matching models for dually diagnosed patients. Psychiatr Clin North Am 16:167–175, 1993.
18. Rounsaville BJ, Dolinsky ZS, Babor TF, Meyer RE. Psychopathology as a predictor of treatment outcome in alcoholics. Arch Gen Psychiatry 44:505–513, 1987.
19. McLellan AT, Alterman AI, Metzger DS, et al. Similarity of outcome predictors across opiate, cocaine, and alcohol treatments: role of treatment services. J Consult Clin Psychol 62:1141–1158, 1994.
20. Weissman MM, Klerman GL, Markowitz JS, Ouelette R. Suicidal ideation and suicide attempts in panic disorder and attacks. N Engl J Med 321:1209–1214, 1989.
21. Ries RK. Assessment and Treatment of Patients with Coexisting Mental Illness and Alcohol and Other Drug Abuse: Treatment Improvement Protocol (TIP) Series 9. Rockville, MD: Center for Substance Abuse Treatment, 1994.
22. Gerstein DR. Evaluating recovery services: the California Drug and Alcohol Treatment Assessment (CALDATA). California Department of Alcohol and Drug Programs, 1994.
23. Beresford TP, Blow KC, EH, Singer K, Lucey MR. Clinical practice: comparison of CAGE questionnaire and computer assisted laboratory profiles in screening for covert alcoholism. Lancet 336:482–485, 1990.
24. Selzer ML. The Michigan alcoholism screening test: the quest for a new diagnostic instrument. Am J Psychiatry 127:1653–1658, 1971.
25. Conigrave KM, Hall WD, Saunders JB. The AUDIT questionnaire: choosing a cut-off score. Addiction 90:1349–1356, 1995.
26. Skinner HA. The drug abuse screening test. Addictive Behaviors 7:363–371, 1982.
27. McLellan AT, Luborsky L, Woody GA, O'Brien CP. An improved diagnostic evaluation instrument for substance abuse patients: the Addiction Severity Index. J Nerv Ment Dis 168:26–33, 1980.
28. Barlow DH. Cognitive-behavioral approaches to panic disorder and social phobia. Bull Menninger Clin 56:27–37, 1992.
29. Monti PM, O'Leary T. Coping and Social Skills training for alcohol and cocaine dependence. In: Psychiatric Clinics of North America. Vol 22. NS Miller, RM Swift, eds. Philadelphia: Saunders, pp 447–470, 1999.
30. Hales RE, Hilty DA, Wise MG. A treatment algorithm for the management of anxiety in primary care practice. J Clin Psychiatry 58:76–80, 1997.

31. Uhlenhuth EH, Balter MD, Ban TA, Yang K. International study of expert judgement on therapeutic use of benzodiazepines and other psychotherapeutic medications: pharmacology of anxiety disorders. J Affect Disord 35:153–162, 1995.
32. Ciraulo DA, Sands BF, Shader RI. Critical review of liability for benzodiazepine abuse among alcoholics. Am J Psychiatry 145:1501–1506, 1988.
33. Kranzler HR, Burleson JA, Del Boca FK, et al. Buspirone treatment of anxious alcoholics: a placebo-controlled trial. Arch Gen Psychiatry 51:720–731, 1994.
34. Malcolm R, Anton RF, Randall CL, et al. A placebo-controlled trial of buspirone in anxious inpatient alcoholics. Alcohol Clin Exp Res 16:1007–1013, 1992.
35. Taylor L, Gorman J. Theoretical and therapeutic considerations for the anxiety disorders. Psychiatr Q 63:319–342, 1992.
36. Schweitzer E. Generalized anxiety disorder: longitudinal course and pharmacologic treatment. Psychiatr Clin North Am 18:843–857, 1995.
37. Mason BJ. Dosing issues in the pharmacotherapy of alcoholism. Alcohol Clin Exp Res 20:10A–16A, 1996.
38. Kranzler HR, Amin H, Modesto-Lowe V, Oncken C. Pharmacologic treatments for drug and alcohol dependence. Psychiatr Clin North Am 22(2):401–423, 1999.
39. Swift RM. Drug therapy of alcohol dependence. New Engl J Med 340(19):1483–1489, 1999.

3
Substance Abuse and Depression

Lauren P. Lehmann
University of Virginia Health Sciences Center
and Salem VA Medical Center
Salem, Virginia

John R. Hubbard*
Vanderbilt University Medical Center
and Nashville VA Medical Center
Nashville, Tennessee

Peter R. Martin
Vanderbilt University Medical Center
Nashville, Tennessee

INTRODUCTION

The relationship between substance abuse and depression has been a focus of interest and inquiry for several decades. Reports suggest that the lifetime prevalence of major depression among patients with substance use disorders is high; estimates vary from approximately 25% (1) to 60% (2–4). The role of substance intoxication, chronic use, and withdrawal in the appearance of depressive symptoms is becoming better recognized, as are apparent gender differences in prevalence and symptom severity (3,5,6). The co-occurrence of depression and substance abuse is far-reaching, affecting social, vocational, health, and interpersonal functioning (7). Depressive symptoms vary with the

---

*Currently in private practice.

type (2) and number (8) of drugs used, as well as with the dose and frequency of drug use (2,5,9). Despite a greater appreciation of comorbid substance use disorders and depression, this problem is still often undiagnosed and undertreated. For example, a recent study of 595 depressed patients showed that less than 10% of those with comorbid substance use disorders had received substance abuse counseling (4).

One of the primary areas still to be clarified is the nature of the relationship between depression and substance-related disorders, and the etiology of the symptom overlap. Meyer (10) and others have proposed multiple potential reasons for observed associations between substance abuse and depression. Psychopathology may be a risk factor for addictive disorders, substance abuse may produce psychiatric symptoms, and psychopathology and substance use may be independent of each other. A possible common underlying neurochemical mechanism for depression and substance abuse has not been clearly identified, but it is an area of great research interest.

This chapter reviews information on the relationship between depressive disorders and the major substances of abuse. Hopefully progress in this area will lead to a better understanding and treatment of patients with these disorders.

ALCOHOL AND DEPRESSION

Although there is considerable epidemiological and neurobiological evidence linking alcohol use and depression, the exact nature of this relationship has yet to be elucidated and may vary between patients. In their review of the substance abuse and depression literature, Swendsen and Merikangas (11) proposed that multiple causal factors and mechanisms probably underlie the association of alcoholism and depression. Neurobiological similarities have been postulated as one of these mechanisms. For example, monoamine, cholinergic, and other neurotransmitter systems have been implicated in both disorders (12,13).

The relationship between depression and both acute alcohol-related states (such as intoxication and withdrawal) and chronic use problems (such as abuse, protracted withdrawal, and chemical dependence) has been studied. All of these alcohol-related conditions have been shown to be associated with dysphoric mood states, but the mechanism of mood depression is not well understood and may differ among various alcohol-related conditions. In addition, the length of time alcohol has been abused, amount of use, predisposing genetic factors, gender, and multiple other variables may influence the mechanism of comorbidity with depression. Likewise, the different depressive states may be caused by different underlying neurochemical mechanisms, and thus could be associated with alcoholism by different processes. Current information must therefore be considered only a beginning in our understanding of this complex problem.

Alcohol is a CNS depressant, and so it is not surprising that acute alcohol intoxication can produce a dysphoric state (14). The dysphoria appears to be related to the amount of use. Alcohol intoxication increases impulsivity and thus raises the risk of self-injury and suicidal behavior. For example, a study by Cornelius et al. (15) found an approximately 40% prevalence of suicide attempts in the week prior to hospitalization, with most involving impulsiveness and heavy drinking. They suggested that heavy alcohol use increased impulsivity rather than induced suicidal ideation.

The association between depression and chronic alcohol use has been another area of interest. Some studies suggest that alcohol and affective disorders occur together at higher rates than would be expected by chance (16,17). In a community sample of over 500 subjects, using the Schedule for Affective Disorders and Schizophrenia (SADS) and Research Diagnostic Criteria (RDC), Weissman and Myers (18) found a 44% lifetime prevalence of major depression in alcoholics and a 15% lifetime prevalence of minor depression. Negative life events, a family history of depression, and neuroticism have been identified as risk factors for depression in alcoholics (19,20).

A family study suggested that a lifetime history of depression and a family history of alcoholism were associated with comorbid alcohol dependence (21). Others, however, reported that depression and alcoholism segregated independently in families (22).

The comorbidity of alcoholism and depression can be clinically very important. In most cases, alcohol and depression negatively influence the comorbid disorder, causing more severe problems than either alone (23). As with intoxication, concurrent chronic alcohol abuse and depressive disorders have been associated with an increased risk for suicide (24–28). In addition, certain areas of performance may be greatly affected by the comorbidity (29,30). Cortical operations known to be affected by both alcohol and depression include learning, memory, and motor function (31). For example, alcohol consumption, depression, and neuropsychological performance have been linked (29,30). In some reports the comorbidity appeared to be less important. For example, Hirschfeld et al. (32) found no differences in either time to recovery from major depression or time to relapse to another episode of depression in two samples, with and without concurrent alcoholism, although the course of the former was worse in terms of social functioning.

Treatment options may also be influenced by detection of comorbidity. Thus, it is generally considered important to treat an alcohol-related disorder if significant progress is to be made with depression. That is, if alcohol abuse or dependence goes undetected or untreated, depressive symptoms may be more resistant to medications and other forms of treatment. Data suggest that remission in alcoholism increased the odds of remission in depression (33).

Similar relationships between depressed mood and alcohol abuse have been reported in adolescents. In a prospective study of over 1000 adolescents, those with depressive symptoms and heavy drinking were more likely to have low levels of functioning, high levels of childhood externalizing problems and stressful life events, low levels of family social support, and high levels of delinquency (34). Alpert et al. (35) found that childhood and adolescent onsets of depression were risk factors in the development of alcohol dependence and abuse in adulthood. King et al. (36) noted that depressed male adolescents had increased risk of later alcohol and drug abuse.

Several studies suggest that the relationship between alcohol and depression is different for men and women. Depressed women alcoholics appear to be more severely depressed than their male counterparts, and that depressive symptoms were predictive for alcoholism in women but that the reverse was true for men (36–39). In a study of 3755 twin pairs, Prescott et al. (40) found major depression to be more common in women and alcoholism in men. About 68% of women with both depression and alcoholism identified depression as preceding alcoholism, whereas the opposite was reported in 61% of the men (39). These results suggested that possible causal relationships may be gender-influenced processes.

Substantial evidence exists that mood changes induced by alcohol diminish with abstinence (41–49). For example, Brown and Schuckit (44) reported that 42% of their 191 alcoholic inpatients had Hamilton Depression Rating Scale (HDRS) scores in the moderately to severely depressed range, but that by the fourth week of abstinence this number had declined to 6%. Furthermore, 3 months after discharge, there was no recurrence of depressive symptoms except in those who relapsed. In a similar study they found that the rate of remission of depressive symptoms consistently followed the course of the primary illness (i.e., either depression or alcohol dependence), and a minimum of 3 weeks of abstinence was necessary to differentiate between the two groups (50). Other data also suggest that relapses are accompanied by the return of previously remitted depressive symptoms (51).

Alcohol withdrawal is a condition that has repeatedly been shown to be associated with dysphoria, but the extent to which this occurs is variable (14,41). Some estimates of withdrawal-related dysphoria are as high as 98% (41). Because of the relationship between depression and alcohol withdrawal, some earlier prevalence studies should be considered in this light (52). For example, Ross et al. (53) reported a lifetime prevalence of about 23% for major depression and approximately 13% for dysthymia in alcoholics; however, 66% of the sample had been drinking within 7 days of the interview. Forty-three percent claimed onset of depressive symptoms before alcohol use and 40% after the onset of alcohol use. Other studies (54,55) estimated secondary depression at 28–70%, depending on the assessment method. Herz et al. (56) found a 16% current prevalence for depression and an 11% current prevalence for dysthymia in 74 patients.

Regarding possible markers for depression in alcoholics, Dackis et al. (57) found thyroid-releasing hormone (TRH) abnormalities in 53% of patients in alcohol withdrawal. Twenty-five percent had a blunted response to the thyroid-stimulating hormone (TSH) test after 3 weeks of sobriety, suggesting that the TRH test is not specific for depression in alcoholics. They also examined the dexamethasone suppression test (DST) and found abnormal results in three of 15 subjects in withdrawal but no abnormalities in 32 subjects after 4 weeks of sobriety, concluding that the DST may have more diagnostic utility as an adjunct in diagnosing depression in alcoholics with some sobriety. One caveat in the use of the DST, however, arose from the work of Nelson et al. (58), who found that advanced age (over 45 years) may confound the results by making patients nonsuppressors.

A major area of interest has been the distinguishing of alcohol-induced transient secondary depression from primary depression with a comorbid alcoholism. Schuckit (59) and others (60) have investigated a primary-secondary depression dichotomy, with secondary depressions being directly attributable to alcohol use and resolving with abstinence (59,61). Schuckit cautioned that prevalence of depressive symptoms in alcoholics must be considered in light of the sample, criteria, timeframe, and duration (14,62). He suggested that about one-third of alcoholics will have lifetime major depression, which will improve with abstinence and supportive treatment, that only about 5% of men and 10% of women will have a current coexisting major depression, and that these patients typically have depressive episodes independent of drinking (59). Schuckit defined primary depression as occurring prior to the onset of first major life problem from alcoholism or after 3 months of abstinence. Secondary depression often disappeared within 1 week of abstinence but may mimic a course similar to that of primary depression (63). Weissman et al. (64) found similar depressive symptoms that were less severe in patients with secondary depression.

In a study of 231 men and 90 women, Hesselbrock et al. (65) identified gender differences as being important in the dichotomy. As in the studies reviewed above (36–40), major depression was most common among females and more often preceded alcohol use compared to males. Hesselbrock and colleagues noted that patients with primary depression reported more "affective disturbances" than did secondary depressives. Powell et al. (66) reported trends suggesting that primary depressives had more psychiatric hospitalizations, more ECT treatments, longer duration of depression, and shorter duration of alcoholism. Raimo and Schuckit (67) postulated that there was no relationship between primary unipolar depression and alcoholism. From a sample of 2945 alcoholic subjects, Schuckit and coworkers also concluded that primary and secondary depressions could be differentiated by demographic and other factors (68). In contrast, Greenfield et al. (69) reported that concurrent major depression, either primary or secondary, was predictive of relapse in their sample of over 100 patients (60 men and 41 women).

Some studies have not found significant correlations between alcoholism and depression. For example, Hodgins et al. (70) reported no direct causal relationship between depression and drinking outcomes in their 84 treatment subjects. Similar results were reported by Davidson and Blackburn (71).

The neurochemical mechanism(s) involved in alcoholism and depression continue to be investigated. The effects of alcohol on the brain are widespread, involving most systems and structures. Mechanisms may differ according to the specific alcohol-related problem of a particular patient (i.e., intoxication, withdrawal, abuse, or dependence). Serotonergic and glutamatergic systems are particularly affected by alcohol, which in turn affects most neurotransmitter systems.

Withdrawal has been associated with various neuropathological alterations (72). Identified abnormalities include decreased serotonin transmission (73–75) that becomes normal on acute alcohol administration (73). Serotonin deficiency may be an important component of alcohol-related disorders and depression. Branchey et al. (76) found significantly elevated tyrosine and phenylalanine levels and decreased tryptophan levels and tryptophan ratios in eight depressed alcoholic patients compared to 26 alcoholics without a history of depression. Badawy's work (77) supports this hypothesis, linking serotonin deficiency to higher liver tryptophan pyrrolase activity and implicating the tryptophan metabolite quinolinate in the development of depressive symptoms. In a study of 58 alcoholic subjects, Swann et al. (78) found a positive correlation among plasma tryptophan, large neutral amino acids (a marker of 5-HT function), symptoms of dysphoria, and later onset of alcoholism.

Heinz et al. (79) compared Beck Depression Inventory (BDI) and HDRS scores with various neurotransmitter metabolite levels in 21 abstinent alcoholics and 11 controls. They found correlations between cerebral spinal fluid (CSF) 3-methoxy-4-hydroxyphenylglycol (MHPG) and 5-hydroxyindoleacetic acid (5-HIAA) concentrations and depressive symptoms, implicating noradrenergic abnormalities as well as serotonergic function in the onset of depressive symptoms. Serotonin deficiency was implicated in the higher suicide rate found among alcoholics with depression (80,81), in memory impairment (82), and in blackouts (83) frequently seen in alcoholics. Other studies suggested that low serotonin levels are associated with increased alcohol preference and consumption (84,85). Some reports suggest no relationship between depression and either postsynaptic alpha$_2$-adrenoceptor function (86) or reduced sensitivity of dopamine receptors (87).

Overall, it appears that primary depression and alcoholism may occur independently, that secondary depression frequently exists in relation to alcohol use and withdrawal, that there are gender differences in the expression of these two disorders, and that serotonin and its precursors as well as other neurochemical systems are implicated in the development of depressive symptoms. Greater understanding of the association between alcoholism and depression may lead to improved methods of prevention and treatment of these important, and common, comorbid disorders.

MARIJUANA AND DEPRESSION

Marijuana, the most frequently used illicit drug in the United States, has been legalized in some states for medical use (88). Because of its frequent use, common comorbidity with depression, and multiple neuropsychiatric actions, the relationship between marijuana exposure and depression is of significant interest. Depression has been associated with chronic marijuana use, as part of the marijuana withdrawal syndrome and as a possible explanation for the reported "amotivational syndrome."

Using the Diagnostic Interview Schedule (DIS), Halikas et al. (89) found signs of depression in 29% of 100 heavy marijuana users. In a follow-up study 6–7 years later (using an instrument similar to the DIS), Weller and Halikas (90) found major depressive episodes to be the most frequent diagnosis (44%) in their population of 97 marijuana users (68% of the group was using marijuana at least weekly and 20% was using daily). This represented an increase of 15% over initial interview and was statistically significant. The authors suggested that marijuana use did not cause psychiatric illness but that the diagnosis was clarified, or that marijuana use in their population may have exacerbated pre-existing psychiatric problems. This conclusion is supported by a longitudinal study involving 101 18-year-olds that showed that, prior to becoming regular marijuana users, subjects were inattentive, labile, inconsiderate, and insecure, and had poor social skills as children (91). Other studies show that heavy marijuana use has been associated with depressed mood in women (92), greater depression during abstinence periods in men (93), and increased suicide rate (94).

Depression may be related to the postulated amotivational syndrome (95–97) that is associated with chronic marijuana use. This syndrome is of considerable concern (especially in children) but remains controversial because of complicating factors that often coexist in people who use marijuana (98,99). Affected individuals are reported to be withdrawn, asocial, apathetic, and easily distracted. In addition, they have poor concentration and impaired judgment and communication skills. The chronic exposure to marijuana may be directly involved in the etiology of this proposed syndrome, or an underlying depression or related personality traits may predate the onset of marijuana use and be a reason for use.

The DSM-IV does not have a diagnosis of cannabinoid withdrawal; however, withdrawal symptoms have been previously reported. During the withdrawal state from marijuana, symptoms of depression often begin a few hours after the last use and persist for 4–5 days. For example, Mendleson et al. (100) published a case report of a 23-year-old woman with a significant increase in depressed mood that peaked 48 hours after withdrawal from 21 days of daily, heavy use. Her symptoms were accompanied by high Profile of Mood States (POMS) depression scores for 96 hours. Other symptoms noted to occur with the withdrawal syndrome and depression include irritability, restlessness, anxiety, decreased appetite, weight loss, and insomnia (88,95,96,100).

The mechanism of action of marijuana is not well understood and may differ between states of chronic use and withdrawal. Data suggest that the major active chemical in marijuana, delta-9-tetrahydrocannabinol (THC), binds to specific endogenous receptors, disrupts cellular metabolism, impedes cellular protein synthesis, affects cell membranes, alters the dopamine system, and affects benzodiazepine receptors (88,101–106). Which, if any, of these neurochemical systems may be involved in depressive symptoms is not known at this time; considerably more work is needed to better understand the association between marijuana abuse and depression.

STIMULANTS AND DEPRESSION

Depression has been associated with acute and chronic use of stimulants, as well as stimulant withdrawal. In attempting to define the comorbidity of stimulant use and depression, Gawin and Kleber (107) studied 70 outpatients, of whom 35 had psychiatric diagnoses. Thirty percent of these patients had depression, which was similar to findings in other studies of patients with stimulant abuse (108,109). Rounsaville et al. (110) found lifetime rates of depressive disorders among 298 treatment-seeking cocaine abusers to be about 60%, which declined to approximately 30% during exclusive cocaine use.

In characterizing their population, Gawin and Kleber (107) found that 33% had depressive disorders—13% with major depression and melancholia and 20% with dysthymia. Symptoms persisted for more than 10 days after last use and were consistent with previous symptoms during abstinence. Interestingly, the group with psychiatric diagnoses used less cocaine than the remainder of the sample but reported that it produced the same effect. It was postulated that the depressed group might have an increased sensitivity to the effects of cocaine, thereby using it to self-medicate dysphoria. Eight of the authors' 70 subjects reported increased severity of depressive symptoms as intensity and duration of cocaine use increased, for which they postulated an acute depletion of catecholamine neurotransmitters and supersensitivity of dopamine (DA) autoreceptors. This is supported by reports of successful treatment with antidepressants of symptoms of stimulant withdrawal (111).

In an attempt to differentiate primary from secondary depression, the TRH test was used for depression in patients with cocaine abuse (109). Forty-seven percent of 17 patients had an inadequate TSH response. However, the TRH test lacked specificity for major depression in cocaine abusers when administered during the first 7 days of abstinence. Nunes et al. (111) gave the Structured Clinical Interview for DSM-III (SCID) to 30 outpatients with cocaine abuse and found that 63% met lifetime criteria for affective disorder. In addition, 17% met lifetime criteria for major depression, 13% met criteria for current depression, 17% met lifetime criteria for depression not otherwise specified (NOS), 13% met criteria for current depression NOS, 27% met criteria for lifetime "atypical depression," and 13% met criteria for current "atypical depression." They also found that the patients with the highest HDRS scores had the lowest levels of cocaine use and a family history of affective disorder. They postulated that the depressed cocaine users may have a heightened pharmacological sensitivity to cocaine and/or may be using cocaine to self-medicate depression.

In their sample of 298 cocaine-abusing inpatients and outpatients, Rounsaville et al. (110) found a lifetime prevalence of about 30% for major depression and approximately 12% for minor depression. In addition, about 5% and 0.7% had current major and minor depression, respectively. For two-thirds of their depressed sample, the onset of the disorders occurred after initiation of drug use. These results are similar to those reported by Mirin et al. (112–114), who also found a rate for affective disorder of about 27% among stimulant abusers' female relatives. In a follow-up study by Weiss et al. (115), however, the prevalence of depression in stimulant abusers declined significantly, which was attributed to changes in the epidemiology of cocaine use.

Kleinman et al. (116) found depression more commonly in crack or freebase cocaine users than in intranasal users and those with a longer duration of use. It appears, then, that depressive symptoms are typically found in early stages of stimulant abstinence, probably due to effects on the same neurotransmitters involved in depression. A significant minority of patients, however—who may have an increased sensitivity to the pharmacological properties of stimulants—likely have an underlying depressive disorder, generally predating the onset of stimulant use.

A pattern of stimulant-abstinence cycle and depression has been described. Watson et al. (117) noted depressed mood, lethargy, hyperphagia, hypersomnia, increased REM sleep, and reduced urinary MHPG in four chronic, high-dose amphetamine users abruptly withdrawn from stimulants. The MHPG levels returned to normal when the depressed mood resolved. Gawin and Kleber (107) further outlined the stimulant-withdrawal cycle: binge use is followed by severe depressive symptoms within 30 minutes of last dose. In their study of 30 chronic cocaine-abusing outpatients, they described three phases. Depression, anhedonia, insomnia, irritability, and anxiety, then hypersomnolence and hyperphagia categorized the crash phase (9 hours–14 days). Longer-term withdrawal (1–10 weeks) has high craving, mild dysphoria, irritability, and anxiety. The final phase of extinction (indefinite) was characterized by euthymic mood.

Both depression and stimulants have been linked to similar effects on brain neurotransmitters. The neurochemical changes in serotonin (5-HT), dopamine (DA), norepinephrine (NE), and peptide systems (corticotropin-releasing factor, neuropeptide Y) induced by stimulant use parallel changes in human and animal models of depression (118). Stimulants act predominantly through blockade of serotonin, dopamine, and NE presynaptic reuptake. Stimulants increase serotonergic activity by inhibiting uptake of 5-HT released in the synaptic cleft, which in turn inhibits 5-HT synthesis with chronic use (119). On cessation of stimulant use, 5-HT levels are decreased, and presumably are associated with onset of depressive symptoms. In addition, the decrease in serotonergic tone may cause the insomnia noted during cocaine intoxication, and the rebound increase in 5-HT during withdrawal may produce the hypersomnia characteristic of that phase of use.

The blockade of catecholamine reuptake (120,121) by stimulants results acutely in an increase in NE synthesis; however, with chronic use, NE and DA depletion act in concert to produce anergia and other depressive symptoms typical of the "crash" (122). Stimulants also block DA reuptake, leaving excess

DA in the synapse and increasing DA synthesis. This has been postulated to lead to changes that are related to anhedonia noted with chronic use. Supersensitivity of DA and beta-adrenergic receptors on postsynaptic neurons in response to synaptic neurotransmitter depletion also parallels the beta-adrenergic receptor supersensitivity in postsynaptic neurons of patients with major depression. Adding to the complexity is the interactions between these neurotransmitters. Serotonin regulates aspects of both NE and DA function (118), such that serotonergic deficits can produce dopaminergic deficits and dysregulated noradrenergic function.

NICOTINE AND DEPRESSION

Nicotine exposure is very common throughout the world. Because it readily crosses the blood–brain barrier, it is able to interact with neurochemical systems, for example, binding to acetylcholine (ACh) receptors in the brain and elsewhere (123). Both nicotine use and withdrawal have been associated with depression.

Studies suggest an association between chronic nicotine use and depression (124–126). Smokers reported mood-elevating effects of smoking, hypothesized to be either relief of the abstinence syndrome or a brain enhancement effect. Several authors have noted both a greater prevalence of smoking among depressed patients (127,128) and a greater prevalence of depression among smokers (129–131). Also, there appears to be a correlation between a history of depression and the onset of smoking (132,133), greater difficulty in smoking cessation (127,130,131,134–137), and relapse to smoking (134,138). For example, Glassman et al. (135) found that 60% of smokers had a history of major depression and were twice as likely to fail in their attempts to stop smoking as those without a history of depression. Female gender might also be a predictor for depression in smokers (131,139,140). Glassman (141) suggested that, for some, nicotine might serve as an antidepressant. In a study involving 1566 female twins, Kendler et al. (142) found that a family history of depression predicted smoking and theorized that the association is due to genetic factors predisposing vulnerable individuals to both depression and smoking. That depression and nicotine use are related has been clearly established. At this point, the factors determining that relationship remain undefined.

Dysphoric or depressed mood, restlessness, irritability, anxiety, drowsiness, confusion, poor concentration, and insomnia generally characterize nicotine withdrawal (123). Hughes et al. (143) and others (144–146) reported that nicotine withdrawal may both induce depressed mood in vulnerable individuals and mimic early depression. Breslau et al. (136) supported earlier reports (147,148) that nicotine-withdrawal symptoms are more severe in smokers with histories of depression. Depression was reported in about 23% of their sample of 239 smokers, who endorsed decreased heart rate, drowsiness, trouble concentrating, and feeling depressed during cessation attempts (136). Depressive symptoms during withdrawal were also associated with failure in cessation attempts (149,150).

Stimulation of possibly presynaptic nicotinic receptors during short-term exposure results in release of ACh, NE, DA, 5-HT, vasopressin, growth hormone, and ACTH in the brain and catecholamines in other sites, e.g., the adrenal medulla and blood vessels (123). Central nervous system effects are due to actions of nicotine on receptors and are dose-related. Cholinergic mechanisms and the interaction of ACh and catecholamines, both implicated in depression, may be a common link here as well (151).

OPIATES AND DEPRESSION

Opiate use has also been associated with depressive symptoms and, paradoxically, with depression treatment (152,153). Acute and chronic opiate use produces an initial mood elevation, but this mood is ultimately replaced by dysphoria (154). A protracted withdrawal syndrome has also been described, wherein depressive symptoms persisted for up to 24 weeks after withdrawal (155,156).

A lifetime prevalence for depression of about 50% was found by Rounsaville et al. (157) in 533 opiate-addicted patients. Using the Schedule for Affective Disorders and Schizophrenia–Lifetime (SADS-L) and RDC, they reported that 24% had a current major depressive episode and 2% had dysthymia. Others have also documented the presence of depressive symptoms in their populations of opiate addicts (158–160). Brooner et al. (161) found a prevalence of about 16% for depression in 716 opiate abusers seeking methadone maintenance. Brewer et al. (162) identified depression as one variable predicting continued opiate use. Maddux et al. (163) reported that the most depressed of his 173 opiate-using subjects were those who were opiate-dependent. About 87% of 67 methadone patients had major depression, and those who had autonomous mood disorders were more likely to complete treatment and less likely to use other drugs (164). Sproule et al. (165,166) found that 125 codeine-dependent patients reported depression related to codeine use, showing modest elevation on the Symptom Checklist-90 (SCL-90) depression subscale.

As with alcohol abstinence, reports exist of remission of depressive symptoms in some patients with opiate abstinence, suggesting that the primary-secondary depression dichotomy may extend to opiates as well. Strain et al. (167) found that self-reported depressive symptoms, as measured by the BDI, declined significantly 7 days after cessation of heroin use, despite continued methadone use. Rounsaville et al. (168) reported that 17% of 157 opiate-dependent subjects had major depression and 60% had some depressive symptoms upon entrance into treatment. These declined to 12% and 31%, respectively, after 6 months of abstinence and were unrelated to specific antidepressant treatment. Rounsaville et al. (169) also correlated depressive symptoms and rates of major depression in 877 primary relatives of 201 opiate abusers, finding significantly higher rates of depression in first-degree relatives of both depressed and nondepressed opiate users. These results indicate a direct depressant effect of opiates. Therefore, careful termination of opiate pain medication use in comorbid patients is the usual first step in treatment.

In his work on brain reward mechanisms involved with opiate use and subsequent withdrawal, Nestler (170) postulated that chronic opiate use elevates levels of G proteins, morphine-regulated and cAMP-regulated phosphoproteins, including tyrosine hydroxylase, the rate-limiting enzyme in catecholamine synthesis. Opiate use may be associated with changes in catecholamine neurotransmitters. In addition, binding at kappa and possibly sigma receptors has been associated with dysphoric effects (171–174), and Extein et al. (174) suggested opiate-receptor dysfunction as a possible factor in depression. Opiate-receptor function, withdrawal symptoms, and dysphoria may also be related, as suggested by the association of opiate-withdrawal severity and the degree of dysphoria (175).

OTHER DRUGS AND DEPRESSION

The relationship between depression and inhalant abuse is not well known. The 1990 lifetime prevalence of solvent and aerosol abuse was 17–19% among high school seniors (43). These substances appear to affect metabolism and syntheses of brain neurotransmitters and may produce mood swings, including dysphoria (43). There are limited data on depression and solvent/aerosol abuse, but Westermeyer (176) reported a case of a 44-year-old woman who developed depression after brief abstinence from inhalation of carbon tetrachloride for several years. The depression increased in severity over a 4-week period but responded to antidepressants. Crites and Schuckit (177), however, found no difference in the incidence of affective symptoms between 120 solvent-abusing adolescents and 636 other drug-abusing adolescents. Dinwiddie et al. (178) reviewed psychiatric diagnoses of 11 chronic solvent abusers, only one of whom was diagnosed with a secondary depression. Overall, the depressive symptoms associated with solvent/aerosol abuse generally appear to be mild and transitory.

Although hallucinogens such as lysergic acid diethylamide (LSD) and phencyclidine (PCP) generally are not associated with severe mood disturbances, reports suggest that use of 3,4-methylenedioxymethamphetamine (MDMA, "Ecstasy"), a hallucinogen with stimulant properties, produces depressive symptoms (179–181), possibly related to damage to serotonergic neurons (182). MDMA has been noted to increase extracellular DA and 5-HT. NE and neuropeptide levels are also affected (182), and tryptophan hydroxylase activity is reduced (183). Peroutka et al. (184) found depression to be one of the untoward side effects the day after MDMA use in 21–36% of their 100 subjects. Curran and Travill (185) found "low mood" 4 days after MDMA use in 12 subjects, and Parrott and Lasky (186) described depressed mood 2 days after MDMA use in 30 subjects. The long-term effects of MDMA on mood are unknown at this point.

Use of sedatives, including benzodiazepines, has been linked to depression (187,188), although few empirical studies of this relationship exist (189). A positive correlation between prewithdrawal depressive symptoms and sedative-withdrawal symptom severity has been reported (190), as has the presence of depressive symptoms in withdrawal as a predictor of withdrawal failure (191). In a prospective study involving 82 alcohol- or benzodiazepine-dependent subjects undergoing detoxification, Charney et al. (192) found that the benzodiazepine-dependent subjects had a worse outcome in terms of abstinence at 3 months but not at 6 months.

Clinical studies of the relationship between sedatives and depression have yielded conflicting results. Steffens et al. (81) found that about 27% of their approximately 300 depressed subjects were sedative users. In their sample of 375 subjects with major depression, Abraham and Fava (82) reported that sedative users were among substance abusers with the fewest lifetime depressive episodes. Likewise, Chutuape et al. (83) found past and present sedative use common among opiate users, but a low prevalence of depression in these subjects. Finally, from a sample of 1874 monozygotic male twin pairs, Lin et al. (85) concluded that the association they found between major depression and sedative abuse or dependence was nonfamilial in origin.

CONCLUSIONS

Substance abuse and depression comorbidity is an active area for research, yet much remains to be learned about the relationship between these common disorders. Depressive symptoms are often found during drug withdrawal and with protracted withdrawal from alcohol, opiates, nicotine, stimulants, and marijuana. Furthermore, depressive symptoms are frequently seen with the chronic use of these same substances. Whether the neurochemical mechanisms are the same in chronic use and withdrawal states differ is not well known.

Exploration of the coexistence of these disorders resulted in the identification of possible gender differences and familial patterns, as well as the differentiation between primary and secondary depressions. Common neurobiological mechanisms have been proposed to link substance abuse and depression. The monoamine systems, particularly serotonin, have been implicated most often. The possible role of serotonin makes use of serotonin-reuptake inhibitors as a first-line medication in the treatment of patients with depression and substance abuse. Other possible systems included a broader role for opiate receptors, peptides, acetylcholine, and other molecules such as ACTH. Although the limbic area has been identified as the primarily affected site, other brain areas may be involved as well.

Substances of abuse appear to be causal factors in depressive symptoms in many patients. In other patients, depression may occur first and promote use of drugs in an attempt at self-medication of symptoms (such as depression) or "numbing" their feelings. Serotonin and other neurochemicals may be involved in the mechanism of both disorders.

Despite the special needs of patients with comorbid substance use disorders and depression, physicians and other medical professionals often overlook the need for substance abuse treatment or miss the comorbidity diagnosis altogether. Careful reevaluation for comorbid substance abuse is advised, especially in cases of treatment-resistant depression. Future work in this area is important to further define pathogenetic processes and predisposing factors, aid in diagnosis, and optimize treatment of patients with comorbid substance abuse and depression.

REFERENCES

1. HE Ross, FB Glaser, T Germanson. The prevalence of psychiatric disorders in patients with alcohol and other drug problems. Arch Gen Psychiatry 45:1023–1031, 1988.

2. NS Miller, D Klamen, NG Hoffmann, JA Flaherty. Prevalence of depression and alcohol and other drug dependence in addictions treatment populations. J Psychoact Drugs 28:111–124, 1996.
3. DA Charney, AM Paraherakis, JC Negrete, KJ Gill. The impact of depression on the outcome of addictions treatment. J Subst Abuse Treat 15:123–30, 1998.
4. ID Montoya, D Svikis, SC Marcus, A Suarez, T Tanielian, HA Pincus. Psychiatric care of patients with depression and comorbid substance use disorders. J Clin Psychiatry 61: 696–705, 2000.
5. BF Grant. Comorbidity between DSM-IV drug use disorders and major depression: results of a national survey of adults. J Subst Abuse 7:481–497, 1995.
6. MQ Wang, CB Collins, RJ DiClemente, G Wingood, CL Kohler. Multiple drug use and depression: gender differences among African-Americans in a high-risk community. J Alcohol Drug Education 43:87–96, 1997.
7. B Donohue, R Acierno, E Kogan. Relationship of depression with measures of social functioning adult drug abusers. Addict Behav 21:211–216, 1996.
8. MQ Wang, CB Collins, RJ DiClemente, G Wingood, CL Kohler. Depressive symptoms as correlates of polydrug use for blacks in a high-risk community. South Med J 90:1123–1128, 1997.
9. J Westermeyer, S Kopka, S Nugent. Course and severity of substance abuse among patients with comorbid major depression. Am J Addictions 6:284–292, 1997.
10. RE Meyer. How to understand the relationship between psychopathology and addictive disorders: another example of the chick and the egg. In: Psychopathology and Addictive Disorders. RE Meyer, ed. New York: Guilford Press, 1986.
11. JD Swendsen, KR Merikangas. The comorbidity of depression and substance use disorders. Clin Psychol Rev 20:173–189, 2000.
12. A Markou, TR Kosten, GF Koob. Neurobiological similarities in depression and drug dependence: a self-medication hypothesis. Neuropsychopharmacology 18(3):135–174, 1998.
13. SC Dilsaver. The pathophysiologies of substance abuse and affective disorders: an integrative model? J Clin Psychopharmacol 7:1–10, 1987.
14. RM Anthenelli, MA Schuckit. Affective and anxiety disorders. In: Principles of Addiction Medicine. NS Miller, ed. Chevy Chase, MD: American Society of Addiction Medicine, 1994.
15. JR Cornelius, IM Salloum, NL Day, ME These, JJ Mann. Patterns of suicidality and alcohol use in alcoholics with major depression. Alcohol Clin Exp Res 20:1451–1455, 1996.
16. MT Lynskey. The comorbidity of alcohol dependence and affective disorders: treatment implications. Drug Alcohol Depend 52:201–209, 1998.
17. BF Grant, TC Harford. Comorbidity between DSM-IV alcohol use disorders and major depression: results of a national survey. Drug Alcohol Depend 39:197–206, 1995.
18. MM Weissman, JK Myers. Clinical depression in alcoholism. Am J Psychiatry 137:372–373, 1980.

19. A Roy. Neuroticism and depression in alcoholics. J Affect Disord 52:243–245, 1999.
20. A Roy. Aetiology of secondary depression in male alcoholics. Br J Psychiatry 169:753–757, 1996.
21. DA Dawson, BF Grant. Family history of alcoholism and gender: their combined effects on DSM-IV alcohol dependence and major depression. J Stud Alcohol 59:97–106, 1998.
22. W Maier, K Merikangas. Co-occurrence and contransmission of affective disorders and alcoholism in families. Br J Psychiatry June (suppl):93–100, 1996.
23. EZ Hanna, BF Grant. Gender differences in DSM-IV alcohol use disorders and major depression as distributed in the general population: clinical implications. Compr Psychiatry 38:202–212, 1997.
24. SJ Waller, JS Lyons, MF Costantini-Ferrando. Impact of comorbid affective and alcohol use disorders on suicidal ideation and attempts. J Clin Psychol 55:585–95, 1999.
25. BF Grant, DS Hasin. Suicidal ideation among the United States drinking population: results from the National Longitudinal Alcohol Epidemiologic Survey. J Stud Alcohol 60:422–429, 1999.
26. A Porsteinsson, PR Duberstein, Y Conwell, C Cox, N Forbes, ED Caine. Suicide and alcoholism: distinguishing alcoholic patients with and without cormorbid drug abuse. Am J Addict 6:304–310, 1997.
27. A Roy, D Lamparski, J DeJong, V Moore, M Linnoila. Characteristics of alcoholics who attempt suicide. Am J Psychiatry 147:761–765, 1990.
28. GE Murphy, RD Wetzel, E Robins, L McEvoy. Multiple risk factors predict suicide in alcoholism. Arch Gen Psychiatry 49:459–463, 1992.
29. K Schaefer, N Butters, T Smith, M Irwin, S Brown, P Hanger, I Grant, M Schuckit. Cognitive performance of alcoholics: a longitudinal evaluation of the role of drinking history, depression, liver function, nutrition and family history. Alcohol Clin Exp Res 15:653–660, 1991.
30. S Glenn, A Errico, O Parsons, A King, S Nixon. The role of antisocial, affective and childhood behavioral characteristics in alcoholics' neurological performance. Alcohol Clin Exp Res 17:162–169, 1993.
31. PN Tariot, H Weingartner. A psychobiological analysis of cognitive failures. Arch Gen Psychiatry 43:1183–1188, 1986.
32. RMA Hirschfeld, T Kosier, MB Keller, PW Lavori, J Endicott. The influence of alcoholism on the course of depression. J Affect Disord 16:151–158, 1989.
33. DS Hasin, WY Tsai, J Endicott, TI Mueller, W Coryell, M Keller. Five-year course of major depression: effects of comorbid alcoholism. J Affect Disord 41:63–70,1996.
34. M Windle, PT Davies. Depression and heavy alcohol use among adolescents: concurrent and prospective relations. Dev Psychopathol 11:823–844, 1999.
35. JE Alpert, M Fava, LA Uebelacker, AA Nierenberg, JA Pava, JJ Worthington III, JF Rosenbaum. Patterns of axis I comorbidity in early-onset versus late-onset major depressive disorder. Biol Psychiatry 15:202–211, 1999.

36. CA King, N Ghaziuddin, L McGovern, E Brand, E Hill, M Naylor. Predictors of comorbid alcohol and substance abuse in depressed adolescents. J Am Acad Child Adolesc Psychiatry 35:743–751, 1996.
37. HM Pettinati, JD Pierce Jr, AL Wolf, RM Rukstalis, CP O'Brien. Gender differences in comorbidly depressed alcohol-dependent outpatients. Alcohol Clin Exp Res 21:1742–1746, 1997.
38. BS Moscato, M Russell, M Zielezny, E Bromet, G Egri, P Mudar, JR Marshall. Gender differences in the relation between depressive symptoms and alcohol problems: a longitudinal perspective. Am J Epidemiol 146:966–974, 1997.
39. JM Bjork, DM Dougherty, FG Moeller. Symptomatology of depression and anxiety in female "social drinkers." Am J Drug Alcohol Abuse 25:173–182, 1999.
40. CA Prescott, SH Agger, KS Kendler. Sex-specific genetic influences on the comorbidity of alcoholism and major depression in a population-based sample of US twins. Arch Gen Psychiatry 57:803–811, 2000.
41. J Solomon. Alcoholism and psychiatric disorders. In: Alcoholism: Biomedical and Genetic Aspects. HW Goedde, PD Agarwal, eds. New York: Pergamon Press, pp 216–227, 1989.
42. MA Schuckit, MG Monteiro. Alcoholism, anxiety and depression. Br J Addiction 83:1371–1380, 1988.
43. MA Schuckit. Drug and Alcohol Abuse: A Clinical Guide to Diagnosis and Treatment. 4th ed. New York: Plenum, 1995.
44. SA Brown, MA Schuckit. Changes in depression among abstinent alcoholics. J Stud Alcohol 49: 412–417, 1988.
45. MA Schuckit. Alcohol and depression: a clinical perspective. Acta Psychiatrica Scandinavica 377:28–32, 1994.
46. MH Keeler, CI Taylor, WC Miller. Are all recently detoxified alcoholics depressed? Am J Psychiatry 136:4B586–588, 1979.
47. B Liskow, D Mayfield, J Thiele. Alcohol and affective disorder: assessment and treatment. J Clin Psychiatry 43:144–147, 1982.
48. HM Pettinati, AA Sugarman, HS Maurer. Four year MMPI changes in abstinent and drinking alcoholics. Alcoholism: Clin Exp Res 6:487–494, 1982.
49. KM Davidson. Diagnosis of depression alcohol dependence: changes in prevalence with drinking status. Br J Psychiatry 166:199–204, 1995.
50. SA Brown, RK Inaba, JC Gillin, MA Schuckit, MA Stewart, MR Irwin. Alcoholism and affective disorder: clinical course of depressive symptoms. Am J Psychiatry 152:45–52, 1995.
51. H Roggla, A Uhl. Depression and relapses in treated chronic alcoholics. Int J Addict 30:337–349, 1995.
52. SL Satel, TR Kosten, MA Schuckit, MW Fischman. Should protracted withdrawal from drugs be included in DSM-IV? Am J Psychiatry 150:695–704, 1993.
53. HE Ross, FB Glaser, T Germanson. The prevalence of psychiatric disorders in

patients with alcohol and other drug problems. Arch Gen Psychiatry 45:1023–1031, 1988.
54. HP Weingold, JM Lachin, HA Bell, et al. Depression as a symptom of alcoholism: search for a phenomenon. J Abnorm Psychol 73:195–197, 1968.
55. AT McLellan, KA Druley. Random relation between drugs of abuse and psychiatric diagnoses. J Psychiatr Res 13: 179–184, 1977.
56. LR Herz, L Volicer N D'Angelo, D Gadish. Additional psychiatric illness by diagnostic interview scechule in male alcoholics. Comp Psychiatry 30:72–79, 1990.
57. CA Dackis, J Bailey, ALL Potash, RF Stuckey, IL Extein, MS Gold. Specificity of the DST and the TRH test for major depression in alcoholics. Am J Psychiatry 141:680–683, 1984.
58. WH Nelson, P Sullivan, A Khan, RN Tamragouri. The effect of age on dexamethasone suppression test results in alcoholic patients. Am J Psychiatry 143:237–239, 1986.
59. MA Schuckit. Genetic and clinical implications of alcoholism and affective disorder. Am J Psychiatry 143:140–147, 1986.
60. JE Helzer, TR Pryzbeck. The co-occurrence of alcoholism with other psychiatric disorders in the general population and its impact on treatment. J Stud Alcohol 49:219–224, 1988.
61. K O'Sullivan, P Williams, M Daly, et al. A comparison of alcoholics with and without co-existing affective disorder. Br J Psychiatry 143:133–138, 1983.
62. MA Schuckit. The clinical implications of primary diagnostic groups among alcoholics. Arch Gen Psychiatry 42:1043–1049, 1985.
63. M Schuckit. Alcoholic patients with secondary depression. Am J Psychiatry 140:711–714, 1983.
64. MM Weissman, M Pottenger, K Kleber, et al. Symptom patterns in primary and secondary depression. Arch Gen Psychiatry 34:854–862, 1977.
65. MN Hesselbrock, RE Meyer, JJ Keener. Psychopathology in hospitalized alcoholics. Arch Gen Psychiatry 42:1050–1055, 1985.
66. BJ Powell, MR Read, EC Penick, NS Miller, SF Bingham. Primary and secondary depression in alcoholic men: an important distinction? J Clin Psychiatry 48:98–101, 1987.
67. EB Raimo, MA Schuckit. Alcohol dependence and mood disorders. Addict Behav 23:933–946, 1998.
68. MA Schuckit, JE Tipp, M Bergman, W Reich. Comparison of induced and independent major depressive disorders in 2,945 alcoholics. Am J Psychiatry 154:948–957, 1997.
69. SF Greenfield, RD Weiss, LR Muenz, LM Vagge, JF Kelly, LR Bello, J Michael. The effect of depression on return to drinking: a prospective study. Arch Gen Psychiatry 55:259–265, 1998.
70. DC Hodgins, N el-Guebaly, S Armstrong, M Dufour. Implications of depression on outcome from alcohol dependence: a 3-year prospective follow-up. Alcohol Clin Exp Res 23:151–157, 1999.

71. KM Davidson, IM Blackburn. Comorbid depression and drinking outcome in those with alcohol dependence. Alcohol Alcohol 33:482–487, 1998.
72. F Fadda, ZL Rossetti. Chronic ethanol consumption: from neuroadaptation to neurodegeneration. Prog Neurobiol 56:385–431, 1998.
73. JC Ballenger, FK Goodwin, LF Major, et al. Alcohol and central serotonin metabolism in man. Arch Gen Psychiatry 36:224–227, 1979.
74. DA Gorelick. Serotonin uptake blockers and the treatment of alcoholism. In: Recent Developments in Alcoholism. Vol 7. M Galanter, ed. New York: Plenum, pp 267–281, 1989.
75. A Roy, M Virkkunen, M Linnoila. Serotonin in suicide, violence, and alcoholism. In: Serotonin in Major Psychiatric Disorders. EF Coccaro, DL Murphy, eds. Washington, DC: American Psychiatric Press, 1990.
76. L Branchey, M Branchey, S Shaw, CS Lieber. Relationship between changes in plasma amino acids and depression in alcoholic patients. Am J Psychiatry 141:1212–1215, 1984.
77. AA Badawy. Tryptophan metabolism in alcoholism. Adv Exp Med Biol 467:265–274, 1999.
78. AC Swann, BA Johnson, CR Cloninger, YR Chen. Relationships of plasma tryptophan availability to course of illness and clinical features of alcoholism: a preliminary study. Psychopharmacology 143:380–384, 1999.
79. A Heinz, H Weingartner, D George, D Hommer, OM Wolkowitz, M Linnoila. Severity of depression in abstinent alcoholics is associated with monoamine metabolites and dehydroepiandrosterone-sulfate concentrations. Psychiatry Res 89:97–106, 1999.
80. LE Hollister. Drug-induced psychiatric disorders and their management. Med Toxicol 1:428–448, 1986.
81. DC Steffens, I Skoog, MC Norton, AD Hgart, JT Tschanz, BL Plassman, BW Wyse, KA Welsh-Bohmer, JC Breitner. Prevalence of depression and its treatment in an elderly population: the Cache County study. Arch Gen Psychiatry 57:601–607, 2000.
82. HD Abraham, M Fava. Order of onset of substance abuse and depression in a sample of depressed outpatients. Compr Psychiatry 40:44–50, 1999.
83. MA Chutuape, RK Brooner, M Stitzer. Sedative use disorders in opiate-dependent patients: association with psychiatric and other substance use disorders. J Nerv Ment Dis 185:289–297, 1997.
84. RB Lydiard, MT Laraia, JC Ballenger, EF Howell. Emergence of depressive symptoms in patients receiving alprazolam for panic disorder. Am J Psychiatry 144:664–665, 1987.
85. N Lin, SA Eisen, JFD Scherrer, J Goldberg, WR True, MJ Lyons, MT Tsuang. The influence of familial and non-familial factors on the association between major depression and substance abuse/dependence in 1874 monozygotic male twin pairs. Drug Alcohol Depend 43:49–55, 1996.
86. C Fahlke, U Berggren, C Lundborg, J Balldin. Psychopathology in alcohol

withdrawal: relationship to alpha2-adrenoceptor function. Alcohol Alcohol 34:750–759, 1999.
87. A Heinz, P Dufeu, S Kuhn, M Dettling, K Graf, I Kurten, H Rommelspacher, LG Schmidt. Psychopathological and behavioral correlates of dopaminergic sensitivity in alcohol-dependent patients. Arch Gen Psychiatry 53:1123–1128, 1996.
88. JR Hubbard, SE Franco, ES Onaivi. Marijuana: medical implications. Am Family Physician 60:2583–2588, 1999.
89. JA Halikas, Goodwin DW, Guze SB. Marijuana use and psychiatric illness. Arch Gen Psychiatry 27:162–165, 1972.
90. RA Weller, JA Halikas. Marijuana use and psychiatric illness: a follow-up study. Am J Psychiatry 142:848–850, 1985.
91. J Shedler, J Block. Adolescent drug use and psychological health: a longitudinal inquiry. Am Psychol 45:612–630, 1990.
92. BW Lex, ML Griffin, NK Mello, Mendleson JH. Alcohol, marijuana, and mood states in young women. Int J Addict 24:405–424, 1989.
93. SM Mirin, LM Shapiro RE Meyer, RC Pillard, S Fisher. Casual versus heavy use of marijuana: a redefinition of the marijuana problem. Am J Psychiatry 127:1134–1140, 1971.
94. S Andreasson, P Allebeck. Cannabis and mortality among young men: a longitudinal study of Swedish conscripts. Scand J Soc Med 18:8–15, 1990.
95. S Schnoll, AN Daghestani. Treatment of marijuana abuse. Psychiatr Annals 16:249–254, 1986.
96. L Grinspoon, JB Bakalar. Marijuana In: Substance Abuse: A Comprehensive Textbook. 3rd ed. J Lowinson, P Ruiz, RB Millman, JG Langrod, eds. Baltimore: Williams & Wilkins, 1997.
97. LE Hollister. Health aspects of cannabis. Pharmacol Rev 38:1–20, 1986.
98. RH Schwartz. Marijuana: an overview. Pediatr Clin North Am 34:305–317, 1987.
99. MC Braude, S Szara. Pharmacology of marihuana. New York: Raven Press, 1976.
100. JH Mendleson, NK Mello, BW Lex, S Bavli. Marijuana withdrawal syndrome in a woman. Am J Psychiatry 141:1289–1290, 1984.
101. LA Matsuda, LJ Lolait, MJ Brownstein, et al. Structure of a cannabinoid receptor and functional expression of the cloned cDNA. Nature 346:561–564, 1990.
102. AC Howlett, M Bidaut-Russell, WA Devane, et al. The cannabinoid receptor: biochemical, anatomical and behavioral characterization. Trends Neurosci 13:420–423, 1990.
103. R Lu, JR Hubbard, BR Martin, MT Kalami. Roles of sulfhydryl and disulfide groups in the binding of CP-55, 940 to rat brain cannabinoid receptor. Mol Cel Biochem 121:119–126, 1993.
104. ES Onaivi, A Chakraborti, G Chaudhuri. Cannabinoid receptor genes. Prog Neurobiol 48:275–305, 1996.
105. G Nahas. Biomedical aspects of cannabis usage. Bull Narc 29:13–27, 1977.

106. BGB Sethi, JK Trivedi, P Kumar, et al. Antianxiety effect of cannabis: involvement of central benzodiazepine receptors. Biol Psychiatry 21:3–10, 1986.
107. FH Gawin, HD Kleber. Abstinence symptomatology and psychiatric diagnosis in cocaine abusers. Arch Gen Psychiatry 43:107–113, 1986.
108. FH Gawin, EH Ellinwood. Cocaine and other stimulants. N Engl J Med 318:1173–1182, 1988.
109. CA Dackis, TW Estroff, DR Sweeney, ALC Pottash, MS Gold. Specificity of the TRH test for major depression in patients with serious cocaine abuse. Am J Psychiatry 142:1097–1099, 1985.
110. BJ Rounsaville, SF Anton, K Carroll, et al. Psychiatric diagnosis of treatment seeking cocaine abusers. Arch Gen Psychiatry 48:43–51, 1991.
111. EV Nunes, FM Quitkin, DF Klein. Psychiatric diagnosis in cocaine abuse. Psychiatry Res 28:105–114, 1989.
112. SM Mirin, RD Weiss. Affective illness in substance abusers. Psychiatr Clin North Am 9:503–514, 1986.
113. SM Mirin, RD Weiss, J Michael, ML Griffin. Psychopathology in substance abusers and their families. Resident & Staff Physician 34:61–65, 1988.
114. SM Mirin, RD Weiss, J Michael. Psychopathology in substance abusers: diagnosis and treatment. Am J Drug Alcohol Abuse 14:139–157, 1988.
115. RD Weiss, SM Mirin, ML Griffin, JL Michael. Psychopathology in cocaine abusers. J Nerv Ment Dis 176:719–725, 1988.
116. PH Kleinman, AB Miller, RM Millman, GE Woody, T Todd, J Kemp, DS Lipton. Psychopathology among cocaine abusers entering treatment. J Nerv Ment Dis 178:442–447, 1990.
117. R Watson, E Hartmann, JJ Schildkraut. Amphetamine withdrawal: affective state, sleep patterns, and MHPG excretion. Am J Psychiatry 129:39–45, 1972.
118. TR Kosten, A Markou, GF Koob. Depression and stimulant dependence: neurobiology and pharmacotherapy. J Nerv Ment Dis 186:737–45, 1998.
119. TA Kosten, TR Kosten, FH Gawin, et al. An open trial of sertraline for cocaine abuse. Am J Addictions 1:349–353, 1992.
120. CA Dackis, MS Gold. New concepts in cocaine addiction: the dopamine depletion hypothesis. Neurosci Biobehav 9:469–477, 1985.
121. WC Hall, RL Talbert, L Ereshefsky. Cocaine abuse and its treatment. Pharmacotherapy 10:47–65, 1990.
122. FH Gawin. New uses of antidepressants in cocaine abuse. Psychosomatics 27(suppl):9, 1986.
123. NL Benowitz. Pharmacologic aspects of cigarette smoking and nicotine addiction. N Engl J Med 319:1318–1330, 1988.
124. HJ Waal-Manning, FA de Hamel. Smoking habit and psychometric scores: a community study. NZ Med J 88: 188–191, 1978.
125. N Breslau, MM Kilbey, P Andreski. Nicotine dependence, major depression, and anxiety in young adults. Arch Gen Psychiatry 48:1069–1074, 1991.
126. M Zimmerman, WH Coryell, DW Black. Cigarette smoking and psychiatric illness In: CME Syllabus and Scientific Proceedings in Summary Form, 144th

Depression

Annual Meeting of the American Psychiatric Association. Washington, DC: American Psychiatric Association, 1991.
127. MG Goldstein, R Niaura, DB Abrambs. Medical and behavioral treatment of nicotine dependence. In: Advances in Medical-Psychiatric Practice. A Stoudemire, BS Fogel, eds. Washington, DC: American Psychiatric Press, 1990.
128. JR Hughes, DK Hatsukami, JE Mitchell, BA Dahlgren. Prevalence of smoking in psychiatric outpatients. Am J Psychiatry 143:993–997, 1986.
129. AH Glassman, LS Covey, F Stetner. Smoking cessation, depression, and antidepressants. Abstract presented at the 142nd Annual Meeting of the American Psychiatric Association, May 1989.
130. SM Hall, R Munoz, V Reus. Smoking cessation, depression, and dysphoria. In: Problems of Drug Dependence. National Institute on Drug Abuse Research Monograph Series. LS Harris, ed. Washington, DC: US Government Printing Office, 1992.
131. AH Glassman, JE Helzer, LS Covey, LB Cottler, F Stetner, JE Tipp, J Johnson. Smoking, smoking cessation, and major depression. JAMA 264:1546–1549, 1990.
132. DB Kandel, M Davies. Adult sequelae of adolescent depressive symptoms. Arch Gen Psychiatry 42:255–262, 1986.
133. JR Hughes. Clonidine, depression and smoking cessation. JAMA 254:2901–2902, 1988.
134. LS Covey, AH Glassman, F Stetner. Depression and depressive symptoms in smoking cessation. Compr Psychiatry 31:350–354, 1990.
135. AH Glassman, F Stetner, PS Walsh Raizman, JL Fleiss, TB Cooper, LS Covey. Heavy smokers, smoking cessation, and clonidine: results of a double-blind, randomized trial. JAMA 259:2863–2866, 1988.
136. N Breslau, MM Kilbey, P Andreski. Nicotine withdrawal symptoms and psychiatric disorders: findings from an epidemiologic study of young adults. Am J Psychiatry 149:464–469, 1992.
137. RF Anda, DF Williamson, LG Escobedo, EE Mast, GA Giovino, PL Remington. Depression and the dynamics of smoking: a national perspective. JAMA 264:1541–1545, 1990.
138. S Shiffman. Relapse following smoking cessation: a situational analysis. J Consult Clin Psychol 50:71–86, 1982.
139. T Frederick, RR Frerichs, VA Clark. Personal health habits and symptoms of depression at the community level. Prev Med 17:173–182, 1988.
140. J Chetwynd. Some characteristics of women smokers. NZ Med J 99:14–17, 1986.
141. AH Glassman. Cigarette smoking: implications for psychiatric illness. Am J Psychiatry 150:546–553, 1993.
142. KS Kendler, MC Neale, CJ MacLean, AC Heath, LJ Eaves, RC Kessler. Smoking and major depression: a causal analysis. Arch Gen Psychiatry 50:36–43, 1993.
143. JR Hughes, ST Higgins, DK Hatsukami. Effects of abstinence from tobacco: a critical review. In: Research Advances in Alcohol and Drug Problems. Vol 10.

LT Kozlowski, H Annis, HD Cappell, et al, eds. New York: Plenum, pp 317–398, 1990.
144. J Flanagan, I Maany. Smoking and depression [letter]. Am J Psychiatry 139:540–541, 1982.
145. AH Glassman, L Covey, F Stetner. Smoking cessation and major depression. In: Proceedings of the 28th Annual Meeting of the American College of Neuropsychopharmacology. Nashville, TN: ACNP, 1989.
146. KO Fagerstrom. Towards better diagnoses and more individual treatment of tobacco dependence. Br J Addict 86:543–547, 1991.
147. LS Covey, AH Glassman, F Stetner. Depression and depressive symptoms in smoking cessation. Compr Psychiatry 31:350–354, 1990.
148. SM Hall, R Munoz, V Reus. Smoking cessation, depression and dysphoria. In: Problems of Drug Dependence. National Institute on Drug Abuse Research Monograph Series. LS Harris, ed. Washington, DC: US Government Printing Office, 1992.
149. RJ West, P Hajek, M Belcher. Severity of withdrawal symptoms as a predictor of outcome of an attempt to quit smoking. Psychol Med 19:981–985, 1989.
150. JR Hughes. Tobacco withdrawal in self-quitters. J Consult Clin Psychol 60:689–697, 1992.
151. PA Newhouse, JR Hughes. The role of nicotine and nicotinic mechanisms in neuropsychiatric disease. Br J Addiction 86:521–526, 1991.
152. JA Bodkin, GL Zornberg, SE Lukas, JO Cole. Buprenophine treatment of refractory depression. J Clin Psychopharmacol 15:49–57, 1995.
153. AL Stoll, S Rueter. Treatment augmentation with opiates in severe and refractory major depression. Am J Psychiatry 156:2017, 1999.
154. SM Mirin, RE Meyer, HB McNamee. Psychpathology and mood during heroin use: acute vs. chronic effects. Arch Gen Psychiatry 33:1503–1508, 1976.
155. WR Martin, DR Jasinski. Physiological parameters of morphine dependence in man—tolerance, early abstinence, protracted abstinence. J Psychiatr Res 7:9–17, 1967.
156. WR Martin, DR Jasinski, CA Haertzen et al. Methadone—a reevaluation. Arch Gen Psychiatry 28:286–295, 1973.
157. BJ Rounsaville, MM Weissman, H Kleber, C Wilber. Heterogeneity of psychiatric diagnosis in treated opiate addicts. Arch Gen Psychiatry 39:151–156, 1982.
158. JL Croughan, JP Miller, D Wagelin, BY Whitman. Psychiatric illness in male and female narcotic addicts. J Clin Psychiatry 43:225–228, 1982.
159. A Dackis, MS Gold. Opiate addiction and depression—cause or effect? Drug Alcohol Depend 11:105–109, 1983.
160. MM Weissman, F Slobetz, B Prusoff, M Mezritz, P Howard. Clinical depression among narcotic addicts maintained on methadone in the community. Am J Psychiatry 133:1434–1438, 1976.
161. RK Brooner, VL King, M Kidorf, CW Schmidt, GE Bigelow. Psychiatric and substance use comorbidity among treatment-seeking opioid abusers. Arch Gen Psychiatry 54:71–80, 1997.

162. DD Brewer, RF Catalano, K Haggerty, RR Gainey, CB Fleming. A meta-analysis of predictors of continued drug use druing and after treatment for opiate addiction. Addiction 93:73–92, 1998.
163. JF Maddux, DP Desmond, R Costello. Depression in opioid users varies with substance use status. Am J Drug Alcohol Abuse 13:375–385, 1987.
164. A Rosenblum, B Fallon, S Magura, L Handelsman, J Foote, D Bernstein. The autonomy of mood disorders among cocaine-using methadone patients. Am J Drug Alcohol Abuse 25:67–80, 1999.
165. BA Sproule, UE Busto, G. Somer, MK Romach, EM Sellers. Characteristics of dependent and nondependent regular users of codeine. J Clin Psychopharmacol 19:367–372, 1999.
166. MK Romach, BA Sproule, EM Sellers, G Somer, UE Busto. Long-term codeine use is associated with depressive symptoms. J Clin Psychopharmacol 19:373–376, 1999.
167. EC Strain, ML Stitzer, GE Bigelow. Early treatment time course of depressive symptoms in opiate addicts. J Nerv Ment Dis 179:215–221, 1991.
168. BJ Rounsaville, MM Weissman, K Crits-Christoph, C Wilber, H Kleber. Diagnosis and symptoms of depression in opiate addicts: course and relationship to treatment outcome. Arch Gen Psychiatry 39:151–156, 1982.
169. BJ Rounsaville, TR Kosten, MM Weissman, B Prusoff, D Pauls, SF Anton, K Merikangas. Psychiatric disorders in relative of probands with opiate addiction. Arch Gen Psychiatry 48:33–42, 1991.
170. E Nestler. Molecular mechanisms of drug addiction. Neuroscience 12:2439–2450, 1992.
171. JH Jaffe, WR Martin. Opioid analgesics and antagonists. In: Goodman and Gilman's The Pharmacological Basis of Therapeutics. 8th ed. AG Gilman, TW Rall, AS Nies, P Taylor, eds. New York: Pergamon Press, pp. 485–521, 1990.
172. JM Musacchia. The psychotomimetic effects of opiates and the sigma receptor. Neuropsychopharmacology 3:191–200, 1990.
173. HM Emrich. A possible role of opioid substances in depression. Adv Biochem Psychopharmacol 32:77–84, 1982.
174. I Extein, AL Pottash, MS Gold. A possible opioid receptor dysfunction in some depressive disorders. Ann NY Acad Sci 398:113–119, 1982.
175. L Handelsman, MJ Aronson, R Ness, KJ Cochrane, PD Kanof. The dysphoria of heroin addiction. Am J Drug Alcohol Abuse 18:275–287, 1992.
176. J Westermeyer. The psychiatrist and solvent-inhalant abuse: recognition, assessment, and treatment. Am J Psychiatry 144:903–907, 1987.
177. J Crites, MA Schuckit. Solvent misuse in adolescents at a community alcohol center. J Clin Psychiatry 40:39–43, 1979.
178. SH Dinwiddie, CF Zorumski, EH Rubin. Psychiatric correlates of chronic solvent abuse. J Clin Psychiatry 48:334–337, 1987.
179. S Williamson, M Gossop, B Powis, P Griffiths, J Fountain, J Strang. Adverse effects of stimulant drugs in a community sample of drug users. Drug Alcohol Depend 44:87–94, 1997.

180. F Schifano, L Di Furia, G. Forza, N Minicuci, R Bricolo. MDMA ("ecstasy") consumption in the context of polydrug abuse: a report on 150 patients. Drug Alcohol Depend 52:85–90, 1998.
181. PK McGuire, H Cope, TA Fahy. Diversity of psychopathology associated with use of 3,4-methylenedioxymethamphetamine ("Ecstasy"). Br J Psychiatry 165:391–395, 1994.
182. SR White, T Obradovic, KM Imel, MJ Wheaton. The effects of methylenedioxymethamphetamine (MDMA, "Ecstasy") on monoaminergic neurotransmission in the central nervous system. Prog Neurobiol 49:455–79, 1996.
183. CJ Schmidt, VL Taylor. Depression of rat brain tryptophan hydroxylase activity following the acute administration of methyledioxymethamphetamine. Biochem Pharmacol 36:4095–4102, 1987.
184. SJ Peroutka, H Newman, H Harris. Subjective effects of 3,4-methylenedioxymethamphetamine in recreational users. Neuropsychopharmacology 1:273–277, 1988.
185. HV Curran, RA Travill. Mood and cognitive effects of +/–3,4-methylenedioxymethamphetamine (MDMA, "ecstasy"): week-end "high" followed by mid-week low. Addiction 92:821–831, 1997.
186. AC Parrott, J Lasky. Ecstasy (MDMA) effects upon mood and cognition: before, during and after a Saturday night dance. Psychopharmacology 139:261–268, 1998.
187. SB Patten, JV Williams, EJ Love. Depressive symptoms attributable to medication exposure in a medical inpatient population. Can J Psychiatry 41:651–654, 1996.
188. NS Miller, BM Belkin, MS Gold. Alcohol and drug dependence among the elderly: epidemiology, diagnosis, and treatment. Compr Psychiatry 32:153–165, 1991.
189. SB Patten, EJ Love. Drug-induced depression. Psychother Psychosom 66:63–73, 1997.
190. K Rickels, E Schweizer, WG Case, DJ Greenblatt. Long-term therapeutic use of benzodiazepines. I. Effects of abrupt discontinuation. Arch Gen Psychiatry 47:899–907, 1990.
191. M Lader. Anxiety or depression during withdrawal of hypnotic treatments. J Psychosom Res 38(suppl 1):113–123, 1994.
192. DA Charney, AM Paraherakis, KJ Gill. The treatment of sedative-hypnotic dependence: evaluating clinical predictors of outcome. J Clin Psychiatry 61:190–195, 2000.

4
Bipolar Disorder and Comorbid Substance Use Disorders

Carlos A. Zarate, Jr.
National Institute of Mental Health
National Institutes of Health
Bethesda, Maryland

Mauricio F. Tohen
Eli Lilly Laboratories
Indianapolis, Indiana
and Harvard Medical School
Boston, Massachusetts

INTRODUCTION

Bipolar disorder is a major public health problem. It is a chronic and recurring severe mental illness affecting approximately 2% of the population. The co-occurrence of alcoholism with other psychiatric disorders has been widely recognized (1), co-occurring mood disorders being one of the most common. Bipolar disorder patients with comorbid substance use disorders (SUDs)—referred to as having "dual diagnoses"—can be a challenge to the clinician, because they may not respond well to conventional treatments. In addition, these patients may have a greater risk for relapse, attrition, and readmission rates, and may manifest symptoms that are more severe, chronic, and refractory (2,3).

In this chapter, we review the literature on the comorbidity of bipolar disorder and SUDs.

PREVALENCE

Prevalence of SUD in Community Surveys

The Epidemiologic Catchment Area (ECA) study found that the lifetime prevalence of DSM-III drug dependence among respondents in the age range of 18 to 44 years was 5.1% (4). In the National Comorbidity Survey (NCS), of the respondents 15–54 years of age, 51.0% were reported to have used either illicit drugs or nonmedical prescription psychotropic drugs or inhalants at some time in their lives, and 15.4% had done so in the past 12 months (5). In the same survey, 7.5% (14.7% of lifetime users) had been dependent at some time in their lives and 1.8% had been dependent in the past 12 months (5).

The prevalence of comorbid bipolar disorder and SUD will vary depending on the type of sample the estimates are calculated on. The prevalences discussed in this chapter are of: 1) SUD in non-treatment-seeking bipolar disorder patients, 2) SUD in bipolar disorder patients seeking treatment, and 3) bipolar spectrum disorder in substance abusing patients presenting for treatment.

Prevalence of SUD Disorders in Non-Treatment-Seeking Bipolar Disorder Patients

The ECA study found that the lifetime prevalence of bipolar I disorder was 0.8% (6). A more recent study suggests that the prevalence of mania may actually be much higher—the National Comorbidity Survey (NCS) reported a lifetime prevalence of 1.6% for mania (7). The NCS examined the lifetime co-occurrence of DSM-III-R alcohol abuse and dependence with other psychiatric disorders (8). Of all Axis I disorders, bipolar was by far the most likely to be associated with comorbid SUD (8). The lifetime prevalence of substance dependence and abuse in the ECA study for patients with mood disorder was estimated to be 60.7% for bipolar I disorder, 48.1% for bipolar II disorder, and 27% for major depression (1). The only other psychiatric disorder with a higher lifetime prevalence for SUD is antisocial personality disorder. Indeed, the ECA study (1) found that the likelihood of an individual with bipolar disorder having an SUD was six times greater than that in the general population and twice that of having an SUD associated with unipolar depression.

Prevalence of SUD in Bipolar Disorder Patients Presenting for Treatment

Studies have reported different rates of SUD depending on whether the estimates are based on the patient's presenting for treatment for his or her first manic episode or one of many. Tohen and colleagues (9) reported fairly low rates of lifetime SUD in first-episode manic patients. The authors reported that the lifetime prevalence of drug abuse or dependence in patients admitted for a first episode of mania was 17.1% (24% among women and 6% among men). In contrast, Keck et al. (10) reported much higher lifetime prevalence of SUD in their patients hospitalized for the first time for treatment of a manic or mixed episode. They reported a 38% prevalence of alcohol use disorders and a 32% prevalence of drug use disorder in their 34 first-episode manic patients. When these patients were compared with the 37 who had had multiple episodes of mania, no differences were found in the prevalence rate of SUDs. In another study (involving predominantly multiple-episode manic patients), Keck and colleagues (11) found that of the 106 bipolar disorder patients admitted for a manic or mixed episode who completed the 12-month follow-up, 55 (52%) met criteria for a substance-related disorder during the interval. These included 16 patients (15%) with drug abuse/dependence syndromes only, 14 (13%) with alcohol abuse/dependence only, and 25 (24%) with both syndromes. A recent study examined the medical records of 204 DSM-III-R bipolar I inpatients to determine the rates of SUD and its effect on outcome of bipolar patients (12). Past substance abuse was present in 34% of the bipolar sample and most often comprised alcoholism (34%), followed by cocaine (30%), marijuana (29%), sedative-hypnotic or amphetamine (21%), and opiate (13%) abuse.

Whether the risk of SUDs in patients with bipolar disorder increases as the course of the affective illness progresses remains to be determined. Future studies will need to prospectively follow a cohort of first-episode manic patients, paying close attention to the use of substances.

Prevalence of Bipolar Spectrum Disorders in Patients Presenting for Treatment of Substance Abuse

Studies of treatment-seeking substance abusers have typically shown prevalence rates of bipolar disorder to range from 2 to 31%, with sample sizes ranging from as low as 30 to as high as 501 patients (13–16).

WHY THE COMMON ASSOCIATION BETWEEN COMORBID SUBSTANCE USE DISORDERS AND BIPOLAR DISORDER?

Several possible explanations for the frequent co-occurrence of bipolar disorder and SUD are described below.

One possibility that has been suggested is that this high association is due to a common causal pathway (e.g., common disturbance in neurotransmitter systems and/or postreceptor signaling pathways, or genetic predisposition) (17,18). Another possibility might be related to the nature of the symptoms of mania. Manic patients may exhibit behavioral disinhibition and engage in high-risk behaviors such as speeding, spending sprees, or excessive use of psychoactive substances. Bipolar disorder patients may engage in excessive use of alcohol even when they usually do not drink during their euthymic periods (19,20). This latter theory rests on the premise that alcoholism is secondary to the affective illness.

A third suggested explanation for the frequent co-occurrence is referral bias (21). This explanation, referred to as Berkson's bias (22), states that patients with two or more concurrent disorders are more likely to seek treatment than those with a single disorder. Because many studies examining the prevalence of SUD and bipolar disorder have been conducted at treatment, and inpatient, tertiary, or academic centers are perhaps more likely to be referred severely ill bipolar patients who commonly abuse alcohol or drugs (23), the prevalence of SUD may be overestimated.

The hypothesis of self-medication and masking of affective symptoms has also received much attention as another plausible explanation for the high co-occurrence of SUD and bipolar disorder (24). It is common belief that the manic patients drink during their manic episodes to "bring their symptoms under control" (23,25,26) and use cocaine or other stimulants during their depressive episodes to bring their mood up. However, not all authors support the self-medication hypothesis. Mirin and colleagues (27) compiled data on 350 hospitalized, drug-dependent patients over a 10-year period. They found that both bipolar disorder and cyclothymia were significantly more frequent among stimulant abusers (17.5%) than among opiate (5.4%) or sedative-hypnotic (6.8%) abusers, and concluded that cocaine abuse during mania was apparently an attempt to increase the "high" rather than improve the depression. In this hypothesis of self-medication or masking of symptoms, it has been suggested that substance abuse may initiate bipolar disorder in certain vulnerable individuals by precipitating early affective episodes (28). However, Strakowski and colleagues (29) found that antecedent substance abuse was associated with a later rather than an earlier age of onset of bipolar disorder.

Winokur et al. (30) have suggested that antecedent alcohol abuse may represent a risk factor for some patients who otherwise have a relatively lower risk of developing bipolar disorder, therefore resulting in a delay in the onset of bipolar disorder until after several years of alcohol abuse. Strakowski and colleagues (31) also found that bipolar patients with antecedent alcohol and drug abuse, compared with those without antecedent substance abuse, demonstrated a shorter period between the onset of the first affective syndrome and hospitalization. In addition, they found that antecedent substance abuse appears to shorten the period between the first affective syndrome and hospitalization. They go on to suggest that if these patients were self-medicating, it was not particularly effective.

RISK FACTORS FOR BIPOLAR AND SUBSTANCE USE DISORDERS

The risk factors that have been associated with comorbidity of SUD in patients with identified bipolar disorder include: age of onset, gender, mixed episode of bipolar disorder, and family history. These risk factors are discussed below.

Early Age of Onset

Some studies have suggested that bipolar disorder patients with comorbid SUD have an earlier age of onset of bipolar disorder (32,33). Feinman and Dunner (32) reported that earlier age of onset was more common among bipolar patients with comorbid substance abuse than among bipolar patients without substance abuse/dependence or among primary substance abuse/dependence patients who subsequently developed bipolar disorder. Winokur et al. (30) found a significantly earlier onset of bipolar alcoholics with primary affective disorder. The risk factor of age of onset is reviewed in more detail below, under "Chronology of Bipolar Disorder and SUD Comorbidity."

Gender

The NCS found that males were significantly more likely than females to have a lifetime history of dependence (9.2% vs 5.9%). In contrast, the ECA Study found that lifetime drug use disorders are equally prevalent among male and female drug users (4). Among patients with bipolar disorder, the data currently available on this issue are conflicting. Some studies have found that substance abuse is higher in males than in females (12,30,32,34). Another study does not support this finding—Tohen and colleagues (9), in a prospective study of patients hospitalized for their first manic or mixed episode, found that women were more than six times as likely as men to have a history of comorbid substance abuse or dependence (10 of 25 [40%] vs. 1 of 16 [6.3%]). Discrepancies in these findings may be due to several factors. The majority of studies with the finding of higher rates of SUD in men than in women were generally cross-sectional investigations of patients who had had multiple episodes. In contrast, the study by Tohen and colleagues (9) involved the prospective follow-up of patients hospitalized for their first manic episode (thus eliminating the confounding factors of chronic illness and long-term exposure to psychotropic medications).

Mixed Mania

The majority of studies in bipolar disorder patients have reported higher rates of SUD in patients with mixed rather than classic episodes (12,33,35–38). Keller et al. (35) reported that bipolar patients with the mixed and rapid-cycling forms of the illness were more likely to abuse alcohol than patients with pure mania and pure depression. Sonne and colleagues (33) also found that bipolar disorder patients who abused substances were more likely to experience rapid cycling and to have dysphoric and irritable mood states than patients who did not abuse substances. Feinman and Dunner (32) noted that "complicated" and "secondary," compared to "primary," bipolar disorder patients had a greater percentage of rapid cycling. Primary bipolar disorder refers to patients with no past or present history of alcohol or substance abuse. Complicated bipolar refers to patients whose primary bipolar disorder was complicated by substance abuse that began after the onset of the bipolar disorder, and secondary bipolar refers to patients whose bipolar disorder began after the onset of alcohol or substance abuse or dependence. Tohen and colleagues (9) found that 60% of patients in their first hospitalization for a mixed episode had comorbid substance use compared to only 27% of those with pure mania. In addition, drug abuse and dependence were found to be higher in persons with mixed mania than those with pure mania (20% vs. 11%, respectively). Not all studies are in agreement with higher rates of SUD in mixed manic-depressive rather than in classic mania. For example, Keck and colleagues (11) found no significant differences in the rates of SUD between patients with pure mania and those with mixed mania of either alcohol abuse/dependence (40% vs. 38%, respectively) or psychoactive drug abuse/dependence (38% vs. 21%, respectively).

Family History

Links in genetic vulnerability for bipolar illness and alcoholism can be seen in family-history data. Research suggests that a family history of alcoholism tends to be higher among alcoholic bipolar patients than among nonalcoholic bipolar patients. Hensel et al. (34) found a fourfold greater morbid risk for alcoholism among relatives of male patients with bipolar disorder complicated by drinking problems as compared with male bipolar patients without drinking problems. Warner et al. (39) found that 60% of the relatives of patients with moderate to severe substance abuse had a history of substance abuse, in contrast to 30.8% substance abuse for relatives of patients without a substance abuse history.

Feinman and Dunner (32) reported that complicated and secondary bipolar disorder patients' relatives had the highest morbid risk for alcohol and drug abuse compared to primary bipolar disorder patients. These observations suggest that bipolar illness and alcoholism are transmitted independently in the bipolar disorder patient who has alcoholism. In contrast, Winokur et al. (30) found that there was no greater risk for the complicated or secondary groups in family history for bipolar disorder, unipolar disorder, or alcoholism. They studied 231 inpatients and outpatients with bipolar disorder (70 with and 161 without alcohol dependence) and their families. The authors hypothesized that alcohol use disorders among bipolar patients are not independently transmitted but rather are often a secondary complication of the bipolar disorder.

CHRONOLOGY OF BIPOLAR DISORDER AND SUD COMORBIDITY

The association between SUD and bipolar disorder remains unclear. Some have suggested that SUD is a consequence of the mood instability inherent in bipolar disorder, others that SUD is a risk factor for precipitating or perpetuating affective episodes, or an attempt at self-medication of symptoms. Studying the temporal relationship between the onset of SUD and bipolar disorder may be one way of addressing this relationship. Goodwin and Jamison (28) have suggested that SUD may initiate bipolar disorder by way of kindling and sensitization (40). In this model, repeated intermittent exogenous stressors (such as abuse of alcohol or cocaine) may initiate progressively more severe and frequent affective responses, eventually culminating in spontaneous mood episodes (40). With this theory in mind, Ananth et al. (41) have speculated that use of cocaine might contribute to a rapid-cycling pattern in bipolar disorder. For this model to hold true, the age of onset of bipolar disorder with antecedent substance abuse should be earlier than in patients without substance abuse (28). However, several studies did not find an earlier age of onset of SUD (30,32,42). Morrison (42) observed that alcoholic bipolar patients had a later age of onset of their bipolar disorder (28 years) than did nonalcoholic bipolar patients (23 years). Winokur et al. (30) observed that the alcoholic bipolar patient does not differ from the nonalcoholic bipolar patient in clinical course. In fact, they found that the patients in whom alcoholism preceded the bipolar illness were less likely to relapse than patients whose bipolar illness preceded the alcoholism.

Feinman and Dunner (32), in a retrospective chart review of 188 bipolar patients, also did not find that SUD preceded bipolar disorder. They found that the complicated group compared to the two other groups had the earliest age of onset of symptoms at 13.3 years. In addition, compared to the other two groups they had the highest percentage of suicide attempts. More recently, Strakowski and colleagues (31), examining the associations of antecedent drug and alcohol abuse with the age of onset of bipolar disorder, studied a sample of 59 patients presenting with their first episode of psychotic mania. Antecedent alcohol abuse was present in 12 patients (20%), and antecedent drug abuse in 19 (32%). Antecedent alcohol abuse was associated with a later age of onset of bipolar disorder but not antecedent drug abuse (31). In another study, Strakowski et al. (29) studied the 12-month outcome of 77 patients who were recruited from consecutive inpatient admissions who met DSM-III-R criteria for bipolar disorder, manic or mixed with psychosis. The authors found that the courses of SUD were separate from those of bipolar disorder. The authors concluded that substance abuse does not result simply from attempts at self-medication or from the impulsivity of mania.

COURSE OF BIPOLAR DISORDER WITH SUD

Although several studies have examined comorbidity of substance abuse and affective disorders (39,43–45), relatively little has been determined about the effect of substance abuse on the course of bipolar disorder. There is some evidence that the coexistence of bipolar disorder and SUD will worsen prognosis by way of producing mixed states, an increased risk of suicide and rehospitalization, and noncompliance. Mayfield and Coleman (26) suggested that rapid cycling might be precipitated by an increased abuse of alcohol.

Himmelhoch et al. (36) reported that in a sample of 84 bipolar disorder patients admitted to an affective disorders clinic, substance abuse was significantly associated with poor outcome. They suggested that the use of alcohol and drugs might induce a mixed state. Keller et al. (35) found that patients who had bipolar disorder with associated alcoholism had an increased likelihood of rapid cycling and a slower time to recovery from affective episodes. They found that 13% of 67 patients with mixed mania or rapid-cycling disorder (both forms of bipolar illness are less likely to respond to treatment) had concurrent alcohol use disorder, and that these patients recovered more slowly than those with pure mania or pure depression.

Morrison (42), Feinman and Dunner (32), and Goldberg and colleagues (12) have all reported a substantially higher rate of suicide attempts among alcoholic patients with bipolar disorder than among nonalcoholic bipolar patients. Morrison (42) reported that alcoholic bipolar patients have almost twice the percentage of suicide attempts as nonalcoholic bipolar patients. Feiman and Dunner (32) also noted that suicide attempts were more common in complicated and secondary than in primary bipolar patients.

Reich et al. (23) and Brady et al. (43) found that patients with coexisting bipolar and substance use disorders were twice as likely as patients with bipolar disorder alone to require hospitalization. Sonne and colleagues (33) studied the onset, course, and features of bipolar disorder in 44 patients. Compared to those without a concurrent SUD, substance-using patients averaged twice as many hospitalizations and had an earlier age of onset of affective disorders. They were also more likely to have other comorbid Axis I disorders and twice as likely to have mixed symptoms at the time of the interview.

Tohen et al. (46), in a 4-year prospective follow-up study of 75 patients who recovered from an index manic episode, reported that a history of alcoholism was a predictor of poor outcome for the bipolar disorder. They found that the presence of SUDs was strongly associated with a shorter time to relapse and poor psychosocial outcome. In addition, in a sample of first-episode patients (9), the median time to recovery was shorter for persons without drug abuse than those with comorbid drug abuse (43 days vs. 55 days, respectively; $p = 0.045$). The presence of comorbid drug abuse was also associated with a lower probability of recovery at 2 years. Recently, Tohen et al. (3) studied the 24-month outcome of 219 patients who were recruited from consecutive inpatient admissions who met DSM-III-R/IV criteria for bipolar disorder manic or mixed or unipolar major depression with psychotic features. The authors did not find that substance use disorder was predictive of either syndromic or functional recovery at 2 years follow-up. Recently, in a retrospective chart review of 204 DSM-III-R bipolar I inpatients, Goldberg and colleagues (12) found that remission during hospitalization was less likely among patients with prior substance abuse, especially alcohol or marijuana abuse.

Several studies (12,29,47–49) have reported that having an SUD increased the likelihood of medication noncompliance in patients with bipolar disorder. In a study examining the 12-month outcome of 134 patients admitted for a DSM-III-R manic or mixed episode of bipolar disorder, Keck and colleagues (11) found that medication compliance was inversely associated with the presence of comorbid SUDs. The authors also found that patients who did not complete the study were more likely to have a history of SUDs (13 [50%] of 26) than those who completed the 12-month follow-up (32 [30%] of 106). However, surprisingly, the presence of comorbid SUDs was not associated with either syndromic, symptomatic or functional recovery (11). In other words, the latter study suggests that substance abuse appears to have an indirect and deleterious effect on the course of bipolar disorder by means of its impact on medication compliance.

Strakowski and colleagues (29) found that substance abuse was independently (because of noncompliance) associated with lower syndromic recovery rates. Weiss and colleagues (49) studied the patterns of medication compliance, and reasons given for noncompliance, among 45 patients with bipolar disorder and SUD. The authors found that patients who were prescribed both lithium and valproate were significantly more likely to report full compliance with valproate than with lithium. Side effects were the most common reason for lithium noncompliance, but were not cited as a reason for valproate noncompliance. Another finding was that patients prescribed benzodiazepines, neuroleptics, and tricyclic antidepressants used more medication than prescribed. With this study, the authors conclude that valproate may have greater acceptability than lithium among patients with bipolar disorder and SUD.

MANAGEMENT OF SUD

Substance abuse and its associated behaviors may lead clinicians and family members to fail to recognize bipolar disorder. Conversely, the diagnosis of SUD may be overlooked in patients who have bipolar disorder. Monitoring SUD in patients dually diagnosed with psychiatric illness and SUD is critical for diagnosis and for evaluation of progress. Weiss et al. (50) studied the validity of substance use self-reports in 55 dually diagnosed outpatients, of whom 15 had a diagnosis of bipolar disorder. The authors concluded that self-reports in nonpsychotic, dually diagnosed outpatients under certain conditions (e.g., when patients are in treatment, when urine samples are collected with patients' prior knowledge) may be highly valid.

DIAGNOSTIC DIFFICULTIES IN PATIENTS WITH BIPOLAR DISORDER AND COMORBID SUDS

There is a marked difficulty in diagnosing bipolar affective disorder in the presence of comorbid SUD because substantial overlap may exist between the symptoms of bipolar disorder and the intoxication and withdrawal states resulting from psychoactive substances. For example, stimulant intoxication can produce a syndrome indistinguishable from mania or hypomania, and substantial depressive symptoms upon withdrawal from the stimulants. In addition, the phenomenological overlap between bipolar disorder and attention deficit disorder is significant. In both disorders patients may experience hyperactivity, impulsivity, agitation, racing thoughts, and distractibility, which often makes it difficult to distinguish between the two syndromes (51).

Psychotherapies

Until recently, psychotherapeutic approaches to patients with bipolar disorder received scant research attention. Jamison et al. (52) found that patients with bipolar disorder were far more likely to value psychotherapy than were physicians who treated bipolar patients, despite the fact that most of the physicians surveyed were practicing psychotherapists. Many different types of psychotherapy for both bipolar disorder and SUD have been utilized (53–59). However, few studies have examined which psychotherapies should be used in bipolar disorder patients with comorbid SUD (60). Treatment of comorbid disorders may occur sequentially (the patient is treated first for SUD and then for the psychiatric disorder) or in parallel (the patient is treated simultaneously for both disorders; usually treatment is delivered for each at different sites in unrelated clinical programs). However, since these forms of treatment have not produced favorable outcomes for patients with coexisting bipolar disorder and SUD, recent research has focused on integrated treatment (61), which consists of 20 sessions of relapse-prevention group therapy. The treatment uses an integrated approach by discussing topics that are relevant to both disorders and by highlighting common aspects of recovery from and relapse to each disorder. Group sessions focus on such topics as identifying and addressing triggers, managing symptoms of bipolar disorder without abusing substances, recognizing early warning signs for both disorders, and taking medications as prescribed.

Pharmacotherapies

Lithium

In naturalistic outcome studies, SUD has been reported to affect response to lithium in bipolar disorder patients (46,62–64). In a 4-year follow-up study of 24 bipolar patients after their first manic episode (46), alcoholism was found to be significantly associated with a shorter time in remission from affective symptomatology. O'Connell and colleagues (62) found the incidence of SUD to be substantially higher in patients with a poor outcome (36%) compared to patients with a good outcome (7%). Two open-label studies with lithium show mixed results in bipolar spectrum disorder patients with comorbid cocaine abuse (65,66). Gawin and Kleber (65), in an open-label study with lithium carbonate, found it to be effective in cocaine abusers with cyclothymia. In contrast, Nunes and coworkers (66) failed to find any benefit of lithium in 10 cocaine abusers with bipolar spectrum disorders.

Anticonvulsants: Valproate and Carbamazepine

Weiss et al. (49) reported that compliance with mood-stabilizer treatment was significantly higher among bipolar patients with SUD when valproate, rather than lithium, was the primary pharmacotherapy. Brady and colleagues (67), in an open-label study with valproate, found it to be safe and effective in nine mixed-manic bipolar patients with concurrent substance dependence who had a history of either intolerance or lack of response to lithium. In addition, this study did not show any changes in liver transaminases at the end of the study compared to baseline values. Goldberg and colleagues (12) found in a retrospective medical chart review that bipolar I inpatients with substance abuse histories who received divalproex or carbamazepine remitted during hospitalization more often than did those who received lithium as the sole mood stabilizer.

CONCLUSION

To understand the relationship between bipolar disorder and comorbid SUD, it is important to know the temporal sequence of onset. Several studies suggest that comorbid SUD in mania co-occurs more frequently with bipolar disorder than is expected by base-rate estimates. Future research will require prospective evaluation of bipolar disorder patients with and without SUD who are followed longitudinally to determine how these co-occurring syndromes develop and interact over time, and how they may affect the response to treatment.

REFERENCES

1. Regier DA, Farmer ME, Rae DS, Locke BZ, Keith SJ, Judd LL, Goodwin FK. Comorbidity of mental disorders with alcohol and other drug abuse: results from the Epidemiologic Catchment Area (ECA) study. JAMA 264:2511–2518, 1990.
2. Sheehan MF. Dual diagnosis. Psychiatr Q 64:107–134, 1993.
3. Tohen MT, Hennen J, Zarate CA Jr, Baldessarini RJ, Strakowski SM, Stoll AL, Faedda GL, Suppes T, Gebre-Medhin P, Cohen BM. The McLean first episode project: two year syndromal and functional recovery in 219 cases of major affective disorders with psychotic features. Am J Psychiatry 1999. In press.
4. Anthony JC, Helzer JE. Syndromes of drug abuse and dependence. In: Psychiatric Disorders in America: The Epidemiologic Catchment Area Study. Robins LN, Regier DA, eds. New York: Free Press, 1991.
5. Warner LA, Kessler RC, Hughes M, Anthony JC, Nelson CB. Prevalence and correlates of drug use and dependence in the United States. Arch Gen Psychiatry 52:219–229, 1995.
6. Robins LN, Helzer JE, Weissman MM, et al. Lifetime prevalence of specific psychiatric disorders in three sites. Arch Gen Psychiatry 949–958, 1984.
7. Kessler RC, McGonagle KA, Zhao S, Nelson CB, Hughes M, Eshleman S, Wittchen H-U, Kendler KS. Lifetime and 12-month prevalence of DSM-III-R psychiatric disorders in the United States: results from the national comorbidity survey. Arch Gen Psychiatry 51:8–19, 1994.
8. Kessler RC, Crum RM, Warner LA, Nelson CB, Schulenberg J, Anthony JC. Lifetime co-occurrence of DSM-III-R alcohol abuse and dependence with other psychiatric disorders in the national comorbidity survey. Arch Gen Psychiatry 54:313–321, 1997.
9. Tohen M, Zarate CA Jr, Zarate SB, Gebre-Medhin P, Pike S. The McLean/Harvard First-Episode Mania Project: pharmacologic treatment and outcome. Psychiatry Ann 26(7 suppl):5444–5448, 1996.
10. Keck PE Jr, McElroy SL, Strakowski SM, West SA, Sax KW, Hawkins JM, Huber TJ, et al. Outcome and comorbidity in first- compared with multiple-episode mania. J Nerv Ment Dis 183:320–324, 1995.
11. Keck PE Jr, McElroy SL, Strakowski SM, West SA, Sax KW, Hawkins JM, Bourne ML, Haggard P. 12-month outcome of patients with bipolar disorder following hospitalization for a manic or mixed episode. Am J Psychiatry 155:646–652, 1998.
12. Goldberg JF, Garno JL, Leon AC, Kocsis JH, Portera L. A history of substance abuse complicates remission from acute mania in bipolar disorder. J Clin Psychiatry 60:733–740, 1999.

13. Hesselbrock M, Meyer R, Keener J. Psychopathology in hospitalized alcoholics. Arch Gen Psychiatry 42:1050–1055, 1995.
14. Ross HE, Glaser FB, Germanson T. The prevalence of psychiatric disorders in patients with alcohol and other drug problems. Arch Gen Psychiatry 45:1023–1031, 1988.
15. Nunes EV, Quitkin FM, Klein DF. Psychiatric diagnosis in cocaine abuse. Psychiatry Res 25:105–114, 1989.
16. Weiss RD, Mirin SM, Michael JL, et al. Psychopathology in chronic cocaine abusers. Am J Drug Alcohol Abuse 12:17–29, 1986.
17. Dilsaver S. The pathophysiologies of substance abuse and affective disorders: an integrative model? J Clin Psychopharmacol 7:1–10, 1987.
18. Luthar SS, Merikangas KR, Rounsaville BJ. Parental psychopathology and disorders in offspring: a study of relatives of drug abusers. J Nerv Ment Dis 181:351–357, 1993.
19. Liskow B, Mayfield D, Thiele J. Alcohol and affective disorder: assessment and treatment. J Clin Psychiatry 43:144–147, 1982.
20. Weiss RD, Mirin SM. Substance abuse as an attempt at self-medication. Psychiatr Med 3:357–367, 1987.
21. Searles JS, Alterman AI. Differential attrition rates alcohol abusing and non-abusing schizophrenic inpatients: a methodological note. Alcohol Clin Exp Res 16:705–707, 1992.
22. Berkson J. Limitations of the application of fourfold table analysis to hospital data. Biometr Bull 2:47–53, 1946.
23. Reich LH, Davies RK, Himmelhoch JM Jr. Excessive alcohol use in manic-depressive illness. Am J Psychiatry 131:83–86, 1974.
24. Kalodner CR, Delucia JL, Ursprung AW. An examination of the tension reduction hypothesis: the relationship between anxiety and alcohol in college students. Addict Behav 14:649–654, 1989.
25. Zisook S, Schuckit MA. Male primary alcoholics with and without family histories of affective disorder. J Stud Alcohol 48:337–344, 1987.
26. Mayfield D, Coleman LL. Alcohol use and affective disorder. Dis Nerv Syst 29:467–474, 1968.
27. Mirin SM, Weiss RD, Griffin ML, Michael JL. Psychopathology in drug abusers and their families. Compr Psychiatry 32:36–51, 1991.
28. Goodwin FK, Jamison KR. Manic-Depressive Illness. New York: Oxford University Press, 1990.
29. Strakowski SM, Sax KW, McElroy SL, Keck PE Jr, Hawkins JM, West SA. Course of psychiatric and substance abuse syndromes co-occurring with bipolar disorder after a first psychiatric hospitalization. J Clin Psychiatry 59:465–471, 1998.
30. Winokur G, Coryell W, Akiskal HS, Masser JD, Keller MB, Endicott J, et al. Alcoholism in manic-depressive (bipolar) illness: familial illness, course of

illness, and the primary-secondary distinction. Am J Psychiatry 152:365–372, 1995.
31. Strakowski SM, McElroy SL, Keck PE Jr, West SA. The effects of antecedent substance abuse on the development of first-episode psychotic mania. J Psychiatr Res 30:59–68, 1996.
32. Feinman JA, Dunner DL. The effect of alcohol and substance abuse on the course of bipolar affective disorder. J Affect Disord 37:43–49, 1996.
33. Sonne SC, Brady KT, Morton WA. Substance abuse and bipolar affective disorder. J Nerv Ment Dis 182:349–352, 1994.
34. Hensel B, Dunner DL, Fieve RR. The relationship of family history of alcoholism to primary affective disorder. J Affect Disord 1:105–113, 1979.
35. Keller MB, Lavori PW, Coryell W, Andreasen NC, Endicott J, Clayton PJ, Klerman GL, Hirschfeld RM. Differential outcome of pure manic, mixed/cycling, and pure depressive episodes in patients with bipolar illness. JAMA 255:3138–3142, 1986.
36. Himmelhoch JM, Mulla D, Neil JF, Detre TP, Kupfer DJ. Incidence and significance of mixed affective states in a bipolar population. Arch Gen Psychiatry 33:1062–1066, 1976.
37. McElroy SL, Strakowski SM, Keck PE Jr, Tugrul KL, West SA, Lonczak HS. Differences and similarities in mixed and pure mania. Compr Psychiatry 36:187–194, 1995.
38. Himmelhoch JM, Garfinkel ME. Sources of lithium resistance in mixed mania. Psychopharmacol Bull 22:613–620, 1986.
39. Warner R, Taylor D, Wright J, Sloat A, Springett G, Arnold S, Weinberg H. Substance use among the mentally ill: prevalence, reasons for use, and effects on illness. Am J Orthopsychiatry 64:30–39, 1994.
40. Post RM. The transduction of psychosocial stress into the neurobiology of recurrent affective disorder. Am J Psychiatry 149:999–1010, 1993.
41. Ananth J, Wohl M, Ranganath V, Beshay M. Rapid cycling patients: conceptual and etiological factors. Neuropsychobiology 27:193–198, 1993.
42. Morrison JR. Bipolar affective disorder and alcoholism. Am J Psychiatry 131:1130–1133, 1974.
43. Brady K, Casto S, Lydiard R, Malcom R, Arana G. Substance abuse in an inpatient psychiatric sample. J Drug Alcohol Abuse 17:389–397, 1991.
44. Russell JM, Newman SC, Bland RC. Drug abuse and dependence. Acta Psychiatr Scand 376(suppl):54–62, 1994.
45. Strakowski SM, Tohen M, Stoll AL, Faedda GL, Goodwin DC. Comorbidity in mania at first hospitalization. Am J Psychiatry 149:554–556, 1992.
46. Tohen M, Waternaux CM, Tsuang MT, Hunt AT. Four-year follow-up of twenty-four first-episode manic patients. J Affect Disord 19:79–86, 1990.
47. Keck P, McElroy S, Strakowski S, Bourne M, West S. Compliance with maintenance treatment in bipolar disorder. Psychopharmacol Bull 33:87–91, 1997.
48. Maarbjerg K, Aagaard J, Vestergaard P. Adherence to lithium prophylaxis. I.

Clinical predictors and patient's reasons for nonadherence. Pharmacopsychiatry 21:121–125, 1988.
49. Weiss RD, Greenfield SF, Najavits LM, Soto JA, Wyner D, Tohen M, Griffin ML. Medical compliance among patients with bipolar disorder and substance abuse disorder. J Clin Psychiatry 59:172–174, 1998.
50. Weiss RD, Najavits LM, Greenfield SF, Soto JA, Shaw SR, Wyner D. Validity of substance use self-reports in dually diagnosed outpatients. Am J Psychiatry 155:127–128, 1998.
51. Blacker D, Tsuang MT. Contested boundaries of bipolar disorder and the limits of categorical diagnosis in psychiatry. Am J Psychiatry 149:1473–1483, 1992.
52. Jamison KR, Gerner RH, Goodwin FK. Patient and physician attitudes toward lithium: relationship to compliance. Arch Gen Psychiatry 36:866–869, 1979.
53. Davenport YB, Ebert MH, Adland ML, Goodwin FK. Couples group therapy as an adjunct to lithium maintenance of the manic patient. Am J Orthopsychiatry 47:495–502, 1977.
54. Basco MR, Rush AJ. Cognitive-Behavioral Therapy for Bipolar Disorder. New York: Guilford Press, 1996.
55. Frank E, Kupfer DJ, Ehlers CL, Monk TH, Cornes C, Carter S, Frankel D. Interpersonal and social rhythm therapy for bipolar disorder: integrating interpersonal and behavioral approaches. Behavior Therapist 17:143–149, 1994.
56. Beck AT, Wright FD, Newman CF, Liese BS. Cognitive Therapy of Substance Abuse. New York: Guilford Press, 1993.
57. Cerbone MJA, Mayo JA, Cuthbertson BA, O'Connell RA. Group therapy as an adjunct to medication in the management of bipolar affective disorder. Group 16(3):174–187, 1992.
58. Miklowitz DJ. Psychotherapy in combination with drug treatment for bipolar disorder. J Clin Psychopharmacol 16(suppl 1):56S–66S, 1996.
59. Najavits L, Weiss R. The role of psychotherapy in the treatment of substance use disorders. Harvard Rev Psychiatry 2:84–96, 1994.
60. Weiss R, Najavits L. Overview of treatment modalities for dual diagnosis patients: pharmacotherapy, psychotherapy, twelve-step programs. In: Dual Diagnosis: Substance Abuse and Comorbid Medical and Psychiatric Disorders. Kranzler H, Rounsaville B, eds. New York: Marcel Dekker, pp 87–105, 1998.
61. Weiss RD, Najavits LM, Greenfield SF. A relapse prevention group for patients with bipolar and substance use disorders. J Subst Abuse Treat 16:47–54, 1999.
62. O'Connell RA, Mayo JA, Flatlow L, Cuthbertson B, O'Brien BE. Outcome of bipolar disorder on long-term treatment with lithium. Br J Psychiatry 159:123–129, 1991.
63. Albanese M, Bartel R, Bruno R. Comparison of measures used to determine substance abuse in an inpatient psychiatric population. Am J Psychiatry 151:1077–1078, 1994.
64. Bowden CL. Predictors of response to divalproex and lithium. J Clin Psychiatry 56(suppl 3):25–30, 1995.

65. Gawin FH, Kleber HD. Cocaine abuse treatment: open pilot trial with desipramine and lithium carbonate. Arch Gen Psychiatry 41:903–909, 1984.
66. Nunes EV, McGrath PJ, Wager S, Quitkin JM. Lithium treatment for cocaine abusers with bipolar spectrum disorders. Am J Psychiatry 147:655–657, 1990.
67. Brady KT, Sonne SC, Anton R, Ballenger JC. Valproate in the treatment of acute bipolar affective episodes complicated by substance abuse: a pilot study. J Clin Psychiatry 56:118–121, 1995.
68. Winokur G, Clayton PJ, Reich T. Manic depressive illness. St Louis: Mosby, 1969.

5
Substance Abuse in Schizophrenia

Biological Factors Mediating Comorbidity
and the Potential Role of Atypical
Antipsychotic Drugs

Myung A. Lee and Herbert Y. Meltzer
Vanderbilt University Medical Center
Nashville, Tennessee

INTRODUCTION

Substance abuse is a common feature of many types of psychiatric disorders. The rate in schizophrenia is one of the highest for all psychiatric disorders (1). Comorbidity for substance abuse in schizophrenia has an important influence on course of illness, relapse, quality of life, morbidity, and compliance. High comorbidity for substance abuse may be related in part to biological factors. This chapter reviews the factors contributing to comorbidity for substance abuse in schizophrenia and the role of atypical antipsychotic drug in the treatment of substance abuse in patients with schizophrenia.

PREVALENCE OF SUBSTANCE ABUSE

In the pivotal U.S. Epidemiologic Catchment Area (ECA) study published in 1990 and covering the period from 1980 to 1984, the lifetime rate of comorbid substance abuse disorders in schizophrenia was 47% ± 4.0 (SE) (1). Recent studies in patients with schizophrenia reported similar prevalence (2–6). There is some evidence that the prevalence of substance abuse in patients with schizophrenia has increased with time (3,7). For example, Fowler et al. (3) have reported that estimates of lifetime alcohol and stimulant abuse/dependence increased twofold from the 1960s and 1970s to the 1990s. However, estimates of cannabis abuse have changed little over time, while estimates of lifetime hallucinogen abuse and dependence have declined (3). Although lifetime prevalence of substance abuse/dependence may have increased over time (3,7), rates of active substance abuse/dependence in cross-sectional studies have changed little, ranging from 20 to 40% (5,8,9). According to the ECA study (1), 33.7% of patients with schizophrenia met criteria for an alcohol disorder and 27.5% for other drug abuse disorders. In addition, they reported that people with schizophrenia are more than three times as likely to have an alcohol disorder (odds ratio 3.3) and more than six times as likely to have drug use disorder (odds ratio 6.2) compared to the general U.S. population. This rate of substance abuse in schizophrenia is higher than those of unipolar depression (27.2%) and any anxiety disorders (23.7%) (1). However, in the ECA study, the rate of substance abuse/dependence problems for bipolar I disorder was higher than that for schizophrenia (60.7%) (1).

The most frequently abused substance in schizophrenia is nicotine. The prevalence of smoking in schizophrenia has been reported to be between 68 and 88% (10–13), which is more than two to three times higher than the U.S. population rate of 30% (14). This prevalence is higher than the prevalence of smoking among patients with mood, anxiety, or other psychiatric disorders (10). The next most frequently abused substances are alcohol and cannabis, followed by stimulants (3–5,15,16).

Drugs of abuse have been reported to be influenced by availability and affordability. However, it has been reported that people with schizophrenia abuse stimulants two to five times more than the general population (5,17,18). The ECA study (1) also reported a higher odds ratio for drug (6.2) than alcohol (3.3) use disorders in schizophrenia. However, when examining lifetime prevalence of schizophrenia in people with drug abuse compared to people with no drug abuse, cocaine and amphetamine abuse did not significantly increase lifetime prevalence of schizophrenia, although alcohol and marijuana abuse did (1). A person who abuses one kind of drug is more likely to abuse other kinds (19). This appears to explain the great proportion (14–49%) of substance-abusing schizophrenics who abuse multiple substances (2,6,15,20,21).

DEMOGRAPHIC AND CLINICAL CORRELATES OF SUBSTANCE ABUSE IN SCHIZOPHRENIA

Factors that have been associated with higher rates of substance abuse in schizophrenia include male gender (3,5,6,20,26), younger age (3,5,6,20), earlier age at onset (5,24), increased number of hospitalizations (20,23, 25,27,28), noncompliance with treatment (20,26), depressive symptoms (6,8,17,22,23,29,30), paranoid subtype (23,24,26), more functional impairment (5,21), increased risk of suicide (25,30,32), and increased violent behavior (33,34) (Table 1). Although most of the studies report no difference in severity of positive symptoms in substance-abusing schizophrenics compared to nonabusing schizophrenics (2,5,22–25), increased positive symptoms have also been reported in alcohol-abusing schizophrenics compared to nonabusing schizophrenics (17,20,27). The severity of negative symptoms has been reported to be lower (2,22,24,25) in substance-abusing schizophrenics than in nonabusing schizophrenics, but there are contrary reports (2,23,36). Regardless of what substance patients used, depression rating was higher in substance abusers (6,8,17,22,23,29,30). However, 4-week (22) and 1-year (8) follow-up studies have reported that depression decreased when substance abuse dimin-

Table 1. Demographic and Clinical Correlates of Substance Abuse in Schizophrenia

	Compare to non–substance abusers
Demographic	Male gender, younger age, increased number of hospitalizations, noncompliant with treatment, more functional impairment
Clinical	
Subtype	Higher rate in paranoid subtype
Positive symptoms	No difference in severity
Negative symptoms	Lower or no difference
Depression	More depression
Suicide	Increased or no difference
Violent behavior	Increased
Tardive dyskinesia	Increased in alcoholics and cannabis abusers
Extrapyramidal symptoms	Lower in smokers, increased dystonic reaction in cocaine abusers, increased akathisia in alcoholics
Cognition	No difference

Source: Refs. 2,3,5,6,8,16,17,20–30,32–36,42–43,45,47–50.

ished. Similarly, Zisook et al. (36) have reported no difference in depressive symptoms between schizophrenics with history of substance abuse and with no substance abuse. In addition, Brady et al. (29) have reported resolution of depressive symptoms in the alcohol-abusing patients with schizophrenia at discharge from the hospital. These studies suggest that any observed differences in the severity of symptoms between abusers and nonabusers reported by numerous studies may have been influenced by the effect of current substance abuse. These differences disappear if the abuser becomes abstinent.

Several studies have reported differences in the effects of various types of abuse on psychopathology, course, outcome, and other various variables. However, since a significant proportion of patients were abusing multiple substances, these differences may not be reliable. Many factors—such as male gender, younger age, increased number of hospitalizations, noncompliance with treatment, and depression—are common to all major types of substance abuse (5,6,20,24,25,31). Furthermore, these findings are not specific for the schizophrenia diagnosis. These same characteristics have also been reported in bipolar affective disorder with substance abuse (37). Therefore, these characteristics appear to represent characteristics of patients with mental illness comorbid with substance abuse in general.

Kovansznay et al. (38) compared the relationship between a history of substance use disorder and early course of psychotic illness in 96 subjects with schizophrenia and 106 subjects with affective psychosis. They reported that lifetime history of substance abuse adversely influence the course of illness at 6 months for subjects with a diagnosis of schizophrenia but not for those with affective psychosis; lower mean Global Assessment of Functioning scores in 42 substance-abusing schizophrenics (42.0 ± 1.79 SE) compared to 54 nonabusing schizophrenics (47.3 ± 1.59 SE) ($p = 0.031$). However, frequency of working or attending school did not differ between groups. In addition, mean Brief Psychiatric Rating Scale (BPRS) (39) total scores at 6 months was higher in the substance-abusing schizophrenics than in nonabusing schizophrenics. However, global scores of Scale for the Assessment of Positive Symptoms (40) and Scale for the Assessment of Negative Symptoms (41) at 6 months were not different between groups, suggesting that the higher BPRS total score in the substance abuse group may be due to greater nonpsychotic symptoms such as depression, anxiety, etc.

Rates of tardive dyskinesia have been reported to be increased (31) or decreased (42) in smokers, and increased in alcoholics (16,42) and cannabis users (43). However, smoking was observed to increase tardive dyskinesia ratings in the laboratory test setting (44). On the other hand, rates of drug-induced parkinsonism were reported to be lower in smokers (45), and not increased in cocaine abusers (46). However, cocaine use was reported as a risk factor for acute dystonic reaction in the psychiatric population treated with neuroleptics (47). Rates of akathisia have been reported to be increased in alcohol abusers (16).

Very few studies have examined the effects of substance abuse on cognitive function. Sevy et al. (48) reported more impairment in conceptual encoding and verbal memory but less impairment in attention in schizophrenic patients who were cocaine abusers compared to nonabusers. On the other hand, Nixon et al. (49) reported no difference in Trail-Making A and B and the Face-Recognition Test between alcohol-abusing and nonabusing schizophrenics. Similarly, Addington and Addington (50) have reported no difference in verbal ability, attention, executive functioning, and verbal and visual memory between abusers and nonabusers. Sandyk (45) reported less cognitive impairment as assessed by Mini-Mental State Examinations in smokers.

We have examined cognitive function in 196 patients with schizophrenia, of whom 66 had current substance abuse of at least moderate severity. A neurocognitive battery that tested attention, working memory, verbal recall memory, verbal fluency, and executive function was administered (51) after at least 3 months of abstinence from substance. No difference was found between those with and without history of substance abuse (Meltzer and Lee, unpublished data). This result is consistent with the reports by Addington and Addington (50) and Nixon et al. (49) and suggests that substance abuse in schizophrenics does not appear to produce long-lasting disturbance on cognitive function when they maintain abstinence from substances.

FACTORS MEDIATING SUBSTANCE ABUSE IN SCHIZOPHRENIA

As previously mentioned, patients with schizophrenia abuse alcohol and drugs at a higher frequency than the general population as well as those with other psychiatric disorders, except for antisocial personality disorder and bipolar I disorder (1). Four hypotheses have been suggested to explain the high rate in schizophrenia:

1. Positive re-enforcing effect (e.g., feeling high) of substances (2,52–58).
2. Self-medication to reduce depression, positive and negative symptoms, or side effects of medications, especially neuroleptic-induced dysphoria, akathisia, and other extrapyramidal symptoms (2,52–58).

3. Chronic treatment with typical neuroleptic drugs may stimulate craving by inducing sensitization (16).
4. Shared underlying pathophysiology between schizophrenia and substance abuse (59).

These will be discussed in detail.

Positive Re-Enforcing Effect and Self-Medication Hypotheses

Several studies (2,52,53) have suggested that patients abuse drugs primarily because of their positive re-enforcing effect, as well as their mood-elevating and calming effects, but less often to alleviate psychotic symptoms or side effects of neuroleptics. In other words, patients with schizophrenia abuse substances for the same reasons that primary substance abusers and those in the general population do. Similarly, Hamera et al. (55) reported that substance abuse was not increased during psychotic symptom exacerbation, which argues against the self-medication hypothesis.

Chronic Typical Neuroleptic Treatment and Substance Abuse

Behavioral sensitization, one of the theories to explain addictive behavior (60–64), is the process whereby intermittent stimulant exposure produces a time-dependent, enduring, and progressively greater behavioral response (60–64). Sensitization is based on mesolimbic dopamine (DA) neurons, with cell bodies in the ventral tegmentum, mediating the positive reinforcing effects of drugs (61–64). Following stimulant exposure, animals sensitized to psychostimulants show enhanced DA turnover in terminal regions such as the nucleus accumbens and decreased DA activity in prefrontal cortex (60–64). However, decreased DA activity in prefrontal cortex has been observed with cocaine but not amphetamine (64). LeDuc and Mittleman (65) have reported that chronic treatment with haloperidol also produced enhanced sensitization of the psychomotor effects of cocaine in rodents. These authors (17) have suggested that neuroleptic treatment may be causally related to increased psychostimulant abuse in schizophrenia by inducing behavioral sensitization. They speculated that the combined effect of chronic neuroleptic treatment and intermittent stimulant abuse might produce behavioral sensitization, which fosters further abuse by enhancing the rewarding properties of abused drugs. Behavioral sensitization has also been reported to be produced by opoids, nicotine, ethanol, and other drugs of abuse (66–71), and involves enhanced mesolimbic DA neurotransmission (67–71).

In agreement with animal studies, Lieberman et al. (72) have reported that schizophrenic patients become psychotic following lower doses of psychostimulants compared to controls. In addition, a higher proportion of schizophrenics with active psychotic symptoms who are receiving neuroleptics became more psychotic when challenged with psychostimulants than those who are challenged without neuroleptics or in a stable state (72). Furthermore, patients receiving neuroleptics were least likely to improve after psychostimulant challenge (72). These findings are consistent with the hypothesis that chronic neuroleptic treatment may produce sensitization to the psychotomimetic effect of psychostimulants.

Shared Underlying Pathophysiology Between Schizophrenia and Substance Abuse

Stress Vulnerability, Substance Abuse, and Schizophrenia

Stress is important to the etiology of schizophrenia as well as craving for abused substances. Studies examining cumulative non-illness-related stressors have reported increased number of stressors a few weeks or months prior to the onset of relapse in schizophrenia, as well as in other psychiatric disorders (73–75). However, Norman and Malla (73) reported that the number of stressful life events in schizophrenia within the defined study period was not different from that in other psychiatric patients. Several clinical and preclinical studies suggest enhanced sensitivity to stress in schizophrenia. For example, patients with schizophrenia have been reported to have enhanced plasma homovanillic acid (HVA) (76), the major metabolite of DA, and greater adrenocorticotropine hormone (ACTH) (77) responses following metabolic stress compared to normal controls. Furthermore, various studies indicate abnormal regulation of the hypothalomic-pituitary-adrenal (HPA) axis in schizophrenia. Patients with schizophrenia, especially inpatients, have higher basal cortisol levels, than normal controls do (78,79). About one-third of schizophrenics show nonsuppression during the overnight 1-mg dexamethasone suppression test (78,80). Recently, we (81) and Mokrani et al. (82) have reported the blunted HPA axis response to challenge with apomorphine, a direct-acting DA-agonist.

A leading hypothesis concerning the pathophysiology of schizophrenia is the contributing neurodevelopmental abnormalities in DA function leading to decreased DA activity in the prefrontal cortical DA system and increased

DA function in the mesolimbic DA system (83). Animal studies have reported that prefrontal dysfunction produced enhanced hormonal and neurochemical responses to stress. Animals with lesions in the medial prefrontal cortex (cingulate gyrus) responded with greater HPA-axis response to restraint stress (84). In addition, in rodents, prefrontal cortical DA depletion has been reported to enhance the responsivity of mesolimbic DA neurons to stress (85). Similarly, birth complications, which have been reported to be significantly more frequent in patients with schizophrenia (86), have been reported to produce enhanced nucleus accumbens DA neuronal responses to repeated stress during adulthood in rodents (87). These clinical and preclinical studies suggest that patients with schizophrenia may have heightened HPA axis and DA responsiveness to stress.

Patients with schizophrenia also showed enhanced sensitivity to psychostimulants. Recent neuroimaging studies (88,89) have reported significantly greater reduction of D2-receptor binding in the striatum after amphetamine challenge in patients with schizophrenia compared to normal controls, suggesting enhanced DA efflux following amphetamine in schizophrenia. This is consistent with the report by Lieberman et al. (72), who reported greater sensitivity to psychostimulant (becoming psychotic with low dose) in patients with schizophrenia compared to normal controls. In addition, schizophrenics who had a transient activation of psychotic symptoms following the psychostimulant challenge had a significantly shorter time to relapse than patients who did not have a symptom exacerbation (90,91). Similarly, substance-abusing schizophrenics have a higher relapse rate than non-substance-abusing schizophrenics (20,23,25,27,28). This enhanced sensitivity to psychostimulants and stress may have a common biological substrate.

Behavioral sensitization also develops following intermittent repeated exposure to stress, which is also mediated via the mesolimbic DA system (92–94). Furthermore, there is cross-sensitization between stress and psychostimulants (and other drugs) (92–94), and the HPA axis appears to mediate this interaction (93,94). Repeated exposure to stress has been reported to increase the behavioral response to psychostimulants and other drugs in rodents (92–94). This stress-induced enhanced sensitivity to addictive drugs is mediated via stress-induced glucocorticoids secretion, which increases the sensitivity of mesolimbic DA neurons to drugs (93,94). For example, metyrapone, an inhibitor of corticosterone, suppressed stress-induced sensitization of the increase of DA in nucleus accumbens induced by cocaine and sensitization of cocaine-induced locomotion (94). Similarly, suppression of stress-induced corticosterone secretion by adrenalectomy abolished stress-induced sensitization of the locomotor effects of amphetamine and morphine (93).

Glucocorticoids at concentrations produced by stress have state-dependent stimulant effects on mesolimbic DA transmission. In rodents, they further enhance DA activity in situations that increase DA activity (e.g., in a dark phase, while eating, and in high responders to novelty), but have little effect in situations with low-normal DA activity (e.g., in a light phase and in low responders to novelty) (95). In summary, patients with schizophrenia may have enhanced HPA axis and DA responses to stress, which may increase the sensitivity to addictive drugs and contribute to the high rate of substance abuse.

Cannabis Abuse and Schizophrenia: Genetic and Environmental Influence

The possibility that substance abuse is a precipitating factor for the psychotic phase of schizophrenia has received considerable attention. Substance abuse may precede the onset of schizophrenia (96,97). Several reports relate cannabis use to the development of schizophrenia (98–102); a summary of the association is presented in the Table 2. Swedish conscripts with a history of cannabis use at age 20—the age of beginning military service—developed schizophrenia 2.4 times more frequently than nonusers (98). The rate was six times higher in heavy users (98). Furthermore, Tien and Anthony (99) examined quantitative relationships between substance use and psychotic diagnosis in a 4994-adult sample from the ECA study. They reported that the risk of developing a psychotic illness in daily users of marijuana was double that for nonusers, after controlling for daily cocaine use and alcohol disorder. Similarly, Linszen et al. (28) have reported significantly more and earlier psychotic relapses in cannabis-abusing schizophrenics, especially in heavy abusers, compared to schizophrenics who did not abuse cannabis, after controlling for other substance abuse. In addition, cannabis abuse was reported to start before the onset of schizophrenia in 69–96% of patients abusing cannabis (28,100). Kovasznay et al. (38) have compared substance abuse in patients during early schizophrenia and affective psychosis. Cannabis was the only substance that showed a difference between groups; more schizophrenics used cannabis than did patients with affective psychosis (69.1% vs. 46.2%; $p = 0.03$). A high comorbid rate of schizophrenia in cannabis abusers, but not in cocaine or amphetamine abusers, was also found in the ECA study (1). Furthermore, Fried (103) has reported that prenatal exposure to marijuana was associated with impairment in verbal ability, memory, and attention in children at age 5 and 6. These areas of cognitive deficit are also present in patients with schizophrenia. The association between cannabis abuse and schizophrenia may be via genetic and/or environmental as well as direct pharmacological effect of cannabis.

Table 2. The Relationship of Cannabis Abuse to Schizophrenia

Prevalence of schizophrenia in cannabis abusers	The higher rate of development of schizophrenia in cannabis abusers compared to nonabusers. The rate was six times higher in heavy abusers.
	Cannabis abuse started before the onset of schizophenia in 69–96% of patients abusing cannabis.
	The higher rate of cannabis abuse in patients with schizophrenia compared to patients with affective psychosis.
Familial risk for cannabis abuse and schizophrenia	Significantly greater familial morbid risk of schizophrenia in patients with acute psychosis abusing cannabis compared to nonabusing patients.
	Increased morbid risks for cannabis abuse in the first-degree relatives of schizophrenics compared to controls.
Effects of cannabis on psychosis	Administration of tetrahydrocannabinol (THC) transiently worsens psychosis in neuroleptic-treated schizophrenics and produces transient psychotic state in controls.

Source: Refs. 28,38,98–102,108.

McGuire et al. (101) examined lifetime morbid risk of psychiatric disorders in the first-degree relatives of 23 patients with acute psychosis and positive cannabis urine screen and sex-matched psychotic controls with negative urine drug screen. They reported significantly greater familial morbid risk of schizophrenia in the positive urine cannabis group (7.1%) than the controls (0.7%), while the risks of other psychoses and nonpsychotic conditions were similar. The same pattern of familial risk was present when the analysis was repeated in patients with DSM-III schizophrenia. In addition, Verma and Sharma (102) reported increased morbid risks for cannabis-use disorder as well as schizoid-schizotypal personality disorder, and paranoid personality disorders in the first-degree relatives of 162 schizophrenics compared to 106 controls. Cannabis abuse has been reported to have a genetic and/or family environmental influence. For example, Kendler and Prescott (104) reported that genetic risk factors have a strong impact on the risk of heavy use, abuse, and probably dependence on cannabis in a population-based sample of female twins. Tsuang et al. (19) reported, in 3372 male twin pairs, influence of a specific family environmental factor for marijuana abuse. Similarly,

Merikangas et al. (105) have reported familial aggregation of cannabis abuse in 231 probands, 61 control probands, and their 1267 first-degree relatives. These studies suggest that cannabis abuse may be a risk factor for the development of schizophrenia, and this association has a genetic as well as a specific family environmental influence.

In contrast with cannabis, the risk in relatives of schizophrenics for alcoholism was reported not to be increased (106). This is in contrast to the study by Lin et al. (107), who reported that association between major depression and alcohol abuse/dependence was influenced by familiar factors. Similarly, intravenous administration of tetrahydrocannabinol (THC), the active ingredient of marijuana, transiently worsens psychosis in neuroleptic-treated schizophrenics and produces transient psychotic state in controls (108). However, ethanol has inconsistent effects on psychosis in schizophrenics (109). Thus, the relationship between cannabis abuse and schizophrenia appears to have some specificity.

Preclinical studies have reported interactions between the cannabinoid and DA system. For example, D_1 and D_2 antagonists block turning behavior induced by cannabinoid agonists injected into the mouse striatum (110). Giuffrida et al. (111) have reported that quinpirol, a D_2-receptor agonist (but not SKF 38393, a D_1-receptor agonist), increased release of anandamide, an endogenous cannabinoid, in the dorsal striatum in rats. They have also reported that the cannabinoid antagonist SR 141716A enhanced the stimulation of motor behavior elicited by systemic administration of quinpirole. On the other hand, Castellano et al. (112) have reported antagonism of the effects of anandamide-induced impairment of memory consolidation by pretreatment with either D_1 (SKF 38393)- or D_2 (quinpirole)-receptor agonists at doses that were ineffective when given alone. Thus, interaction between the cannabinoid and the DA system may differ in different regions of the brain and needs further study. In addition, studies on interactions between the cannabinoid and various other neurotransmitter systems are needed to understand the biological underpinnings involved in cannabis abuse and schizophrenia.

Nicotine and Schizophrenia

Similar to other psychostimulant abuse, nicotine addiction involves the mesocorticolimbic DA mechanism. Pich et al. (68) have reported that cocaine and nicotine produced specific overlapping patterns of activation in the shell and the core of the nucleus accumbens, medial prefrontal cortex, and medial caudate areas in rats trained to self-administer intravenous cocaine and nicotine. Similarly, Pontieri et al. (71) have reported that intravenous administration of nicotine to the rat stimulated local energy metabolism and DA transmission in the shell of the nucleus accumbens.

Nicotinic receptors are divided into high- and low-affinity receptors for nicotine. Nicotinic receptors contain alpha and beta subunits (113). However, the low-affinity nicotinic receptor, which also binds alpha-bungalotoxin, the snake neurotoxin, is composed exclusively of alpha$_7$ subunits (114). Freedman et al. (115) have reported that alpha-bungalotoxin binding in the hippocampus of schizophrenics was significantly decreased in both the dendate gyrus and CA3 region of the hippocampus as compared to matched controls. Another piece of evidence suggesting the alpha$_7$ nicotinic receptor abnormality in schizophrenia comes from the study of sensory gating (116). The regulation of gating of auditory stimulation has been reported to be mediated via hippocampal alpha$_7$ nicotinic receptors (117). Normally, the evoked response to the second auditory stimulus (P50) is lower than the response to the first auditory stimulus because of inhibitory circuits activated by the first stimulus. However, this inhibitory gating effect was impaired in 91% of the schizophrenics (118) as well as 50% of their first-degree relatives who did not have the illness (117). Thus, the P50 deficit may be a risk factor for schizophrenia. Interestingly, prenatal exposure to nicotine produced impairment in auditory processing in children between 1 and 11 years old (103). Nicotine transiently reversed the auditory gating deficit in smoking schizophrenics (118) as well as nonsmoking relatives of schizophrenia (119). Treatment with clozapine has been reported to normalize the P50 deficit (120) as well as decreasing smoking (121,122) in schizophrenics, but typical neuroleptic treatment did not improve either P50 deficit (123) or smoking (124). Whether this abnormality in the nicotinergic neurotransmission is related, in part, to the high rate of smoking in patients with schizophrenia requires further study.

TREATMENT: A ROLE OF ATYPICAL ANTIPSYCHOTIC DRUGS

It has been reported that schizophrenics with and without substance abuse/dependence responded equally to drug treatment, with either typical (2,22,25) or atypical antipsychotic drugs (125,126). However, typical neuroleptics do not diminish substance abuse. Rather, clinical and preclinical studies suggest that typical neuroleptic treatment may *increase* substance abuse. For example, typical neuroleptic treatment has been reported to produce depression, secondary negative symptoms, and extrapyramidal side effects (127,130). These are, as discussed earlier, clinical factors mediating substance abuse in a subgroup of schizophrenics. Haloperidol treatment has been reported to increase smoking in schizophrenia (124) and normals (131). Furthermore, as previously mentioned, chronic treatment with haloperidol enhanced sensitization of the psychomotor effects of cocaine in rodents (65).

Atypical antipsychotic drugs have been reported to be more effective than typical neuroleptics to treat positive, as well as negative and depressive symptoms (128–130). In addition, atypical antipsychotics produce significantly fewer extrapyramidal side effects than typical antipsychotic drugs do (130). Furthermore, treatment with atypical antipsychotic drugs reduces frequency of hospitalization (132,133), and treatment with clozapine has been reported to reduce suicidal attempts (134). In addition, atypical antipsychotic drugs have been reported to decrease substance abuse. For example, use of clozapine in substance-abusing schizophrenics has been reported to reduce smoking (121,122), and there have been case reports of abstinence from alcohol (135) and cocaine (136) following clozapine treatment. Lee et al. (137) have reported that reduction of substance abuse in schizophrenics was significantly higher in the clozapine-treated group than in the group treated with other antipsychotic drugs ($p = 0.01$). Similarly, risperidone has been reported to decrease craving for cocaine in cocaine addicts (138) and for methamphetamine in patients with methamphetamine-induced psychosis (139). In addition, risperidone has been reported to improve the selective cognitive function (psychomotor/motor speed) in a small group of cocaine-withdrawn patients with cocaine dependence (140).

Pharmacologically, atypical antipsychotic drugs differ from typical neuroleptics in several ways. Most atypical antipsychotic drugs affect multiple receptors besides the D_2 receptor, most commonly the 5-HT_{2A} receptor (126 for review). In addition, some atypical antipsychotic drugs, such as clozapine, have higher affinity to D_1 and/or 5-HT_{2A} receptors than D_2 receptors (125). The fewer extrapyramidal side effects of atypical antipsychotic drugs compared to typical neuroleptics have been attributed in part to selectivity for mesolimbic compared to nigrostriatal DA neurotransmission (130). Atypical antipsychotic drugs stimulate c-fos, an immediate early gene, in the prefrontal cortex preferentially to the striatum, but haloperidol, a typical neuroleptic, has the reverse profile (130). Both stimulate c-fos activation in the nucleus accumbens. This pharmacological profile of atypical antipsychotic drugs may benefit substance abuse in schizophrenia (see below).

The biological basis for the greater beneficial effects of atypical antipsychotic drugs for substance abuse in schizophrenia may relate to the sensitization hypothesis previously discussed. Behavioral sensitization has been reported to be mediated via dopamine D_1- and D_2-receptor mechanisms in the forebrain (141). In addition, supersensitive 5-HT$_{2A/2C}$ receptors (142) and subsensitive 5-HT$_{1A}$ receptors (143,144) following cocaine treatment have been reported in rodents. Clozapine is able to antagonize 5-HT$_{2A}$ receptors and is a partial agonist at the 5-HT$_{1A}$ receptor (145,146). Furthermore, clozapine treatment has been reported to attenuate the development of cocaine-conditioned place preference (147) and to produce a partial blockade of both the reinforcing and discriminative stimulus effects of cocaine in rodents (148). However, clozapine treatment was also reported to increase motivation to self-administration of cocaine in rodents (149). Amperozide, another atypical antipsychotic drug with high affinity for the 5-HT$_{2A}$ receptor but low affinity for D$_1$ and D$_2$ receptors, has been reported to suppress ethanol (150,151) and cocaine (152) intake in rodents, suggesting involvement of 5-HT$_{2A}$-receptor mechanism in alcohol and cocaine addiction.

In addition to drug treatment, psychosocial treatment is an important component of treatment of substance abuse. It has been reported that schizophrenic patients with substance abuse may fare better in the integrated dual diagnosis program than in regular substance abuse rehabilitation program (153,154), because schizophrenics have low tolerance to critical and confrontational environments, which is one of the characteristics of regular substance abuse rehabilitation programs. In addition, psychosocial programs should recognize the cognitive deficit of schizophrenics (51,155,156) when designing psychosocial programs for substance-abusing schizophrenics. Obviously, specifically tailored psychosocial programs for patients with dual diagnosis are needed to deal with the high prevalence of substance abuse in schizophrenia. There is a report of successful treatment programs that incorporated substance abuse programs into the psychiatric inpatient, day-hospital, and outpatient programs instead of treating this population in a regular substance abuse program (153). More studies are needed to develop effective psychosocial treatment programs for substance-abusing schizophrenics.

SUMMARY AND FUTURE DIRECTIONS OF RESEARCH

Substance abuse in schizophrenia occurs with a higher prevalence than in all other psychiatric disorders. Its impact on psychopathology appears to be transient, with no significant effect on response to drug treatment and cognitive function. However, substance-abusing schizophrenics have more hospitalizations, and are more noncompliant with treatment and more functionally impaired. Multiple factors appear to be involved in the high prevalence of substance abuse in schizophrenia, such as pleasurable effects of drug ingestion and self-medication of symptoms and side effects of neuroleptics. The biological mechanisms underpinning both substance abuse and schizophrenia appear to be a significant factor in the high rate of comorbidity. In contrast to typical neuroleptics, some atypical antipsychotic drugs, such as clozapine and amperozide, appear to decrease drug intake in rodents. In addition, clozapine was reported to improve abuse of alcohol, cocaine, and smoking in schizophrenics, and risperidone was reported to reduce methamphetamine and cocaine craving in nonschizophrenic patients. Future research is needed on biological mechanisms of both substance abuse and schizophrenia, and on effects of atypical antipsychotic drugs in substance-abusing schizophrenics. In addition, substance abuse treatment programs specific for schizophrenic patients need to be developed.

REFERENCES

1. DA Regier, ME Farmer, DS Rae, BZ Locke, SJ Keith, LL Judd, FK Goodwin. Cormorbidity of mental disorders with alcohol and other drug abuse: results from the Epidemiologic Catchment Area (ECA) study. JAMA 264:2511–2518, 1990.
2. L Dixon, G Haas, PJ Weiden, J Sweeney, AJ Frances. Drug abuse in schizophrenic patients: clinical correlates and reasons for use. Am J Psychiatry 148:224–230, 1991.
3. IL Fowler, VJ Carr, NT Carter, TJ Lewin. Patterns of current and lifetime substance use in schizophrenia. Schizophrenia Bull 24:443–455, 1998.
4. JG Barbee, PD Clark, MS Crapanzano, GC Heintz, CE Kethoe. Alcohol and substance abuse among schizophrenic patients presenting to an emergency psychiatric service. J Nerv Ment Dis 177:400–407, 1989.
5. KT Mueser, PR Yarnod, DF Levinson, H Singh, AS Bellack, K Lee, RL Morrison, KG Yadalam. Prevalence of substance abuse in schizophrenia: demographic and clinical correlates. Schizophrenia Bull 16:31–56, 1990.
6. BJ Cuffel, KA Heithoff, W Lawson. Correlates of patterns of substance abuse among patients with schizophrenia. Hosp Community Psychiatry 44:247–251, 1993.
7. BJ Cuffel. Prevalence estimates of substance abuse in schizophrenia and their correlates. J Nerv Ment Dis 180:589–592, 1992.
8. BJ Cuffel, P Chase. Remission and relapse of substance use disorders in schizophrenia: results from a one-year prospective study. J Nerv Ment Dis 182:342–348, 1994.
9. SJ Bartels, RE Drake, MA Wallach. Long-term course of substance use disorder among patients with severe mental illness. Psychiatr Serv 46:248–251.
10. JR Hughes, DK Hatsukami, JE Mitchell, LA Dahlgren. Prevalence of smoking among psychiatric outpatients. Am J Psychiatry 143:993–997, 1986.

11. DM Ziedonis, TR Kosten, WM Glazer, RJ Frances. Nicotine dependence and schizophrenia. Hosp Community Psychiatry 45:204–206, 1994.
12. J deLeon. Smoking and vulnerability for schizophrenia. Schizophrenia Bull 22:405–409, 1996.
13. GW Dalack, DJ Healy, JH Meador-Woodruff. Nicotine dependence in schizophrenia: clinical phemomena and laboratory findings. Am J Psychiatry 155:1490–1501, 1998.
14. MC Fiore, P Newcombe, P McBride. Natural history and epidemiology of tobacco use and addiction. In: Nicotine Addiction: Principles and Management. CT Orleans, J Slade, eds. New York: Oxford University Press, pp 89–104, 1993.
15. FT Miller, JH Tanenbaum. Drug abuse in schizophrenia. Hosp Community Psychiatry 40:847–849, 1989.
16. P J Duke, C Pantelis, TRE Barnes. South Westminster schizophrenia survey: alcohol use and its relationship to symptoms, tardive dyskinesia and illness onset. Br J Psychiatry 64: 630–636, 1994.
17. PA LeDuc, G Mittleman. Schizophrenia and psychostimulant abuse: a review and reanalysis of clinical evidence. Psychopharmacology 121:407–427, 1995.
18. FR Schneier, SG Siris. A review of psychoactive substance use and abuse in schizophrenia: patterns of drug choice. J Nerv Ment Dis 175:641–650, 1987.
19. MT Tsuang, MJ Lyons, JM Meyer, T Doyle, SA Eisen, J Goldberg, W True, N Lin, R Toomey, L Eaves. Co-occurrence of abuse of different drugs in men: The role of drug-specific and shared vulnerabilities. Arch Gen Psychiatry 55:967–972, 1998.
20. RE Drake, FC Osher, MA Wallach. Alcohol use and abuse in schizophrenia: a prospective community study. J Nerv Ment Dis 177:408–414, 1989.
21. M Shumway, TL Chouljian, WA Hargreaves. Patterns of substance use in schizophrenia: a Markov modeling approach. J Psychiatr Res 28:277–287, 1994.
22. MR Serper, M Alpert, NA Richardson, S Dickson, MH Allen, A Werner. Clinical effects of recent cocaine use on patients with acute schizophrenia. Am J Psychiatry 152:1464–1469, 1995.
23. K Brady, R Anton, JC Ballenger, RB Lydiard, B Adinoff, J Selander. Cocaine abuse among schizophrenic patients. Am J Psychiatry 147:1164–1167, 1990.
24. P Lysaker, M Bell, J Beam-Goulet, R Milstein. Relationship of positive and negative symptoms to cocaine abuse in schizophrenia. J Nerv Ment Dis 182:109–112, 1994.
25. JP Seibyl, SL Satel, D Anthony, SM Southwick, JH Krystal, DS Charney. Effects of cocaine on hospital course in schizophrenia. J Nerv Ment Dis 181:31–37, 1993.
26. D Kozaric-Kovacic, V Folengovic-Šmale, Z Folengovic, A Marušic. Influence of alcoholism on the prognosis of schizophrenic patients. J Stud Alcohol 56:622–627, 1995.
27. FC Osher, RE Drake, DL Noordsy, GB Teague, SC Hurlbut, JC Biesanz, MS Beaudett. Correlates and outcomes of alcohol use disorder among rural outpatients with schizophrenia. J Clin Psychiatry 55:109–113, 1994.

28. DH Linszen, PM Dingemans, ME Lenior. Cannabis abuse and the course of recent-onset schizophrenic disorders. Arch Gen Psychiatry 51:273–279, 1994.
29. KT Brady, T Killeen, P Jarrell. Depression in alcoholic schizophrenic patients. Am J Psychiatry 150:1255–1256, 1993.
30. SJ Bartels, RE Drake, GJ McHugo. Alcohol abuse, depression, and suicidal behavior in schizophrenia. Am J Psychiatry 149:394–395, 1992.
31. DC Goff, DC Henderson, BS Amico. Cigarette smoking in schizophrenia: relationship to psychopathology and medication side effects. Am J Psychiatry 149:1189–1194, 1992.
32. LJ Cohen, MA Test, RL Brown. Suicide and schizophrenia: data from a prospective community treatment study. Am J Psychiatry 147:602–607, 1990.
33. P Räsänen, J Tiihonen, M Isohanni, P Rantakallio, J Lehtonen, J Moring. Schizophrenia, alcohol abuse, and violent behavior: a 26-year followup study of an unselected birth cohort. Schizophrenia Bull 24:437–441, 1998.
34. ME Rice, T Harris. Psychopathy, schizophrenia, alcohol abuse and violent recidivism. Int J Law Psychiatry 18:333–342, 1995.
35. B Kirkpatrick, XF Amador, M Flaum, SA Yale, JM Gorman, WT Carpenter, M Tohen, T McGlasham. The deficit syndrome in the DSM-IV field trial. I: Alcohol and other drug abuse. Schizophrenia Res 20:69–77, 1996.
36. S Zisook, R Heaton, J Moranville, J Kuck, T Jernigan, D Braff. Past substance abuse and clinical course of schizophrenia. Am J Psychiatry 149:552–553, 1992.
37. SC Sonne, KT Brady, WA Morton. Substance abuse and bipolar affective disorder. J Nerv Ment Dis 182:349–352, 1994.
38. B Kovasznay, J Fleischer, M Tanenberg-Karant, L Jandorf, AD Miller, E Bromet. Substance use disorder and the early course of illness in schizophrenia and affective psychosis. Schizophrenia Bull 23:195–201, 1997.
39. JE Overall, DR Gorham. The brief psychiatric rating scales. Psychological Reports 10:799–812, 1962.
40. NC Andreasen. Scale for the Assessment of Positive Symptoms (SAPS). Iowa City: University of Iowa, 1983.
41. NC Andreasen. Scale for the Assessment of Negative Symptoms (SANS). Iowa City: University of Iowa, 1981.
42. L Dixon, PJ Weiden, G Haas, J. Sweeney, AJ Frances. Increased tardive dyskinesia in alcohol-abusing schizophrenic patients. Compr Psychiatry 33:121–122, 1992.
43. A Zaretsky, NA Rector, MV Seeman, X Fornazzari. Current cannabis use and tardive dyskinesia. Schizophrenia Res 11:3–8, 1993.
44. WC Wirshing, J Engle, E Levin, JL Cummings, J Rose. The acute effects of smoking on tardive dyskinesia. In: New Research Program and Abstracts. Washington, DC: American Psychiatric Association, p 89, 1989.
45. R Sandyk. Cigarette smoking: effects in cognitive functions and drug-induced parkinsonism in chronic schizophrenia. Intern J Neurosci 70:193–197, 1993.
46. V Dhopesh, A Macfadden, I Maany, G Gamble. Absence of parkinsonism among

patients in long-term neuroleptics therapy who abuse cocaine. Psychiatr Serv 48:95–97, 1997.
47. AM Hegarty, RB Lipton, AE Merriam, K Freeman. Cocaine as a risk factor for acute dystonic reaction. Neurology 41:1670–1672, 1991.
48. S Sevy, SR Kay, LA Opler, HM van Praag. Significance of cocaine history in schizophrenia. J Nerv Ment Dis 178:642–648, 1990.
49. SJ Nixon, HG Hallford, RD Tivis. Neurocognitive function in alcoholic, schizophrenic, and dually diagnosed patients. Psychiatry Res 64:35–45, 1996
50. J Addington, D Addington. Substance abuse and cognitive functioning in schizophrenia. J Psychiatry Neurosci 22:99–104, 1997.
51. JT Kenney, HY Meltzer. Attention and higher cortical functions in shcizophrenia. J Neuropsychiatry 3:269–275, 1991.
52. J Addington, V Duchak. Reasons for substance use in schizophrenia. Acta Psychiatr Scand 96:329–333, 1997.
53. MF Brunette, KT Mueser, H Xie, RE Drake. Relationships between symptoms of schizophrenia and substance abuse. J Nerv Ment Dis 185:13–20, 1997.
54. LNP Voruganti, RJ Heslegrave, AG Awad. Neuroleptic dysphoria may be the missing link between schizophrenia and substance abuse. J Nerv Ment Dis 185:463–465, 1997.
55. E Hamera, JK Schneider, S Deviney. Alcohol, cannabis, nicotine, and caffeine use and symptom distress in schizophrenia. J Nerv Ment Dis 183:559–565, 1995.
56. J Smith, S Hucker. Schizophrenia and substance abuse. Br J Psychiatry 165:13–21, 1994.
57. JA Selzer, JA Lieberman. Schizophrenia and substance abuse. Psychiatr Clin North Am 16:401–412, 1993.
58. KT Mueser, AS Bellack, JJ Blanchard. Comorbidity of schizophrenia and substance abuse: implication for treatment. J Consult Clin Psychol 60:845–856, 1992.
59. JA Lieberman, BB Sheitman, BJ Kinon. Neurochemical sensitization in the pathophysiology of schizophrenia: deficits and dysfunction in neuronal regulation and plasticity. Neuropsychopharmacology 17:205–229, 1997.
60. J Altman, BJ Everitt, S Glautiern, A Markou, D Nutt, R Oretti, GD Phillips, TW Robbins. The biological, social and clinical bases of drug addiction: commentary and debate. Psychopharmacology 125:285–345, 1996.
61. RA Wise, DC Hoffman. Localization of drug reward mechanisms by intracranial injections. Synapse 10:247–263, 1992.
62. TW Robbins, M Cador, JR Taylor, BJ Everitt. Limbic-striatal interactions in reward-related processes. Neurosci Biobehav Rev 13:155–162, 1989.
63. T Nishikawa, N Mataga, M Takashima, M Toru. Behavioral sensitization and relative hyperresponsivness of striatal and limbic dopaminergic neurons after repeated methamphetamine treatment. Eur J Pharmacol 88:195–203, 1983.
64. RC Pierce, PW Kalivas. A circuitry model of the expression of behavioral sensitization to amphetamine-like psychostimulants. Brain Res Brain Res Rev 25:192–216, 1997.

65. PA LeDuc, G Mittleman. Interactions between chronic haloperidol treatment and cocaine in rats: an animal model of intermittent cocaine use in neuroleptic treated populations. Psychopharmacology 110:427–436, 1993.
66. PW Kalivas, S Taylor, JS Miller. Sensitization to repeated enkephalin administration into the ventral tegmental area of the rat. I. Behavorial characterization. J Pharmacol Exp Ther 235:537–543, 1985.
67. PW Kalivas. Sensitization to repeated enkephalin administration into the ventral tegmental area of the rat. II. Involvement of the mesolimbic dopamine system. J Pharmacol Exp Ther 235:544–550, 1985.
68. EM Pich, SR Pagliusi, M Tessari, D Talabot-Ayer, RH van Huijsduijnen, C Chiamulera. Common neural substrates for the addictive properties of nicotine and cocaine. Science 275:83–86, 1997.
69. KR Goldstein, DJ Knapp, EI Saiff, LA Pohorecky, D. Benjamin. Sensitization to ethanol demonstrated in place-preference and locomotor activation. Soc Neurosci Abstr 18:107, 1992.
70. G DiChiara, A Imperato. Drugs abused by humans preferentially increase synaptic dopamine concentrations in the mesolimbic system of freely moving rats. Proc Natl Acad Sci USA 85:5274–5278, 1988.
71. FE Pontieri, G Tanda, F Orzi, G Dichiara. Effects of nicotine on the nucleus accumbens and similarity to those of addictive drugs. Nature 382:255–257, 1996.
72. JA Lieberman, JM Kane, J Alvir. Provocative tests with psychostimulant drugs in schizophrenia. Psychopharmacology (Berl) 91:415–433, 1987.
73. RMG Norman, AK Malla. Stressful life events and schizophrenia. I: A review of the research. Br J Psychiatry 162:161–166, 1993.
74. H Anisman, R Zachark. Depression: the predisposing influence of stress. Behav Brain Sci 5:89–137, 1982.
75. C Hammen, M Gitlin. Stress reactivity in bipolar patients and its relation to prior history of disorder. Am J Psychiatry 154:856–857, 1997.
76. A Breier, OR Davis, RW Buchanan, LA Moricle, RC Munson. Effects of metabolic perturbation on plasma homovanillic acid in schizophrenia: relationship to prefrontal cortex volume. Arch Gen Psychiatry 50:541–550, 1993.
77. I Elman, CM Adler, AK Malhotra, C Bir, D Pickar, A Breier. Effect of acute metabolic stress on pituitary-adrenal axis activation in patients with schizophrenia. Am J Psychiatry 155:979–981, 1998.
78. C Altamura, G Guercetti, M Percudani. Dexamethasone suppression test in positive and negative schizophrenia. Psychiatry Res 30:69–75, 1989.
79. HY Meltzer. Dopamine, serotonin and glucocorticoids and the psychopathology of schizophrenia. In: Schizophrenia. Alfred Benzon Symposium 38. R Fog, J Gerlach, R Hemmingsen, eds. Copenhagen: Munksgaard, pp 74–91, 1995.
80. R Tandon, C Mazzara, J DeQuardo, KA Graig, JH Meaddor-Woodruff, R Goldman, JF Greden. Dexamethasone suppression test in schizophrenia: relationship to symptomatology, ventricular enlargement, and outcome. Biol Psychiatry 29:953–964, 1991.
81. HY Meltzer, MA Lee, K Jayathilake. The blunted plasma cortisol response to

apomorphine and its relationship to treatment response in patients with schizophrenia. Neuropsychopharmacology 2001 (in press).
82. MC Mokrani, F Duval, MA Crocq, PE Bailey, JP Macher. Multihormonal responses to apomorphine in mental illness. Psychoneuroendocrinology 20:365–375, 1995.
83. DR Weinberger, BK Lipska. Cortical maldevelopment, antipsychotic drugs, and schizophrenia: a search for common ground. Schizophrenia Res 16:87–110, 1995.
84. D Diorio, V Viau, MJ Meaney. The role of the medial prefrontal cortex (cingulate gyrus) in the regulation of hypothalamic-pituitary-adrenal responses to stress. J Neurosci 13:3839–3847, 1993.
85. AY Deutch, WA Clark, RH Roth. Prefrontal cortical dopamine depletion enchances the responsiveness of the mesolimbic dopamine neurons to stress. Brain Res 521:311–315, 1990.
86. H Verdoux, JR Geddes, N Takei, SM Lawrie, P Bovet, JM Eagles, R Heun, RG McCreadie, TF McNeil, E O'Callaghan, G Stober, MU Willinger, P Wright, RM Murray. Obstetric complications and age at onset in schizophrenia: an international collaborative meta-analysis of individual patient data. Am J Psychiatry 154:1220–1227, 1997.
87. WG Brake, MB Noel, P Boksa, A Gratton. Influence of perinatal factors on the nucleus accumbens dopamine response to repeated stress during adulthood: an electrochemical study in the rat. Neuroscience 77:1067–1076, 1997.
88. M Laruelle, A Abi-Dargham, CH van Dyck, R Gil, CD D'Souza, J Erdos, E McCance, W Rosenblatt, C Fingado, SS Zoghbi, RM Baldwin, JP Seibyl, JH Krystal, DS Charney, RB Innis. Single photon emission computerized tomography imaging of amphetamine-induced dopamine release in drug-free schizophrenic subjects. Proc Natl Acad Sci USA 93:9235–9240, 1996.
89. A Breier, T-P Su, R Saunders, RE Carson, BS Kolachana, A deBartolomeis, DR Weinberger, N Weisenfeld, AK Malhotra, WC Eckelman, D Pickar. Schizophrenia is associated with elevated amphetamine-induced synaptic dopamine concentrations: evidence from a novel positron emission tomograph method. Proc Natl Acad Sci USA 94:2569–2574, 1997.
90. JA Lieberman, J Alvir, S Geisler, J Ramos-Lorenzi, M Woerner, H Novarenko, T Cooper, JM Kane. Methylpheridate response, psychopathology and tardive dyskinesia as predictors of relapse in schizophrenia. Neuropsychopharmacology 11:107–118, 1994.
91. DP Van Kammen, JP Docherty, SR Marder, JN Royner, WE Bunney Jr. Long-term pimozide treatment differentially affects behavioral responses to dextroamphetamine in schizophrenia: further exploration of the dopamine hypothesis of schizophrenia. Arch Gen Psychiatry 39:275–281, 1982.
92. PV Piazza, JM Deminiere, M Le Moal, H Simon. Stress- and pharmacologically induced behavioral sensitization increases vulnerability to acquisition of amphetamine self-administration. Brain Res 514:22–26, 1990.
93. V Deroche, M Marinelli, S Maccari, M Le Moal, H Simon, PV Piazza.

Stress-induced sensitization and glucocorticooids. I. Sensitization of dopamine-dependent locomotor effects of amphetamine and morphine depends on stress-induced corticosterone secretion. J Neurosci 15:7181–7188, 1995.
94. F Rouge-Pont, M Marinelli, M Le Moal, H Simon, PV Piazza. Stress-induced sensitizaion and glucocorticoid. II. Sensitization of the increase in extracellular dopamine induced by cocaine depends on stress-induced corticosterone secretion. J Neurosci 15:7189–7195, 1995.
95. PV Piazza, F Rouge-Pont, V Deroche, S Maccari, H Simon, M Le Moal. Glucocorticoids have state-dependent stimulant effects on the mesencephalic dopaminergic transmission. Proc Natl Acad Sci USA 93:8716–8720, 1996.
96. H Silver, E Abboud. Drug abuse in schizophrenia: comparison of patients who began drug abuse before their first admission with those who began abusing drugs after their first admission. Schizophrenia Res 13:57–63, 1994.
97. M Hambrecht, H Hafner. Substance abuse and the onset of schizophrenia. Biol Psychiatry 40:1155–1163, 1996.
98. S Andreasson, P Allebeck, A Engstrom, V Rydberg. Cannabis and schizophrenia: a longitudinal study of Swedish conscripts. Lancet ii:1483–1485, 1987.
99. AY Tien, JC Anthony. Epidemiological analysis of alcohol and drug use as risk factors for psychotic experiences. J Nerv Ment Dis 178:473–480, 1990.
100. P Allebeck, C Adamsson, A Engstrom, U Rydberg. Cannabis and schizophrenia: a longitudinal study of cases treated in Stockholm County. Acta Psychiatr Scand 88:21–24, 1993.
101. PK McGuire, P Jones, I Harvey, M Williams, P McGuffin, RM Murray. Morbid risk of schizophrenia for relatives of patients with cannabis-associated psychosis. Schizophrenia Res 15:277–281, 1995.
102. SL Verma, I Sharma. Psychiatric morbidity in the first-degree relatives of schizophrenic patients. Br J Psychiatry 162:672–678, 1993.
103. PA Fried. Prenatal exposure to marihuana and tobacco during infancy, early and middle childhood: effects and an attempt at synthesis. Arch Toxicol Suppl 17:233–260, 1995.
104. KS Kendler, CA Prescott. Cannabis use, abuse, and dependence in a population-based sample of female twins. Am J Psychiatry 155:1016–1022, 1998.
105. KR Merikangas, M Stolar, DE Stevens, J Goulet, MA Preisig, B Fenton, H Zhang, SS O'Malley, BJ Rounsaville. Familial transmission of substance use disorders. Arch Gen Psychiatry 55:973:981, 1998.
106. KS Kendler, L Karkowski-Shuman, D Walsh. The risk for psychiatric illness in siblings of schizophrenics: the impact of psychotic and non-psychotic affective illness and alcoholism in parents. Acta Psychiatr Scand 94:49–55, 1996.
107. N Lin, SA Eisen, JF Scherrer, J Goldberg, WR True, NJ Lyons, MT Tsuang. The influence of familial and non-familial factors on the association between major depression and substance abuse/dependence in 1874 monozygotic male twin pairs. Drug Alcohol Depend 43:49–55, 1996.
108. DC D'Souza, A Belger, L Zimmerman, S Adams, R Gil, M Sernyak, JH Krystal. Cannabinoid sensitivity in schizophrenia: dose-response of tetrahydrocannabinol

effects in schizophrenics and healthy controls [abstr]. Proceedings of the 36th Annual Meeting of the American College of Neuropsychopharmacology, Kona, HI. P 286, 1997.
109. E Zuzarte, DC D'Souza, R Gil, A Genovese, L Trevisan, J White, DS Charney, JH Krystal. Dose-related ethanol effects in schizophrenic patients [abstr]. Alcohol Clin Exp Res 21(133A):779, 1997.
110. J Souilhac, M Poncelet, M Rinaldi-Carmona, G Le Fur, P Soubrie. Intrastriatal injection of cannabinoid receptor agonists induced turning behavior in mice. Pharmacol Biochem Behav 51:3–7, 1995.
111. A Giuffrida, LH Parsons, TM Kerr, F Rodriguez de Fonseca, M Navarro, D Piomelli. Dopamine activation of endogenous cannabinoid signaling in dorsal striatum. Nat Neurosci 2:358–363, 1999.
112. C Castellano, S Cabib, A Palmisano, V DiMarzo, S Puglisi-Allegra. The effects of amandamide on memory consolidation in mice involve both D1 and D2 dopamine receptors. Behav Pharmacol 8:707–712, 1997.
113. ES Deneris, J Connoly, SW Rogers, R Duvoisin. Pharmacological and functional diversity of neuronal nicotinic acetylcholine receptors. Trends Pharmacol Sci 12:34–40, 1991.
114. P Séguéla, J Wadiche, K Dineley-Miller, JA Dani, JW Patrick. Molecular cloning, functional properties, and distribution of rat brain alpha 7: a nicotinic cation channel highly permeable to calcium. J Neurosci 13:596–604, 1993.
115. R Freedman, M Hall, LE Adler, S Leonard. Evidence in post-mortem brain tissue for decreased numbers of hippocampal nicotinic receptors in schizophrenia. Biol Psychiatry 38:22–33, 1995.
116. MC Waldo, E Cawthra, LE Adler, S Dubester, M Staunton, HT Nagamoto, N Baker, A Madison, J Simon, A Scherzinger, C Drebing, G Gerhardt, R Freedman. Auditory sensory gating, hippocampal volume, and catecholamine metabolism and schizophrenics and their siblings. Schizophrenia Res 12:93–106, 1994.
117. MC Waldo, G Carey, M Myles-Worsley, E Cawthra, LE Adler, HT Nagamoto, P Wender, W Byerley, R Plaetke, R Freedman. Codistribution of a sensory gating deficit and schizophrenia in multi-affected families. Psychiatry Res 39:257–268, 1991.
118. LE Adler, LD Hoffer, A Wiser, R Freedman. Normalization of auditory physiology by cigarette smoking in schizophrenic patients. Am J Psychiatry 150:1856–1861, 1993.
119. LE Adler, LJ Hoffer, J Griffith, MC Waldo, R Freedman. Normalization by nicotine of deficient auditory sensory gating in the relatives of schizophrenics. Biol Psychiatry 32:607–616, 1992.
120. HT Nagamoto, LE Adler, RA Hea, JM Griffith, KA McRae, R Freedman. Gating of auditory P50 in schizophrenics: unique effects of clozapine. Biol Psychiatry 40:181–188, 1996.
121. TP George, MJ Sernyak, DM Ziedonis, SW Woods. Effects of clozapine on smoking in chronic schizophrenic outpatients. J Clin Psychiatry 56:344–346, 1995.

122. J McEvoy, O Freudenreich, M McGee, C Vander Zwaag, E Levin, J Rose. Clozapine decreases smoking in patients with chronic schizophrenia. Biol Psychiatry 37:550–552, 1995.
123. LE Adler, GA Gerhardt, R Franks, N Baker, H Nagamoto, C Drebing, R Freedman. Sensory physiology and catecholamine in schizophrenia and mania. Psychiatry Res 31:297–309, 1990.
124. JP McEvoy, O Frendenreich, ED Levin, JE Rose. Haloperidol increased smoking in patients with schizophrenia. Psychopharmacology (Berl) 119:124–126, 1995.
125. P Buckley, P Thompson, L Way, HY Meltzer. Substance abuse among patients with reatment-resistant schizophrenia: characteristics and implications for clozapine therapy. Am J Psychiatry 151:385–389, 1997.
126. RR Conley, DL Kelly, EA Gale. Olanzapine response in treatment-refractory schizophrenic patients with a history of substance abuse. Schizophrenia Res 33:95–101, 1998.
127. J Gauldi. The causality of depression in schizophrenia. Br J Psychiatry 142:621–624, 1983.
128. Collaborative Working Group on Clinical Trial Evaluations. Assessing the effects of atypical antipsychotics on negative symptoms. J Clin Psychiatry 59(suppl 12):28–34, 1998.
129. Collaborative Working Group on Clinical Trial Evaluations. Atypical antipsychotics for treatment of depression in schizophrenia and affective disorders. J Clin Psychiatry 59:(suppl 12):41–45, 1998.
130. J Arnt, T Skarsfeldt. Do novel antipsychotics have similar pharmacological characteristics?: a review of the evidence. Neuropsychopharmacology 18:63–101, 1998.
131. S Dawe, C Gerada, MAH Russell, JA Gray. Nicotine intake in smokers increases following a single dose of haloperidol. Psychopharmacology (Berl) 117:110–115, 1995.
132. P Weiden, R Aguila, J Standard. Atypical antipsychotic drugs and long-term outcome in schizophrenia. J Clin Psychiatry 57:53–60, 1996.
133. HY Meltzer, P Cola, L Way PA Thompson, B Bastani, MA Davis, B Snitz. Cost effectiveness of clozapine in neuroleptic-resistant schizophrenia: impact on risk-benefit assessment. Am J Psychiatry 150:1630–1638, 1993.
134. HY Meltzer, G Okayli. The reduction of suicidality during clozapine treatment in neuroleptic-resistant schizophrenia: impact on risk-benefit assessment. Am J Psychiatry 152:183–190, 1995.
135. MJ Albanese, EJ Khantzian, SL Murphy, AI Green. Decreased substance use in chronically psychotic patients treated with clozapine. Am J Psychiatry 151:780–781, 1994.
136. Y Yovell, LA Opler. Clozapine reverses cocaine craving in a treatment-resistant mentally ill chemical abuser: a case report and a hypothesis. J Nerv Ment Dis 182:591–592, 1994.
137. ML Lee, RA Dickson, M Campbell, J Oliphant, H Gretton, JT Dalby. Clozapine

and substance abuse in patients with schizophrenia. Can J Psychiatary 43:855–856, 1998.
138. DA Smelson, A Roy, M Roy. Risperidone diminishes cue-elicited craving in withdrawn cocaine-dependent patients. Can J Psychiatry 42:984, 1997.
139. L Misra, L Kofoed. Risperidone in the treatment of methamphetamine psychosis. Am J Psychiatry 154:1170, 1997.
140. DA Smelson, A Roy, M Roy. Risperidone and neuropsychological test performance in cocaine-withdrawn patients. Can J Psychiatry 42:431, 1997.
141. DW Self, WJ Barnhart, DA Lehman, EJ Nestler. Opposite modulation of cocaine-seeking behavior by D_1- and D_2-like dopamine receptor agonists. Science 271:1586–1589, 1996.
142. AD Levy, Q Li, MC Alvarez Sanz, PA Rittenhouse, MS Brownfield, LD Van de Kar. Repeated cocaine modifies the neuroendocrine responses to the 5-HT_{1c}/ 5-HT_2 agonist DOI. Eur J Pharmacol 221:121–127, 1992.
143. AD Levy, Q Li, LD Van de Kar. Repeated cocaine exposure inhibits the adrenocorticotropic hormone response to the serotonin releaser d-fenfluramine and the 5-HT_{1A} agonist, 8-OH-DPAT. Neuropharmacology 33:335–342, 1994.
144. G Perret, JH Schlunger, EM Unterwald, J Kreuter, A Ho, MJ Kreek. Down regulation of 5-HT_{1A} receptors in rat hypothalamus and dentate gyrus after "binge" pattern cocaine administration. Synapse 30:166–171, 1998.
145. A Newman-Tancredi, S Gavaudan, C Conte, C Chaput, M Touzard, L Verriele, V Audinot, MJ Millan. Agonist and antagonist actions of antipsychotic agents at 5-HT1A receptors: a [35S]GTPgammaS binding study. Eur J Pharmacol 355:245–256, 2998.
146. H Rollema, Y Lu, AW Schmidt, SH Zorn. Clozapine increases dopamine release in prefrontal cortex by 5-HT1A receptor action. Eur J Pharmacol 338:R3–5, 1997.
147. TA Kosten, EJ Nestler. Clozapine attenuates cocaine conditioned place preference. Life Sci 55:PL 9–14, 1994.
148. KE Vanover, MF Piercey, WL Woolverton. Evaluation of the reinforcing and discriminative stimulus effects of cocaine in combination with (+)-AJ76 or clozapine. J Pharmacol Exp Ther 266:780–789, 1993.
149. EA Loh, T Fitch, G Vickers, DCS Roberts. Clozapine increases breaking points on a progressive-ratio schedule reinforced by intravenous cocaine. Pharmacol Biochem Behav 42:559–562, 1992.
150. RD Myers, MF Lankford. Suppression of alcohol preference in high alcohol drinking rats: efficacy of amperozide versus naltrexone. Neuropsychopharmacology 14:139–149, 1996.
151. BA McMillen, S Walter, HL Williams, RD Myers. Comparison of the action of the 5-HT_2 antagonists amperozide and trazodone on preference for alcohol in rats. Alcohol 11:203–206, 1994.
152. BA McMillen, EA Jones, LJ Hill, HL Williams, A Bjork, RD Myers. Amperozide, a 5-HT_2 antagonist, attenuates craving for cocaine by rats. Pharmacol-Biochem-Behav 46:125–129, 1993.

153. JW Tsuang, AP Ho, TA Eckman, A Shaner. Dual diagnosis treatment for patients with schizophrenia who are substance dependent. Psychiatr Serv 48:887–889, 1997.
154. S Hansell. Treatment for comorbid schizophrenia and substance abuse disorders. New Direction for Mental Health Services 73:65–73, 1997.
155. AL Hoff, H Riordan, DW O'Donnell, L Morris, LE DeLisi. Neuropsychological functioning of first-episode schizophreniform patients. Am J Psychiatry 149:898–903, 1992.
156. AJ Saykin, DL Shtasel, RE Gur, DB Kester, LH Mozley, P Stafiniak, RC Gur. Neuropsychological deficits in neuroleptic naive patients with first-episode schizophrenia. Arch Gen Psychiatry 51:124–131, 1994.

6
Substance Abuse and Personality Disorders

The Impact of Three Personality Clusters on Prevalence, Course, and Treatment

Lisa A. Ottomanelli and Bryon Adinoff
*University of Texas Southwestern Medical Center
and VA North Texas Health Care System
Dallas, Texas*

INTRODUCTION

Personality governs our way of thinking about ourselves, relating to others, and interacting with our environment. Behavior patterns, cognitive styles, and disposition toward certain emotions are all influenced by personality. It is precisely because personality influences every aspect of one's approach to life that personality disorders are particularly disabling conditions. Indeed, by definition, a personality disorder is characterized by "an enduring pattern of inner experience and behavior that deviates markedly from the expectations of the individual's culture, is pervasive and inflexible, has an onset in adolescence or early adulthood, is stable over time, and leads to distress or impairment" (1).

The heavy use of alcohol or other drugs is often exhibited among individuals with personality disorders. When these two conditions co-occur, the level of impairment is particularly severe. Because of the high prevalence of comorbidity and the serious impairment that results, the interactions between personality disorders and substance abuse warrant specific consideration. Excellent reviews of this area have been published in past years (2,3). This chapter incorporates new findings in the area and discuss how they advance the understanding of the relationship between substance abuse and personality disorders.

The Three Clusters

The *Diagnostic and Statistical Manual of Psychiatric Disorders-IV* (DSM-IV) (1) groups the various personality disorders into three clusters. Although each personality disorder has a unique flavor, personality disorders from the same cluster share some common features. Cluster A includes personality disorders characterized by odd or eccentric personality traits. The personality disorders in this cluster are paranoid, schizoid, and schizotypal. Persons with these particular personality disorders have a reduced capacity for developing and maintaining healthy relationships with other people. Undue suspiciousness, aloof detachment, or intense feelings of discomfort color their social interactions. Cluster B includes personality disorders characterized by dramatic, emotional, or erratic personality styles. Antisocial, borderline, narcissistic, and histrionic personality disorders make up Cluster B. Persons with Cluster B disorders have problems conforming to social norms, difficulties with impulsivity, affective lability, and/or an extreme need for attention. Anxious and fearful traits characterize the Cluster C personality disorders: avoidant, dependent, and obsessive-compulsive. Earlier versions of DSM also included a passive-aggressive personality disorder in this cluster. Individuals with avoidant or dependent personality disorders demonstrate marked impairment in their interpersonal relationships, are bothered by feelings of inadequacy, and are overly sensitive to social rejection. Those with obsessive-compulsive disorder find themselves preoccupied with obtaining perfection and maintaining control across many areas of their lives. The commonality among the three clusters is that the individual's personality traits are inflexible and maladaptive; hence, they cause the individual to experience marked functional impairment and/or subjective distress across a variety of domains.

Chapter Overview

The first part of this chapter focuses on the epidemiology of substance abuse and personality disorders, discussing the prevalence rates of personality disorders among different populations of substance abusers as well as some of the methodological difficulties involved in attempting to determine comorbidity rates. The second section deals with the relationship between personality disorders and substance abuse, exploring some of the proposed theories regarding which disorder came first. In the third section, the impact of personality disorders on the course and treatment of substance abuse is addressed. The effect of personality disorders on treatment outcome is reviewed and treatment recommendations for substance abusers with personality disorders are considered. Finally, future directions for research are discussed.

Before proceeding further, some terminology needs clarification. First, the chapter is a review of personality disorders and substance abuse, not of normal personality functioning and addiction. The emphasis of the review is on *pathological* personality processes as represented by the personality disorder diagnoses in DSM-IV. Individual personality characteristics (e.g., extraversion, conscientiousness, impulsivity, antagonism, etc.) are not considered in and of themselves but only in terms of their relationship to the personality disorders (i.e., as symptoms of the personality disorders). Additionally, the broad term "substance abuse" is used to refer to all substance misuse disorders, including both conditions of substance abuse and substance dependence. "Substance" refers to all psychoactive drugs, including alcohol, but excludes nicotine and caffeine.

EPIDEMIOLOGY OF SUBSTANCE ABUSE AND PERSONALITY DISORDERS

Rates of personality disorders among substance abusers vary widely depending on the population studied, the diagnostic classification system, the assessment method, and even the drug of abuse. We begin this section by providing the reader with an overview of the prevalence rates of personality disorders among substance abusers.

Substance Abuse and Personality Disorders in the General Population

A high degree of co-occurrence between personality disorders and substance abuse is seen in the general population, particularly with regard to antisocial personality disorder (ASPD) and alcoholism. In the Epidemiologic Catchment Area survey, the co-occurrence of alcoholism with other psychiatric conditions was examined among five community samples of approximately 20,000 people (4). Psychiatric disorders studied included the Axis I disorders of mania, schizophrenia, somatization, anorexia, affective disorders, and anxiety disorders and the Axis II disorder ASPD. Of all the psychiatric diagnoses investigated, the highest comorbidity rate observed was between alcoholism and ASPD. In the general population, male alcoholics were four times more likely to have a diagnosis of ASPD than nonalcoholics, and female alcoholics were 12 times more likely to be diagnosed with ASPD then nonalcoholic females. In 1997, Kessler and colleagues (5) examined the lifetime co-occurrence of alcohol use disorders and other psychiatric disorders among a nationally representative household sample. They found that persons with alcohol dependence had higher rates of comorbidity with ASPD than with Axis I Anxiety or Affective disorders. In both of these studies, ASPD was the only personality disorder investigated along with selected Axis I disorders. Thus, a comprehensive picture of the comorbidity rates of the various personality disorders and substance abuse in the general population is lacking.

Drake and Vaillant (6) conducted a longitudinal investigation of the comorbidity of alcoholism with the entire range of DSM-III personality disorders in a community sample. The sample consisted of inner-city adolescent nondelinquent males who had served as a control group for a separate study that investigated juvenile delinquency. Subjects were matched for ethnicity, and no African-Americans were included in the study. At the 33-year follow-up, they found that among alcohol-dependent men, 37% met criteria for an Axis II personality disorder by age 47. The prevalence rates of the personality disorder diagnoses associated with alcoholism were skewed toward the interpersonally withdrawn disorders (e.g., schizoid, dependent, and avoidant) rather than acting-out disorders (e.g., antisocial, borderline). As the authors note, this distribution probably reflects the sample-selection characteristics of including only nondelinquent early-adolescent males. Even so, information about the association between personality disorders and alcoholism can be gleaned from this study. *All* the subjects with ASPD were also alcoholics, while almost none of the subjects with schizoid personality disorders were alcohol-dependent.

Thus, in the general population a strong association has been demonstrated between alcoholism and ASPD. However, a comprehensive and methodologically sound assessment of the comorbidity rates between alcoholism and the full range of personality disorders remains lacking. Furthermore, information on the comorbidity between the personality disorders and drug dependence other than alcohol dependence in the general population is also unavailable at the present time.

Substance Abuse and Personality Disorders Among Treatment Populations

Comorbidity rates of substance abuse and personality disorders among clinical samples (e.g., patients currently engaged in inpatient or outpatient substance abuse treatment) are even higher than those seen in community-based populations. Among treatment populations, at least 50% of substance abusers typically meet criteria for an Axis II diagnosis. Comorbidity rates vary somewhat depending on the particular sample characteristics in these populations, and range from 56% to as high as 91% when the full spectrum of personality disorders is examined (Table 1) (7–16).

In an inpatient substance abuse treatment population, Nace and colleagues (9) found that 57% of substance abusers had an Axis II personality disorder. ASPD was the most frequently diagnosed personality disorder in this sample. When a sample of cocaine-dependent inpatients was studied, 70% of patients met criteria for at least one personality disorder (10). Comorbidity rates were highest for borderline personality disorder (BPD) (34%), followed by ASPD (28%) and narcissistic personality disorder (28%). In outpatient substance abuse patients, the prevalence rate of personality disorders was at least 60% in alcoholics (13,14) and 48% in cocaine addicts (15).

Consistently, the most frequently diagnosed personality disorders among substance abuse treatment populations are ASPD and BPD. Admittedly, these two personality disorders, which are characterized by impulsive behavior, have considerable diagnostic overlay with substance dependence. Substance abuse is even listed as one of the criteria used to diagnose BPD and many of the criteria for ASPD can be direct consequences of substance abuse (arrest, disregard for safety of others, irresponsibility, etc.).

Some studies have attempted to deal with the problem of overlapping criteria when making personality disorder diagnoses by employing diagnostic rules that exclude behaviors that occur in combination with substance use. Even when such conservative assessment methods are employed, however, high rates of these particular personality disorders among substance abusers are still observed. For example, 41% of hospitalized alcoholics had ASPD even when symptoms that were directly related to alcohol use (e.g., alcohol intoxication before age of 15, drunk driving) were excluded in making ASPD diagnoses (7). Using structured interviews to distinguish general behavioral characteristics from those that were consequences of substance use, ASPD and BPD still emerge as the most frequently diagnosed personality disorders (9,10). Of course, making such distinctions is especially difficult in those with an early onset of substance abuse, which is not infrequent. Furthermore, some

Table 1. Treatment Samples Prevalence Rates

Study	Hesselbrock et al., 1985 (7)	Nace et al., 1983 (8)	Nace et al., 1991 (9)	Kranzler et al., 1994 (10)	Morgenstern et al., 1997 (11)	Kosten, et al., 1982 (11a)
Setting	Inpatient	Inpatient	Inpatient	Inpatient	Inpt and outpt	Inpt and outpt
Population	Alcohol	Alcohol	Subst. abuse	Cocaine	Subst. abuse	Opiate
Measure	DIS	DIB	SCID-II	SCID-II	SCID-II	SADS
Criteria	DSM-III	NA	DSM-III-R	DSM-III-R	DSM-III-R	DSM III
N	321	94	100	50	366	389
Any PD			57%	70%	56%	68%
Cluster A						
Paranoid			7%	22%	20%	1%
Schizotypal			0%	2%	3%	2.4%
Schizoid			0%	4%	1%	2%
Cluster B						
Histrionic			6%	4%	4%	5%
Narcissistic			4%	28%	6%	2%
Borderline		13%	3%	34%	19%	12%
Antisocial	41%		17%	28%	26%	55%
Cluster C						
Avoidant			2%	22%	18%	1%
Dependent			4%	10%	4%	3%
Compulsive			2%	16%	10%	NA
Passive-aggressive			5%	8%	10%	0.50%
Mean No. of PDs				2.54	2.3	
>1 PD					>50%	24%

literature indicates that such distinctions not only may be unnecessary but may actually obscure the clinical significance of comorbidity. When diagnosing ASPD, for example, using restrictive criteria that require independence of antisocial behavior and substance abuse results in a reduction in diagnostic reliability as well as prognostic significance (17,18). On the other hand, diagnosing ASPD without respect to substance abuse status increases the

DeJong et al., 1993 (12)		Nurnberg et al., 1993 (13)	Smyth and Washousky, 1995 (14)	Barber et al., 1996 (15)	Cacciola et al., 1996 (16)
Inpatient	Inpt TC	Outpatient	Outpatient	Outpatient	Outpatient
Alcohol	Polydrug	Alcohol	Alcohol	Cocaine	Opiate
SIDP DSM-III-R 178	86	SCID-II DSM-III-R 50	SCID-II DSM-III-R 48	SCID-II DSM-III-R 289	SIDP-R DSM-III-R 210
78%	91%	64%	60%	48%	66%
14%	27%	22%	31%	7%	4%
17%	47%	1%	6%	1%	1%
4%	7%	6%	2%	1%	5%
34%	64%	3%	6%	4%	8%
7%	13%	3%	15%	6%	6%
17%	65%	8%	31%	11%	8%
5%	48%	10%	15%	20%	38%
19%	27%	10%	29%	9%	8%
29%	35%	5%	13%	2%	3%
19%	26%	4%	13%	3%	4%
14%	49%	9%	19%	6%	6%
1.8	4	2.6	3.2	—	—
50%	80%	62%	40%	18%	—

reliability of the diagnosis without adversely affecting its validity (18). Finally, when ASPD is diagnosed using less restrictive criteria, an association with greater treatment involvement (number of days in inpatient or outpatient treatment) and poorer treatment outcome is observed (17). Thus, using a less restrictive diagnostic system may be more clinically and prognostically meaningful.

EXPLORING CAUSAL RELATIONSHIPS

Trying to unravel which came first—the personality disturbance or the substance use—is a daunting challenge. Indeed, the term "dual diagnosis" is often employed in order to circumvent the issue of cause and merely state that both disorders occur concurrently. We recognize that a discussion of which-came-first causal association can be simplistic. Clearly, multiple factors can contribute to the development of both of these disorders. That is, overlapping genetic predispostions and environmental experiences can increase or decrease the risk for the development of a personality and/or substance abuse disorder. However, this linear construct provides an organizing framework in which to examine causal relationships between substance abuse and personality disorders. Therefore, the following discussion is limited to a review of the empirical literature that most carefully examines the temporal relationship of personality disorders and substance abuse.

Does Chronic Substance Abuse Cause Personality Disorders?

One etiological pathway that has been proposed asserts that the pharmacological effects of chronic substance use results in a drug-induced personality state, a syndrome that is considered diagnostically compatible with the personality disorders (2). This model suggests that the effects of alcohol and drugs on the brain, combined with the immediate gratification of needs that occurs with drug use, results in a variety of traits that are common features of many personality disorders. Stimulants, for example, can result in paranoid symptoms, alcohol is associated with impulsive and aggressive behaviors, and marijuana can reportedly produce an "amotivational" syndrome. Other drug-induced personality traits include impulsivity, decreased frustration tolerance, self-centeredness, grandiosity, passivity-withdrawal, and affect intolerance.

There is some evidence supporting this construct. For example, an examination of data from Drake and Vaillant's (6) longitudinal study suggests that alcoholic men with personality disorders display disturbances in personality functioning primarily due to their drinking rather than the persistence of early problems with adaptation. In this study, nonalcoholic men with personality disorders showed early-childhood problems in a variety of behavioral domains, whereas alcoholic men with personality disorders did not demonstrate these difficulties in early childhood. In fact, the alcoholic men with personality disorders were comparable to the men *without* personality disorders on these childhood domains. The findings may not, however, apply to all personality disorders, as this was a nonsociopathic sample. Indeed, only six of the 86 men with alcohol dependence and personality disorders had ASPD, and there were no subjects with BPD in this sample. Thus, these alcoholic men with primarily interpersonally withdrawn personality disorders, rather than acting-out or impulsive personality disorders, may have experienced normal character development until they became alcohol-dependent. Whether character structure returns to premorbid levels during periods of protracted abstinence was not addressed by this data.

In general, it appears that most substance-specific personality symptoms (e.g., stimulant-associated paranoia) resolve relatively quickly with the cessation of substance use. As noted in the subsequent section, empirical studies suggest that when symptoms consistent with a personality disorder persist without diminishing following the cessation of substance use, the presence of a personality disorder is likely.

Do Personality Disorders Lead to Substance Abuse?

There are several lines of evidence that suggest that the personality disturbance *precedes* the substance abuse. Examination of the individual characteristics that are considered risk factors for substance abuse may serve to illuminate the relationship between substance misuse and personality disorders. A growing body of evidence has identified impulsivity and conduct disturbance as risk factors for the development of a substance use disorder. For example, cross-sectional studies show that impulsive, antisocial, and aggressive traits, broadly termed "behavioral disinhibition", distinguishes between children of alcoholics as compared with children of nonalcoholics (19). Moreover, prospective studies have demonstrated that higher levels of behavioral disinhibition are present among people who then go on to develop alcohol or drug problems (20–22). Behavioral disinhibition is a common feature of the Cluster B ASPDs and BPDs that co-occur frequently with substance use disorders. Such studies imply that impulsivity and conduct disturbance act as predisposing factors for later substance abuse, suggesting that early character disturbance precedes the development of substance use disorders.

Morgenstern and colleagues (11) addressed this issue by examining the temporal continuity of character disorder symptoms assessed in adult alcoholics with either BPD or paranoid personality disorder (PPD). They examined the predictive power of a cumulative measure of early maladjustment that included measures of childhood impulsivity/hyperactivity, conduct disturbance, and presence of Axis I disorders in childhood. They found that early maladjustment predicted personality disorder symptoms in adult alcoholics, even after partialing out the current and cumulative effects of alcohol use. Maladjustment in childhood was significantly related to character pathology in adulthood, independent of the effects of alcohol use. These data suggest that personality disorders in substance abusers reflect a persistence of behavior problems across time, rather then being a consequence of substance use itself—at least for BPD and PPD. Although ASPD was included in other analyses in Morgenstern and coworkers' study, it was not included in the latter analysis, perhaps because childhood conduct disturbance is one of the criteria for this disorder. It would be interesting to assess whether this same relationship can be generalized to other personality disorders such as avoidant, dependent, or narcissistic personality disorders.

Weiss et al. (23) explored whether hospitalized cocaine addicts had different personality disorder diagnoses during drug-free periods vs. drug-use periods. They found that the majority of personality disorder diagnoses were present during both drug use *and* abstinence, whereas only 8% of the personality disorder diagnoses were made exclusively under conditions of drug use. The data revealed that personality disorders typically were stable irrespective of patients' current drug use patterns and conflicted with the supposition that addiction causes personality disturbance. Of course, some may argue that once the drug use starts it alters personality so dramatically that even during periods of abstinence the personality disturbance persists. That is, it could be said that the personality patterns of drug users become so ingrained that maladaptive personality traits remain even when substance use is discontinued.

While considering the ability of substance abuse and ASPD to influence the development of each other, it is important to keep in mind that they are two distinct disorders. Adoption studies indicate that ASPD and alcohol dependence show specificity of inheritance (e.g., 24–26). These studies have demonstrated that adoptees with biological relatives having antisocial behaviors had high frequencies of ASPD but did not have higher frequencies of alcoholism. Those adoptees whose biologic relatives were alcoholics were prone toward alcoholism but not ASPD. Such data point out that a predisposition toward one disorder does not necessarily imply a predisposition to the other.

An Interactive Model? Yes and No.

In clinical practice, substance abuse and personality disorders are generally assumed to operate in an interactive and interdependent manner, rather than a straightforward causal model. The research supports this supposition but only as applied to the acting out, antisocial, and/or impulsive personality disorders.

The studies heretofore discussed collectively provide evidence that some personality disorders, such as BPD, ASPD and PPD, in adulthood can be traced to childhood characteristics and persist over time, regardless of whether substance abuse enters into the clinical picture. These particular personality disorders may represent an increased vulnerability to substance abuse, which then exacerbates underlying maladaptive character traits. In essence, when both disorders are present, each may modify the expression of the other and affect response to treatment. (Treatment response will be discussed further in a subsequent section.) From a biological perspective, it may be hypothesized that a particular disturbance in neurophysiological circuitry results in a personality characteristic associated with a personality disorder (i.e. impulsivity), increasing the vulnerability to substance abuse. The subsequent chronic use of substances then exacerbates the pre-existing biologic imbalance, increasing the severity of the personality-disordered symptom, which furthers the substance abuse. For the interpersonally withdrawn personality disorders (Clusters A and C), however, there is no strong evidence that there is an interaction between personality disorders and substance abuse. It is plausible that for these other personality disorders there is no increased incidence of personality disorders, as compared to the general population, and no increased incidence of individuals with these personality disorders having substance abuse.

IMPACT OF PERSONALITY DISORDERS ON THE COURSE OF SUBSTANCE ABUSE

There is little question that the presence of certain personality disorders affects the course and presentation of substance use disorders. This observed relationship is most valid for substance abusers with Cluster B disorders, as most studies have either compared substance abusers with personality disorders (the majority of which are Cluster B disorders) to those without personality disorders, or have examined specific personality disorders such as ASPD or BPD. The evidence suggests that these personality disorders are associated with a more severe course of substance abuse characterized by early onset of addiction, greater addiction severity, poorer psychosocial functioning, and high degrees of psychiatric impairment.

A multitude of studies have demonstrated that ASPD is associated with an earlier age of onset for alcohol use and dependence (7,27–29) and for cocaine use and dependence (17). Severity of drug dependence is also affected by the coexistence of a personality disorder. Alcoholics with ASPD, for example, exhibit a higher alcohol symptom count and longer duration of alcoholism (4). A distinct pattern of alcohol use characterized by compulsive use, drinking to manage moods and enhance functioning, and pervasive use of alcohol in one's life is seen among alcoholics with personality disorders as compared with those without personality disorders (9). BPD was the largest personality disorder group represented in this study; hence, this particular pattern of alcohol use may pertain more to BPD than other personality disorders. Polydrug use, another indicator of severity, is also more likely among substance abusers with a personality disturbance. For example, alcohol-dependent patients with BPD are more likely to use illegal drugs than alcohol-dependent patients without BPD (27), and cocaine addicts with ASPD have higher rates of alcohol dependence than those without ASPD (15–17). The patients with coexisting ASPD or BPD and substance abuse described in these studies are probably the individuals commonly referred to as the "Type II alcoholic" in Cloninger and colleagues' (26) nomenclature or the "Type B alcoholic" in Babor and colleagues' (30) nomenclature. These subtypes reportedly show an increased genetic load for alcohol dependence, have an earlier onset of substance use and abuse, are more impulsive, demonstrate a more severe course of substance abuse, and are more resistant to treatment than others with substance abuse disorders. Whether the patients in these identified subtypes actually demonstrate a higher incidence of personality disorders has not, to our knowledge, been examined.

Not all personality disorders have an equal capacity to influence the course of addiction. For instance, examination of severe personality disorders—borderline, antisocial, and paranoid—by Morgenstern et al. (11) showed that they were not all consistently related to indicators of the course of alcoholism. In this study, ASPD and BPD were consistently related to age of onset, lifetime severity, and number of alcohol treatments, while PPD was related only to number of alcohol treatments. Examining current patterns of drinking through regression analysis determined that the individual disorders were unique predictors of drinking patterns. Both ASPD and BPD predicted dependence severity. ASPD and PPD uniquely predicted cumulative quantity of drinking, and BPD uniquely predicted psychological problems related to drinking. Thus, no single personality disorder diagnosis was related to all the course variables studied. ASPD and BPD were consistently related to course variables, but PPD was not.

In general, greater psychosocial, psychiatric, and medical impairment is seen among substance abusers with personality disorders than among those without an additional Axis II diagnosis. Increased impairment in the areas of social functioning, employment, legal problems, and marital and educational status is seen among both alcoholics and opiate addicts with ASPD compared to those without ASPD (7,31,32). Additionally, substance abusers with personality disorders experience more medical problems and complications than do non-personality-disordered substance abusers (31,32). Compared to cocaine-dependent patients without personality disorders, cocaine-dependent patients with personality disorders are likely to have higher rates of anxiety and mood disorders (15,17) and significantly higher levels of psychiatric severity (15). Specifically, these patients have higher Psychiatry Severity scores on the Addiction Severity Index (ASI) and more overall psychopathology as determined by the Global Severity Index of the Brief Symptom Inventory (BSI). Depression is also frequently seen in narcotic addicts with personality disturbance (33). Alcoholics with personality disorders demonstrate a variety of psychiatric problems, including anxiety, depression, mania, and schizophrenia (29). Alcoholics with personality disorders report more dissatisfaction with their quality of life overall, social life, emotional health, relationships, and job and school performance, in particular, compared to alcoholics without personality disorders (9,34).

Although overall greater levels of psychiatric symptomatology can be expected among substance abusers with personality disorders, there is some heterogeneity with regard to particular psychiatric symptoms expressed. In alcoholics, ASPD was associated with greater sensation seeking, aggressiveness, lack of empathy, and less distress, while BPD was associated with greater distress, rejection concerns, dependency needs, early attentional and social withdrawal problems, and more impaired coping (11). Therefore, overall greater levels of psychopathology can be expected among substance abusers with personality disorders, and the particular psychiatric symptom presentation is likely to vary depending on the particular Axis II diagnosis.

Triggers and Coping Styles

Another angle from which to explore the influence of personality disorders on substance abuse is to assess situations, or triggers, that stimulate cravings for alcohol or drugs and how personality disorders affect the ability to cope with them. When the full range of personality disorders is examined, three broad groups of triggers emerge as prominent: unpleasant emotions, testing personal control, and conflict with other people (14). Triggers associated with BPD, however, include both positive (e.g., feeling good) and negative situations (e.g., negative emotional and physical states, tension, and social rejection) (8,35). These results suggested that patients with BPD may be at higher risk for relapse than other substance abusers when life is going well (8). Considering that most addicts in recovery initially experience a decrease in negative consequences associated with substance abuse, BPD addicts may begin craving early in recovery as life begins to stabilize.

The coping styles that personality-disordered substance abusers rely on to handle common trigger situations are important. Not surprisingly, they often choose methods of coping that are less effective in meeting the challenge of these triggers than those chosen by non–Axis II patients. For example, substance abusers with BPD used more avoidance to cope with triggers and less problem-solving and positive appraisal than non-BPD patients (35). Within the entire range of personality disorders, emotion-oriented—rather than task-oriented or even avoidant—styles of coping were most often employed (14). A resultant hypothesis is that the behavioral deficits associated with personality disorders influence the pattern of drinking, which then becomes the coping style (14). Once use of substances dominates as the preferred coping mechanism, it interferes with the already limited abilities of patients with personality disorders to develop alternative coping methods of dealing with unpleasant situations and emotions. In essence, the early onset of substance abuse prevents the acquisition of a range of coping responses, because of impaired development. Thus, these individuals are particularly susceptible to relapse following treatment because they do not have an established repertoire of other coping strategies.

IMPACT OF PERSONALITY DISORDERS ON SUBSTANCE ABUSE TREATMENT

Effects of Axis II Diagnosis on Treatment Outcome

The common assumption that personality disorders have a negative impact on treatment outcome has been supported in the literature, although not consistently. Multiple studies have demonstrated that alcoholics and opiate addicts with an additional diagnosis of a personality disorder are more likely to have a negative response to substance abuse treatment (13,33,36,37). Axis II diagnoses from Cluster B (ASPD, BPD, histrionic personality disorder), in particular, have been identified as risk factors that predict the poorest overall treatment response (16). Additionally, substance abusers with personality disorders are more likely to drop out of treatment prematurely; those with ASPD have the highest attrition rates (16). The negative outcomes associated with ASPD have been emphasized in several studies (31,32).

Some investigators maintain that the relationship between poor treatment outcome and ASPD has not been consistently demonstrated (38,39). Cacciola et al., in a comparison of addicts with ASPD to addicts with personality disorders other than ASPD, found no significant differences in drug use at 7-month follow-up (16). Both of these personality-disordered groups showed improvement across a number of areas studied, including employment, social, psychiatric, and legal status. The "other" personality group excluded patients with ASPD; however, the ASPD group did not exclude patients with other personality disorders. Hence, comorbid personality disorders in the ASPD group may have resulted in a failure to detect differences between the two groups. In Cacciola and coworkers' study (40), ASPD was not a negative predictor of treatment response in alcohol- and cocaine-dependent men at 7-month follow-up. Among these patients, ASPD substance abusers and non-ASPD substance abusers showed comparable rates of treatment response in several areas.

The work of Longabaugh and colleagues (39) suggests that pessimistic generalizations of negative outcomes for ASPD substance abusers may be due to a failure to account for the effects of treatment matching. These investigators assessed drinking outcomes for both antisocial and non-antisocial alcoholics receiving either extended cognitive-behavior therapy (CBT) for 16 sessions or relationship enhancement (RE) for up to 20 sessions, both delivered in a group format. The CBT sessions included functional analysis of drinking antecedents and consequences, and cognitive restructuring that focused on topics such as stimulus control, rearranging consequences, assertion training, problem solving, and dealing with slips and relapses. The RE treatment also included six sessions of functional analysis, but the remaining sessions focused on patients' relationships, with the participation of significant others in some of the sessions. No difference was found between the two treatment groups on overall measures of alcohol consumption during the year following treatment. However, the ASPD alcoholics who received extended CBT drank less intensely (average number of drinks per drinking day) than either the non-ASPD alcoholics who received extended CBT or the ASPD alcoholics treated with RE. Longabaugh et al. (39) therefore suggest that ASPD alcoholics respond as well as, if not more favorably than, other alcoholics to abstinence-oriented CBT. Studies have also shown that patients can be matched to treatment based on the severity of sociopathy (41,42). In these studies, treatment response to either a CBT group or an interactional therapy group was compared for alcoholics who differed on a continuous measure of sociopathy (the California Psychological Inventory Socialization Scale). The CBT, emphasizing skills training in the areas of problem solving, interpersonal skills, relaxation, and dealing with negative moods, was more effective in reducing relapse for patients who were higher in sociopathy. On the other hand, interactional therapy that focused on fostering insight in order to improve interpersonal functioning was more effective in reducing relapse for patients with lower levels of sociopathy. Interestingly, when treatment response was examined using a dichotomous variable of presence or absence of ASPD diagnosis, there was no association with outcome measures. Thus, the personality trait of sociopathy, rather than ASPD diagnosis per se, may be the critical attribute in matching these patients to these types of treatments.

The relationship discussed above may not apply to matching patients to other forms of treatments. Project Match was a large-scale study that assessed the benefits of matching alcohol-dependent patients to different treatments with respect to a variety of patient characteristics, including sociopathy (43). Patients were randomly assigned to one of three individually delivered treatment approaches: cognitive-behavioral coping skills therapy (CBT), 12-Step facilitation (TSF), or motivational enhancement therapy (MET). CBT focused on remediating skill deficits and teaching patients how to cope more effectively with situations that lead to relapse. TSF emphasized the disease-recovery model of alcoholism and assisted patients in working through the 12 Steps of Alcoholics Anonymous. MET was based on the principles of motivational psychology and focused on increasing patients' motivation to change their behavior. The study did not find robust matching effects for any of the patient variables studied. In regard to personality disturbance, sociopathy did not predict treatment response when CBT was compared to MET or TSF therapy.

Perhaps sociopathy is a relevant patient characteristic to consider when matching patients to substance abuse treatment groups but not as important when considering individual therapy approaches. Substance abusers with antisocial characteristics may be able to benefit from coping skills groups because they are usually more didactic and structured than other types of therapy groups. In contrast, antisocial characteristics may be disruptive to the group process in interpersonal therapy groups, which typically are less structured and use an open-discussion format. It may not be necessary to take antisocial personality disturbance into account when assigning patients to individually delivered treatment approaches, since an individual therapist is able to impose as much structure as the patient needs in individual sessions. Another explanation of the discrepant findings may be that CBT, MET, and TSF are comparable treatments for sociopathic patients whereas treatments that focus specifically on relationship issues, such as the RE therapy or interactional therapy described previously, are a poorer treatment choice for sociopathic substance abusers, perhaps because these patients lack empathy and improving relationships is not important to them.

Depression can also be a modifying variable in determining response to treatment in some substance abusers. Both alcoholics and opiate addicts with

ASPD in addition to a lifetime diagnosis of depression showed greater improvement following treatment than did addicts with ASPD alone (32,44).

Categorical vs. Dimensional Approaches to Understanding Treatment Response

Most studies that examine treatment response use a categorical approach to personality disturbance—that is, they compare substance abusers who meet DSM criteria for personality disorders with those who do not. This approach has shown some prognostic value, as discussed above. However, it may also obscure the clinical picture because the relationship of particular personality characteristics to treatment outcome is overlooked. For example, Marlowe and colleagues (45) have shown that categorical diagnoses alone are not sufficient predictors of response to behaviorally based treatment for cocaine dependence. Rather, a dimensional approach that takes into account the number of personality disorder symptoms and the specific traits of various personality disorders yields greater prognostic significance. In this study, substance abusers with a diagnosis of Axis II disorders did not differ significantly on outcome measures from those without additional Axis II diagnoses. When the number of Axis II symptoms were considered, however, there was a significant association with outcome. Specifically, borderline personality symptoms (e.g., impulsivity, affective liability) were negatively correlated and dependent personality symptoms were positively correlated with measures of treatment tenure and abstinence. Symptoms of antisocial (e.g., antisocial tendencies, egocentricity), paranoid (e.g., paranoid ideation), and compulsive (e.g., rigidity) personality disorders also showed negative associations with various indices of treatment response.

Thus, there is a complex relationship between personality disorders and treatment outcome for substance abusers. Although there is substantial evidence in the literature of negative outcomes for antisocial substance abusers, there is also evidence of equivalent and even positive responses to treatment. This is particularly true when other variables are considered, such as treatment type or presence of depression. The literature therefore suggests that when ASPD patients receive general substance abuse treatment and depression is not considered, they do worse in treatment than non-ASPD substance abusers. However, if they are offered CBT they fare better than other substance abusers. Moreover, many, but not all, traits of personality disturbance are negative prognostic indicators for substance abuse treatment. Personality characteristics of impulsivity, antisocial tendencies, rigidity, and paranoia are associated with worse treatment outcome. Dependent characteristics, though, are good treatment indicators in substance abusers.

TREATMENT RECOMMENDATIONS

General Guidelines for the Diagnosis of Comorbid Personality Disorders in Substance Abusers

The careful assessment and diagnosis of personality disorders are important so that treatment interventions can be targeted toward the specific deficits the patient manifests. A careful assessment is critical since labeling of substance abusers with personality disorders is to be avoided (14,46). Once a diagnosis of a personality disorder has been made and become part of patients' permanent medical records, it is extremely difficult for patients to escape or erase this stigma. Such a diagnosis is quite powerful—although it has the potential to inform, it can also negatively color how future treatment providers may view the patient. Personality disorders often garner intense negative reactions from members of the treatment team, and can interfere with the effective treatment of the patient (3). When communicating with other members of the treatment team, it is typically more therapeutic to describe the maladaptive personality traits that are present, how they are likely to be exhibited during treatment, and how they may affect recovery, than to offer a specific diagnosis. This approach speaks directly to the deficits the patient manifests, helping providers focus on resources that the patient needs to develop in treatment in order to be successful.

When contemplating a diagnosis of personality disorder in a patient with substance abuse, several potentially mitigating factors should be considered (Table 2). Since personality disorders represent an "enduring pattern" of behavior (1), a diagnosis of personality disorder should generally require evidence of both behavioral pathology *before* the onset of substance abuse and *persistence* of behaviors following the cessation of substance use. As noted in a previous section, substance-induced specific personality changes, such as marijuana-induced passivity or alcohol-induced impulsivity, generally resolve soon after the cessation of substance use. If there is no lessening of these symptoms following the avoidance of substances, or these symptoms were present prior to the onset of a problematic substance use, or a *complex* of symptoms consistent with a personality disorder is present, then a diagnosis of personality disorder should be strongly considered.

The presence of non–substance abuse Axis I disorders can also complicate the diagnostic picture. For example, many patients with mania appear to

Table 2. Special Considerations in Diagnosing Comorbid Personality Disorders in Substance Abuse Patients

1. Avoid labeling.
2. Dysfunctional personality traits may be a result of chronic substance use. These behaviors typically resolve with several days or weeks of abstinence.
3. Consider evidence of behavioral pathology *prior* to the onset of substance abuse and *persistence* of behaviors following the cessation of substance use to confirm diagnosis of personality disorders.
4. Consider Axis I disorders as the cause of behavioral pathology.
5. Despite need to consider substance-induced or Axis I etiologies, early diagnosis of personality disorder is important.
6. Focus on specific behavioral deficits and their implications for treatment.

have ASPD, patients with depression can seem similar to those with dependent PD, patients with social phobia can be almost indistinguishable from those with avoidant personality disorder, and schizophrenia shares many features with paranoid or schizotypal personality disorder. Since the Axis I disorders are far more responsive to pharmacological intervention (see below) and constitute behaviors (by definition) less engrained and enduring than the personality disorders, it is critical that all Axis I disorders be identified prior to the personality disorders. It should be remembered, however, that non–substance abuse-related Axis I disorders do not preclude the diagnosis of a personality disorder, and that a patient frequently presents with behaviors consistent with both an Axis I and an Axis II disorder.

General Guidelines for the Treatment of Substance Abusers with Comorbid Personality Disorders

No matter what form of substance abuse treatment is implemented, following some basic guidelines for treating patients with personality disorders will help treatment proceed smoothly and enhance the likelihood of positive outcomes (see Table 3). Incorporating limit setting and structure into treatment is particularly important for patients with personality disorders (3,46,47). These parameters help balance the lack of internal controls manifested as impulsivity, decreased frustration tolerance, and difficulty tolerating negative affect. Confronting maladaptive behavior and assisting patients in accepting responsibility for their behavior are also essential components of treatment (46,47). Clinicians need to be able to demonstrate empathy for the pain patients' experience while holding them responsible for the consequences of behaviors

Table 3. General Treatment Guidelines for Substance Abuse Patients with Comorbid Personality Disorders

1. Early assessment and diagnosis of personality disorders.
2. Incorporation of limit setting and structure.

Psychosocial Interventions

1. Treatment interventions targeted toward specific deficits.
2. Confrontation of maladaptive behavior.
3. Demonstration of empathy.
4. Promotion of patient responsibility for consequences of behavior.
5. Promotion of active coping to deal with uncomfortable feelings and difficult situations.
6. Provide stimulating treatment environment.
7. Utilization of self-help groups.
8. Avoidance of insight-oriented approaches early in treatment.

Pharmacological Interventions

1. Consider potential toxicity of pharmacological treatment and substance use in case of relapse.
2. Recognize that medication treatment effects are modest, at best.
3. Cluster A: low-dose neuroleptics for suspiciousness, paranoia, thought disorders.
4. Cluster B: a) mood stabilizers (carbamazepine or sodium valproate), lithium, SSRIs for affective instability, b) mood stabilizers, SSRIs, atypical antipsychotics for impulsivity and/or aggression.
5. Cluster C: target associated Axis I disorders.

and attitudes (46,47). Self-help support groups are often helpful, as peers can provide social support and assist in confronting behaviors that reinforce addiction (2,3,46). Insight-oriented approaches should not be used in the beginning stages of treatment because personality-disordered patients cannot tolerate the uncomfortable feelings that may arise as a result (47). Instead, treatment that promotes active coping to handle difficult feelings and situations is recommended. Finally, ensuring that treatment is stimulating enough to satisfy the novelty-seeking needs of these patients is also important (46).

Cognitive-Behavioral Approaches

There is a growing recognition that skills-training approaches are particularly well suited to the needs of substance abusers with personality disorders.

Mood-management modules and cognitive-behavioral therapies for personality disorders (48–50) are increasingly being applied to the treatment of substance abusers with personality disorders. These cognitive-behaviorally oriented approaches teach substance-dependent patients how to manage feelings, tolerate distress, negotiate interpersonal situations, and challenge irrational thinking that leads to substance use. Essentially, the goal of treatment is to assist the patient in developing more adaptive coping mechanisms.

For example, relapse prevention is one cognitive skills-training approach that has been suggested as being appropriate for use with personality disorder–substance abuse patients (3). It is based on the premise that relapse to substance abuse is often associated with interpersonal conflict, negative emotional states, and social pressure (51). The goal of relapse prevention is to teach patients to cope effectively with these situations rather than drink or use drugs. Recent research (14) indicating that unpleasant emotions and conflict with others are two of the three common triggers for substance use in personality-disordered patients indicates that this approach may be particularly well suited to these patients' needs.

Several studies support the use of CBT in the treatment of substance abuse for patients with personality disorders. For example, outpatient treatment with CBT was superior to the disease and recovery (i.e., 12-Step) model in reducing alcohol use, increasing socialization, and improving psychological functioning in alcoholics with personality disorders (52). Cognitive-behavioral approaches may be especially beneficial for substance abusers with antisocial behavior. As discussed previously, research indicates that addicts with ASPD—or even those who don't meet criteria but have sociopathic personality traits—respond more favorably to CBT than to a relationship-focused treatment approach (39,41,42).

Traditional 12-Step Approach

Nace (2) has discussed how already established treatment interventions can be readily generalized to treating patients with personality disorders. Specifically, Nace maintains that participation in substance abuse rehabilitation in combination with the traditional 12-Step model of Alcoholic Anonymous inadvertently affects personality disorders among substance abusers. These treatment modalities include many of the basic principles recommended for treatment of personality disorders. For example, substance abuse rehabilitation usually occurs in a highly structured environment in which order, scheduled activities, and rules and regulations are natural elements of the treatment setting. Such an environment is based on limit setting and emphasizes adaptation. Moreover, Nace points out that while the 12-Step model focuses on abstinence from alcohol it also emphasizes relationships. Specifically, there is an emphasis on maintaining healthy relationships with others (Steps 5, 8, 9, and 12), relating to oneself in a responsible fashion (Steps 4 and 10), and addressing spiritual relationships (Steps 2 and 3). Additionally, maladaptive character traits are directly mentioned in Steps 6 and 7. Thus, Nace maintains that focusing on treating the substance abuse with a blend of rehabilitation and 12-Step principles will indirectly lead to restructuring of character disturbance. Unfortunately, research studies have not addressed to what extent 12-Step treatment is effective with personality disorders. Considering that 12-Step treatment usually takes place in a highly structured group format, it may be appropriate for use with personality disorders. However, to the extent that it focuses on relationship issues it may be less effective with ASPD substance abuse patients.

Interpersonal Therapy

O'Malley et al. (3) have reviewed the application of interpersonal therapy to the treatment of substance abuse for patients with personality disorders. The use of interpersonal therapy in the treatment of substance abuse is based on the belief that people use alcohol and drugs to cope with problematic interpersonal relationships. The goal of this treatment modality is to focus on patients' relationships in order to assist them in finding ways to relate more effectively and develop satisfying relationships rather than turning to alcohol or drugs. This approach may have applications to many personality disorders, especially those in which difficulty relating to others is a central feature, as seen in avoidant or dependent personality disorders. However, the recent work on treatment matching with substance abusers with personality disorders (39,42) suggests that relationship-focused treatment approaches may be contraindicated for addicts with antisocial behavior. Thus, the particular personality disorder needs to be taken into consideration before broadly applying this treatment intervention to substance abusers with personality disorders.

Pharmacological Approaches

The treatment of personality disorders with pharmacological interventions remains an inexact science, with limited empirical studies (for reviews see Refs. 53–55). For example, Soloff (55) reports that a search of the Medline database (1984–1995) revealed 83 studies dealing with the pharmacotherapy of the personality disorder—64 in borderline and 10 in schizotypal personality disorder. The pharmacological treatment of personality disorder with substance abuse has received even less attention. Some particular considerations to bear in mind when considering a pharmacological approach in the personality-disordered patient with substance abuse include 1) the interactions between the substance of choice and the pharmacological treatment may be toxic, since a return to substance use would not be uncommon, 2) the combination of personality disorder and substance abuse results in a particularly difficult population to pharmacologically treat, with noncompliance, problems in evaluating medication efficacy, distorted psychological meanings ascribed to the medication, intolerance of side effects, and unreasonable expectations being the norm, and 3) medication effects for personality disorder are modest, at best. Consequently, clear goals and expectations for the patient and physician should be discussed before the medication is prescribed. In general, the same limit setting and structure recommended above for the psychosocial therapies should be used in the prescribing of medication.

Gitlin (53) comments that pharmacological treatment of personality disorders can be directed to 1) an associated Axis I disorder, 2) the personality disorder itself, or 3) symptom clusters within and across disorders (i.e. impulsivity, paranoia, or aggression). It is therefore useful to identify exactly which model is being used when personality disorders are being treated with pharmacological interventions. The first model (treating an associated Axis I disorder) is most relevant for Cluster C personality disorders (avoidant, dependent, obsessive-compulsive), as these patients often demonstrate Axis I disorders of depression and/or panic disorder. However, Cluster C disorders are not prominent among substance abuse patients, so models 2) and 3) are the focus of the subsequent discussion.

Both Gitlin (53) and Soloff (54) offer practical algorithms for the treatment of personality disorders. In general, it is most useful to take into account the cluster (i.e., A, B, or C) when a medication for a personality disorder is considered. This guideline is consistent with our understanding of the biological basis of personality disorders. In general, specific neurotransmitters are related to particular personality *dimensions*, not the personality *disorders*. Neurotransmitter and neurohormonal disturbances are therefore best conceptualized as affecting personality dimensions, or characteristics, rather than clusters of multiple discrete behaviors. There is a well-documented relationship between impulsive and aggressive disorders and low serotonin, for example, as well as alterations in GABAergic, noradrenergic, dopaminergic, glutaminergic, glucocorticoid, and opioid neurotransmitter and neurohormonal systems (see Ref. 56 for review). Thus, it is reasonable to infer that pharmacological agents, many of which target relatively specific neurotransmitter functions, would optimally treat specific behaviors. Model 3, in which symptoms common to a personality disorder cluster are pharmacologically treated, would therefore be the paradigm most useful in the treatment of personality disorders.

For the treatment of Cluster A personality disorders, typified by suspiciousness, paranoia, and thought disorders, low-dose neuroleptics are the treatment of choice. Given the difficulty in maintaining an alliance with this population, the atypical antipsychotics, with their lower risk of extrapyramidal symptoms and dystonias, are strongly recommended. Cluster B personality disorders should be treated based on their primary disturbance, which can be dichotomized into affective dysregulation or instability and impulsivity-behavioral dyscontrol/aggression. Mood stabilizers, such as valproic acid or carbamazepine (56), are a useful and well-tolerated intervention for affective instability. Lithium may also be beneficial, although it has a higher risk of toxicity and monitoring levels in this population can be problematic. The selective serotonin-reuptake inhibitors (SSRIs) are particularly useful when depression is the primarily affective disturbance, and all have wide margins of safety. Mood stabilizers and the SSRIs are also useful with symptoms of impulsivity and aggression, and low-dose neuroleptics have reportedly been beneficial with these latter symptoms as well. As noted above, the atypical neuroleptics are recommended. Kranzler et al. (57) reported that fluoxetine, an SSRI, actually worsened treatment response in Type B (see above) alcohol-dependent patients compared to placebo. Although it was not noted whether these patients had a Cluster B personality disorder, this study would suggest that SSRIs may actually *aggravate*, not improve, symptoms in patients with impulsivity and substance abuse. The pharmacological treatment of Cluster C disorders, as addressed previously, is best approached by attending to the associated Axis I disorders.

In addition to weighing the potential interaction between the drug of choice and a pharmacological treatment for a personality disorder, the possible addition of a drug treatment for the substance abuse disorder should be considered. The interactions between drug treatments for both personality and substance abuse disorders do not currently pose a major problem. Naltrexone, for the treatment of alcoholism, and methadone and LAAM, for opioid-replacement therapy, are the only medications with demonstrated efficacy in the treatment of substance abuse disorders. Other than potential elevations in liver enzymes by both naltrexone and the mood stabilizers, concomitant pharmacological interventions for both personality disorders and substance abuse can be prescribed with no more than standard caution.

CONCLUSIONS AND FUTURE DIRECTIONS

The existing literature provides a wealth of information about the nature of the relationship between Cluster B personality disorders, particularly ASPD or BPD, and substance abuse. There is a high rate of comorbidity of these personality disorders with substance abuse both in the general population and among patients being treated for substance abuse. Individuals with ASPD or BPD have an increased likelihood of having a substance abuse disorder, which then exacerbates their maladaptive personality features and complicates the course and treatment of their addiction.

In contrast, considerably less research is available with which to draw solid conclusions about the relationship between substance abuse and personality disorders other than ASPD and BPD. The possibility exists that patients with other personality disorders (not ASPD or BPD) are more similar to substance abusers without personality disorders than they are different. There may not be an interaction between these other personality disorders and substance abuse. That is, there is no greater risk of substance abuse in persons with other personality disorders and no higher incidence of substance abusers having these other personality disorders compared with the general population. When these conditions do co-occur, they do not have the same potential to influence the course and response to treatment as when ASPD and BPD co-occur with substance abuse. To substantiate these hypotheses, the full spectrum of personality disorders needs to be studied with the same intensity with which ASPD and BPD have been investigated in this population. Research that combines the various personality disorders or examines one personality disorder in isolation (e.g., ASPD vs. non-ASPD) offers only limited information to advance our understanding of how the different personality disorders influence addiction.

However, focusing on the dynamic interplay between pathological personality characteristics and addiction may be a more fruitful line of research than examining the personality disorders as discrete entities. A growing body of research has begun to investigate the relationship between particular personality traits and substance abuse (e.g., 11,20,45,58–61), and more work in a similar vein is needed. Alhough the presence of pervasive and inflexible maladaptive personality traits is a shared feature of all the personality disorders, the particular symptoms of each personality disorder are unique and emerging findings suggest that there is variability in their potential to influence the course of addiction and response to treatment. The importance of discrete personality traits, or symptoms, as opposed to personality disorders, is also evident in patterns of inheritance, neurochemical disturbances, and pharmacological treatments. Clinicians and researchers need to develop a greater awareness that all pathological personality traits are not created equal when it comes to addiction.

REFERENCES

1. American Psychiatric Association. Diagnostic and Statistical Manual of Mental Disorders. 4th ed. Washington, DC: American Psychiatric Press, 1994.
2. EP Nace. Substance abuse and personality disorder. Special issue: managing the dually diagnosed patient: current issues and clinical approaches. J Chem Dependency Treatment 3:183–198, 1990.
3. SS O'Malley, TR Kosten, JA Renner. Dual diagnoses: substance abuse and personality disorders. New Directions for Mental Health Services 47:115–137, 1990.
4. JE Helzer, TR Pryzbeck. The co-occurrence of alcoholism with other psychiatric disorders in the general population and its impact on treatment. J Stud Alcohol 49:219–224, 1988.
5. RC Kessler, RC Crum, LA Warner, CB Nelson, J Schulenber, JC Anthony. Lifetime co-occurrence of DSM-III-R alcohol abuse and dependence with other psychiatric disorder in the national comorbidity sample. Arch Gen Psychiatry 54:313–321, 1997.
6. RE Drake, GE Vaillant. A validity study of Axis II of DSM-III. Am J Psychiatry 142:553–558, 1985.
7. MN Hesselbrock, R Meyer, JJ Keener. Psychopathology in hospitalized alcoholics. Arch Gen Psychiatry 42:1050–1055, 1985.
8. EP Nace, JJ Saxon, N Shore. A comparison of borderline and nonborderline alcoholic patients. Arch Gen Psychiatry 40:54–56, 1983.
9. EP Nace, CW Davis, JP Gaspari. Axis II comorbidity in substance abusers. Am J Psychiatry 148:118–120, 1991.
10. HR Kranzler, S Satel, A Apter. Personality disorders and associated features in cocaine-dependent inpatients. Compr Psychiatry 35:335–340, 1994.
11. J Morgenstern, J Langenbucher, E Labouvie, KJ Miller. The comorbidity of alcoholism and personality disorders in a clinical population: prevalence and relation to alcohol typology variables. J Abnorm Psychol 106:74–84, 1997.
11a. TR Kosten, BJ Rounsaville, HD Kleber. DSM-III Personality Disorders in Opiate Addicts. Compr Psychiatry 23:572–581, 1982.
12. CA DeJong, W Van den Brink, FM Harteveld, EG Van der Wielen. Personality disorders in alcoholics and drug addicts. Compr Psychiatry 34:87–94, 1993.
13. HG Nurnberg, A Rifkin, S Doddi. A systematic assessment of the comorbidity of DSM-III-R personality disorders in alcoholic outpatients. Compr Psychiatry 34:447–454, 1993.

Personality Disorders

14. NJ Smyth, RC Washousky. The coping styles of alcoholics with Axis II disorders. J Subst Abuse 7:425–435, 1995.
15. JP Barber, A Frank, RD Weiss, J Blaine. Prevalence and correlates of personality disorder diagnoses among cocaine dependent outpatients. J Personality Disord 10:297–311, 1996.
16. JS Cacciola, MJ Rutherford, AI Alterman, JR McKay, EC Snider. Personality disorders and treatment outcome in methadone maintenance patients. J Nerv Mental Dis 184:234–239, 1996.
17. KM Carroll, SA Ball, BJ Rounsaville. A comparison of alternate systems for diagnosing antisocial personality disorder in cocaine abusers. J Nerv Mental Dis 181:436–443, 1993.
18. SH Dinwiddie, T Reich. Attribution of antisocial symptoms in coexistent antisocial personality disorder and substance abuse. Compr Psychiatry 34:235–242, 1993.
19. KJ Sher, K Walitzer, P Wood, E Brent. Characteristics of children of alcoholics: putative risk factors, substance use and abuse, and psychopathology. J Abnorm Psychol 100:427–448, 1991.
20. CR Cloninger, S Sigvardsson, M Bohman. Childhood personality predicts alcohol abuse in young adults. Alcoholism Clin Exp Res 12:494–505, 1988.
21. M Kammeier, H Hoffman, R Loper. Personality characteristics of alcoholics as college freshmen and at time of treatment. J Stud Alcohol 34:390–399, 1973.
22. R Loper, H Hoffman, M Kammeier. MMPI characteristics of college freshman males who later became alcoholics. J Abnorm Psychol 82:159–162, 1973.
23. RD Weiss, SM Mirin, ML Griffin, JG Gunderson, C Hufford. Personality disorders in cocaine dependence. Compr Psychiatry 34:145–149, 1993.
24. RJ Cadoret, TW O'Gorman, E Troughton, E Heywood. Alcoholism and antisocial personality. Arch Gen Psychiatry 42:161–167, 1985.
25. M Bohman, S Sigvardsson, CR Cloninger. Maternal inheritance of alcohol abuse: cross-fostering analysis of adopted women. Arch Gen Psychiatry 38:965–969, 1981.
26. CR Cloninger, M Boman, S Sigvardsson. Inheritance of alcohol abuse: cross-fostering analysis of adopted men. Arch Gen Psychiatry 38:861–868, 1981.
27. EP Nace, JJ Saxon, N Shore. Borderline personality disorder and alcoholism treatment: a one-year follow-up study. J Stud Alcohol 47:196–200, 1986.
28. MN Hesselbrock, VM Hesselbrock. Depression and Antisocial Personality Disorder in Alcoholism: Gender Comparison [references]. Norwood, NJ: Ablex Publishing, p ix, 1993.
29. EC Penick, BJ Powell, E Othmer. Subtyping Alcoholics by Co-Existing Psychiatric Syndromes: Course, Family History, Outcome. Longitudinal Research in Alcoholism. Hingham, MA: Kluwer-Nijhoff, pp 167–196, 1984.
30. TF Babor, M Hofman, FK DelBoca, VM Hesselbrock, R Meyer, ZS Dolinsky, BJ Rounsaville. Types of alcoholics. I: Evidence for empirically derived typology based on indicators of vulnerability and severity. Arch Gen Psychiatry 49:599–608, 1992.

31. BJ Rounsaville, ZS Dolinsky, TF Babor, R Meyer. Psychopathology as a predictor of treatment outcome in alcoholics. Arch Gen Psychiatry 44:505–513, 1987.
32. GE Woody, AT McLellan, L Luborsky, CP O'Brien. Sociopathy and psychotherapy outcome. Arch Gen Psychiatry 42:1081–1086, 1985.
33. EJ Khantzian, C Treece. DSM-III psychiatric diagnosis of narcotic addicts. Arch Gen Psychiatry 42:1067–1071, 1985.
34. EP Nace, CW Davis. Treatment outcome in substance-abusing patients with a personality disorder. Am J Addictions 2:26–33, 1993.
35. N Kruedelbach, RA McCormick, SC Schulz, R Grueneich. Impulsivity, coping styles, and triggers for craving in substance abusers with borderline personality disorder. J Personality Disord 7:214–222, 1993.
36. SM Griggs, P Tyrer. Personality disorder, social adjustment and treatment outcome in alcoholics. J Stud Alcohol 42:802–805, 1981.
37. TA Kosten, TR Kosten, BJ Rounsaville. Personality disorders in opiate addicts show prognostic specificity. J Subst Abuse Treatment 6:163–168, 1989.
38. AI Alterman, JS Cacciola. The antisocial personality disorder diagnosis in substance abusers: problems and issues. J Nerv Mental Dis 179:401–409, 1991.
39. R Longabaugh, A Rubin, P Malloy, M Beattie. Drinking outcomes of alcohol abusers diagnosed as antisocial personality disorder. Alcoholism Clin Exp Res 18:778–785, 1994.
40. JS Cacciola, AI Alterman, MJ Rutherford, EC Snider. Treatment response of antisocial substance abusers. J Nerv Mental Dis 183:166–171, 1995.
41. RM Kadden, NL Cooney, H Getter, MD Litt. Matching alcoholics to coping skills or interactions therapies: posttreatment results. J Consulting Clin Psychol 57:698–704, 1989.
42. NL Cooney, RM Kadden, MD Litt, H Getter. Matching alcoholics to coping skills or interactional therapies: two-year follow-up results. J Consult Clin Psychol 59:598–601, 1991.
43. Project Match Research Group. Matching alcoholism treatments to client heterogeneity: Project MATCH posttreatment drinking outcomes. J Stud Alcohol 58:7–29, 1997.
44. B Liskow, BJ Powell, EJ Nickel, E Penick. Diagnostic subgroups of antisocial alcoholics: outcome at 1 year. Compr Psychiatry 31:549–556, 1990.
45. DB Marlowe, KC Kirby, D Festinger, S Husband, JJ Platt. Impact of comorbid personality disorders and personality disorder symptoms on outcomes of behavioral treatment for cocaine dependence. J Nerv Mental Dis 185:483–490, 1997.
46. GE Vaillant. A developmental view of old and new perspective of personality disorders. J Personality Disord 1:146–156, 1987.
47. R Walker. Substance abuse and B-cluster disorders. II. Treatment recommendations. J Psychoactive Drugs 24:233–241, 1992.
48. AT Beck, A Freeman. Cognitive Therapy of Personality Disorders. New York: Guilford Press, 1990.
49. KM Abram. The effect of co-occurring disorders on criminal careers: interaction

of antisocial personality, alcoholism, and drug disorders. Special issue: mental disorder and the criminal justice system. Int J Law Psychiatry 12:133–148, 1989.
50. M Linehan. Dialectical behavior therapy for borderline personality disorder: theory and method. Bull Menninger Clinic 51:261–276, 1987.
51. G Marlatt, J Gordon. Relapse Prevention: Maintenance Strategies in the Treatment of Addiction Behaviors. New York: Guilford Press, 1985.
52. MS Fisher, KJ Bentley. Two group therapy models for clients with a dual diagnosis of substance abuse and personality disorder. Psychiatr Serv 47:1244–1250, 1996.
53. MJ Gitlin. Pharmacotherapy of personality disorders: conceptual framework and clinical strategies. J Clin Psychol 13:343–353, 1993.
54. PH Soloff. Algorithms of pharmacological treatment of personality dimensions: symptom-specific treatments for cognitive-perceptual, affective, and impulsive-behavioral dysregulation. Bull Menninger Clinic 62:195–214, 1998.
55. PH Soloff. Special feature: psychobiologic perspectives on treatment of personality disorders. J Personality Disord 11:336–344, 1997.
56. KT Brady, H Myrick, S McElroy. The relationship between substance use disorders, impulse control disorders, and pathological aggression. Am J Addictions 7:221–230, 1998.
57. HR Kranzler, JA Burleson, P Korner, FK DelBoca, MJ Bohn, J Brown, N Liebowitz. Placebo-controlled trial of fluoxetine as an adjunct to relapse prevention in alcoholics. Am J Psychiatry 152:391–397, 1995.
58. RK Brooner, CWJ Schmidt, JH Herbst. Personality Trait Characteristics of Opioid Abusers With and Without Comorbid Personality Disorders [references]. Washington, DC: American Psychological Association, p viii, 1994.
59. LA Fisher, JW Elias, K Ritz. Predicting relapse to substance abuse as a function of personality dimensions. Alcoholism Clin Exp Res 22:1041–1047, 1998.
60. M McGue, W Slutske, J Taylor, WG Iacono. Personality and substance use disorders. I. Effects of gender and alcoholism subtype. Alcoholism Clin Exp Res 21:513–520, 1997.
61. SW Quirk, RA McCormick. Personality subtypes, coping styles, symptom correlates, and substances of choice among a cohort of substance abusers. Assessment 5:157–169, 1998.

7
Comorbid Mental Disorders in Adolescents with Substance Use Disorders

Duncan B. Clark and Jeanette Scheid
*Pittsburgh Adolescent Alcohol Research Center
and University of Pittsburgh
Pittsburgh, Pennsylvania*

INTRODUCTION

At least one in 20 adolescents has substance abuse or dependence (1–3). The development and course of an adolescent substance use disorder (SUD) can be viewed as a life-history trajectory, with many influences toward or away from SUD (4). Models of SUD subtypes typically include consideration of psychopathology dimensions (e.g., mental disorders not defined by substance-related problems), particularly those involving antisocial behaviors and affective characteristics. For example, Zucker (5) proposed a developmentally based alcoholism model with four subtypes: 1) antisocial alcoholism, characterized by early onset, a history of antisocial behaviors, and early treatment entry; 2) developmentally cumulative alcoholism, a cumulative extension of adolescent problem drinking into adulthood; 3) developmentally limited alcoholism, an extension of adolescent problem drinking that offsets in early adulthood; and 4) negative-affect alcoholism, characterized by depression and use of alcohol to cope with or enhance interpersonal relationships. Consideration of the relationships among SUD and other mental disorders is essential for understanding adolescent SUD origins, pathways, and outcomes, as well as for planning and implementing preventive and therapeutic interventions (6).

Earlier onset of alcoholism, compared with later onset, has been found to be associated with more antisocial characteristics and, in some studies, more depression and anxiety symptoms (7–13). These studies do not necessarily apply specifically to the adolescent SUD population, however, as the age defining early-onset SUD typically includes subjects with adult onset—e.g., up to 25 years old (9) or up to 30 years old (14). In a study on the unique influence of adolescent age of onset on SUD characteristics in males, Clark, Kirisci, and Tarter (15) (Table 1) compared SUD adolescents and three groups of SUD adults: 1) adolescent-onset, 2) early-adult-onset (age 18 through 24 years), and 3) late-adult-onset (age 25 years or older). Adolescent-onset SUD males, whether adolescents or adults, had higher lifetime rates of cannabis and hallucinogen use disorders, shorter times from first use to dependence, shorter times between the first and second substance dependencies, higher disruptive behavior disorder rates, and higher major depression rates. These results suggest that adolescent-onset SUD is a distinct and rapidly developing subtype that is more often accompanied by psychopathology than is adult-onset SUD.

The adolescent developmental trajectory toward or away from SUD can be influenced by several specific forms of psychopathology, including disorders defined by antisocial or disinhibited behavior (e.g., conduct disorder, oppositional defiant disorder, attention deficit hyperactivity disorder, and antisocial personality disorder) and disorders defined by negative affect (e.g., major depression, posttraumatic stress disorder, and other anxiety disorders). Childhood antisocial behaviors, particularly behaviors defined diagnostically as conduct disorder, predict the development of early-adolescent substance use (16), adolescent substance-related problems (17), and later SUD (18). Atten-

Table 1. Lifetime SUD and Mental Disorders in Adolescent and Adult Males with SUD

	Adolescents (%)	Adults (%) Adolescent onset	Adults (%) Early-adult onset	Adults (%) Late-adult onset
Alcohol use disorders	79	80	82	74
Cannabis use disorders	96	87	58	25
Hallucinogen use disorders	26	15	11	0
Disruptive behavior disorders	98	56	38	43
Major depression	16	10	1	0

Source: Data from Ref. 15.

tion deficit hyperactivity disorder may also predict SUD (19). A commonly cited motivation for alcohol and drug consumption is the belief that these substances reduce depression and anxiety (20,21; see Ref. 22 for review). Escape from negative emotional states has been found to be a motivation for alcohol consumption in adolescents (23), and is associated with more pathological alcohol consumption (24). High rates of major depression and posttraumatic stress disorder have been consistently demonstrated in samples of adolescents with SUD. Controversy continues about the etiological importance of these disorders because of the observation that SUD can cause or exacerbate mood and anxiety disorders. Regardless, these mental disorders change the trajectory of, and treatment considerations for, adolescent SUD.

This chapter is presented in five sections: 1) antisocial behavior and related disorders, including conduct disorder (CD) and oppositional defiant disorder (ODD); 2) attention deficit hyperactivity disorder (ADHD); 3) mood disorders; 4) posttraumatic stress disorder (PTSD); and 5) other anxiety disorders. Each section briefly defines the considered mental disorders, describes findings on the association between the area of psychopathology and adolescent SUD, considers possible causal relationships, and discusses the implications the form of psychopathology has on adolescent SUD treatment. Adolescents with SUD often have multiple comorbid mental disorders. The relationships among the reviewed disorders, as well as recommendations for assessment, treatment, and future research directions, are discussed in a concluding section.

ANTISOCIAL BEHAVIOR AND RELATED DISORDERS
Definitions

Adolescents with antisocial behaviors fail to conform to social norms in school, work, family and other interpersonal relationships (25). Antisocial behaviors characterize ODD, CD, and antisocial personality disorder (ASPD). ODD is defined by negativistic, hostile, and defiant behavior. Relevant behaviors include losing temper, arguing, defying rules, deliberately annoying others, blaming others for one's behavior, and displaying anger or vindictiveness. CD is characterized by more extreme antisocial behaviors than ODD, and is defined by behaviors classified into four categories: aggression to people and animals, destruction of property, deceitfulness or theft, and serious violations of rules. The DSM criteria for CD have undergone several revisions intended to improve sensitivity and specificity, and to reflect current understanding of the natural history of the disorder (26). ASPD is characterized by a pervasive pattern of disregard for, and violation of, the rights of others occurring since adolescence (e.g., age 15), defined by repeated illegal acts, lying, impulsivity, aggressiveness, disregard for others' safety, irresponsibility, and lack of remorse. While an individual must be at least eighteen for ASPD to be diagnosed, some children diagnosed with ODD progress to CD, and to ASPD in adulthood (25,27,28).

Relationships with Substance Use Disorders

Many studies have documented comorbidity between adolescent SUD and antisocial behaviors, including CD. Among adolescents with SUD, elevated rates of CD have been reported in samples from community (3), clinical (29), and criminal justice (30) sources. CD has been found to be associated with substance dependence in many types of adolescent samples, including teenage mothers (31), incarcerated adolescents (30), adolescents in hospital-based treatment programs (29), a school sample (3), and a large epidemiological birth cohort (32,33).

The Pittsburgh Adolescent Alcohol Research Center (PAARC) is a longitudinal study which compares adolescents with alcohol abuse or dependence with community control adolescents. In a comparison of adolescents with alcohol dependence and community controls from PAARC (34) (Table 2), those with alcohol dependence had increased odds over community controls for CD (adjusted odds ratio = 7.1) and ODD (adjusted odds ratio = 2.0). The association between CD and adolescent SUD was stronger than for any other comorbid mental disorder, a finding consistent with other studies.

Causal Models

Antisocial characteristics often predate and predict substance use and SUD symptoms, as would be expected if antisocial behaviors are indicative of characteristics which cause SUD. The Center for Education and Drug Abuse Research (CEDAR) is a longitudinal study, which compares children of SUD fathers—i.e., high average risk (HAR)—with children of fathers without SUD—i.e., at low average risk or (LAR). HAR boys have higher rates of CD than LAR boys (35), preadolescent CD predicts early adolescent marijuana use (16), and CD predicts adolescent SUD symptoms (17).

The diagnosis of CD often predates substance use in adolescent SUD cases (19,36,37). For example, in the PAARC adolescents with alcohol dependence, most adolescents with comorbid CD and alcohol dependence had

CD prior to alcohol abuse or dependence (63% of females, 65% of males), with the remainder having an approximately simultaneous onset (20% females, 28% males) and few having alcohol abuse or dependence first (17% females, 7% males). Furthermore, CD severity has been found to predict SUD severity (33,36).

Antisocial behaviors and ADHD may, in some individuals, indicate a fundamental characteristic, which has been described as "disinhibitory psychopathology" (38). In possible mechanisms for antisocial behaviors predicting SUD, antisocial behaviors may be indicative of poor behavioral inhibition and increased novelty seeking leading to a propensity toward substance use and an increased SUD risk (9,39). Adolescents with antisocial characteristics have been found to expect that use of alcohol and drugs will enhance their cognitive, affective, and social functioning (40,41), a fact which may be particularly salient given data showing that adolescents with CD tend to have social deficits.

Antisocial behavior may also be facilitated by substance use. For example, though Reebye and colleagues (42) showed that while CD symptoms generally preceded SUD in their clinical sample, the presence of SUD was associated with increased severity of CD. Similarly, Johnson and colleagues (43) found that the number of conduct disorder symptoms at baseline and the increase in number of symptoms over time were greater in youths with early unsanctioned alcohol use than in those who abstained from alcohol. Brown and colleagues (44) reported that while 95% of adolescents entering SUD treatment programs had a history of CD-related behavior, in about half of these adolescents CD behaviors were judged to be primarily related to alcohol and drug involvement. Substance use results in poor judgment and increased association with delinquent peers, both of which would increase the likelihood of engaging in illegal activities, aggressive behaviors, and other characteristics included in defining CD. Additional studies are needed to examine the interacting influences of these characteristics over critical developmental periods (45,46).

A third view of the relationship between antisocial behavior disorders and SUD is that each reflects the presence of common etiological factors. Jessor and Jessor (47) formulated problem behavior theory to explain the relationships among adolescent behaviors such as criminal behavior, alcohol and drug use, risky driving, and early sexual activity. According to this theory, the etiology of such deviant behaviors can be accounted for by a combination of environmental characteristics, including family socioeconomic and parent factors, and psychological variables, such as personality and the perceived environment. In several longitudinal studies with adolescent and young adult samples (47–52), results have supported problem behavior theory. Loeber and colleagues (53) have come to similar conclusions.

Treatment

Although clinical observation suggests that adolescents who have comorbid SUD and antisocial behavior disorders have a worse prognosis and are more difficult to treat than adolescents with SUD without antisocial characteristics, only a limited number of studies are available to support this hypothesis. Kaminer and colleagues (54) showed that adolescents who had CD and SUD, in contrast to those with major depression and SUD, had a significantly higher early dropout rate from a dual diagnosis treatment program. The presence of CD comorbid with SUD decreases adolescents' perceived efficacy to avoid heavy drinking (55). Brown and colleagues (37,44) found that a history of CD independent of alcohol and drug involvement was related to greater posttreatment alcohol consumption and the later development of ASPD.

Behavioral treatments for antisocial behavior disorders include family therapy, parent management training, and multisystemic therapy. There are data to suggest that family therapy is effective for antisocial behavior disorders (56). A meta-analysis by Shadish and colleagues (57) showed a significant treatment effect of family therapy on CD. There are some indications, however, that for more serious conduct problems, more intensive treatment strategies are needed (58). Parent management training has been shown to improve antisocial behaviors (see Ref. 59 for review). Limitations of parent management training include high attrition (59), a decline in effect over time (60), and difficulties in applying the techniques with parents having limited education (61). Multisystemic treatment is a multidimensional approach devised by Henggeler and colleagues (62,63) combining family, peer, school, and community interventions with individual treatment. When compared to "usual treatment" for juvenile offenders, multisystemic treatment was superior as measured by arrest and incarceration rates, self-reported antisocial behaviors, family cohesion, and affiliation with aggressive peers.

Similar approaches have been suggested as effective for adolescent SUD. Studies indicate that family systems therapy (64), adolescent group therapy with a pretreatment module using a cognitive-behavioral approach (65), and multidisciplinary inpatient treatment (66) can be effective approaches for treating adolescent SUD. Family therapy has been shown to improve SUD outcomes whether used alone or in conjunction with other approaches (67).

Given the close interrelationship between SUD and antisocial behavior disorders and the similarity of approaches to treating these conditions, one would expect that effective treatment focused on either disorder would yield an improvement in the comorbid condition. A limited literature indicates that this is the case. In antisocial adolescents, multisystemic treatment may be effective in reducing substance-related arrests and self-reported frequency of substance use (68). Inpatient treatment for adolescent SUD may reduce antisocial behaviors as well as alcohol and drug use (66), although controlled studies are needed.

Future Directions

A diagnostic distinction between antisocial behaviors exclusively associated with substance use and persistent antisocial characteristics independent of substance use may be clinically useful. Moffitt (69) has suggested that a distinction be made between adolescent-limited and life-course-persistent antisocial behavior. This developmentally informed distinction may be useful in considering the relationship between antisocial behavior and substance use disorders and in evaluating whether these groups are different in treatment outcome. CD has recently been found to be treatable through pharmacological intervention, e.g., with methylphenidate (70). The potential advantages and disadvantages of testing such pharmacological treatment for adolescents with CD and SUD need to be considered. Treatment studies need to address cost-effectiveness, determine whether gains made during supervised treatment generalize to other settings such as home or school, and examine the interactive benefits for treating CD and SUD (71,72). Future studies should also focus on the influence of gender on the CD-SUD relationship—although the prevalence of antisocial behavior disorders and alcohol-related problems is higher in males, females with antisocial behavior disorders may have more problematic outcomes (73).

ATTENTION DEFICIT HYPERACTIVITY DISORDER

Definitions

ADHD is defined in the DSM-IV system by two classes of symptoms: 1) inattention and 2) hyperactivity and impulsivity. Inattention is indicated by characteristics such as making careless mistakes in schoolwork, having difficulty organizing tasks and activities, and being easily distracted by extraneous stimuli. Hyperactivity is indicated by characteristics such as fidgeting with hands or feet, having difficulty playing or engaging in leisure activities quietly, and talking excessively. Impulsivity is indicated by blurting out answers before questions have been completed, having difficulty waiting one's turn, or interrupting or intruding on others. Persistence and severity must be evident from an onset of some symptoms prior to age 7 years, persistence for at least 6 months, and clinically significant impairment. Attention and impulse control have long been considered critical to understanding both normal function and psychopathology. The etiology of attentional problems and impulsivity is thought to be multifaceted, with genetic and environmental components (74,75).

Relationships with Substance Use Disorders

In adults with ADHD histories, higher rates of SUD have been reported compared with control groups or expected rates from epidemiological studies (e.g., Refs. 76–78). In an adult sample, Wilens and colleagues (19) found that ADHD cases without other comorbid mental disorders had SUD rates higher than those of controls. Adults with SUD typically have relatively high ADHD rates (e.g., Refs. 79–81). Tarter and others (13) found that a group of "primary" alcoholics were more likely to have ADHD-type symptoms than the following groups: 1) secondary alcoholics, 2) reference cases with other mental disorders, and 3) normal controls. The retrospective diagnostic method used with adult samples, however, limits diagnostic accuracy primarily because of the absence of information from collateral sources such as parents and teachers. High rates of ADHD have also been reported in SUD adolescents (82,83). In the PAARC sample (34), adolescents with alcohol dependence, compared to controls, had higher ADHD rates (adjusted odds ratio 2.8) (Table 2). SUD adolescents with ADHD, compared to those without ADHD, tend to have earlier and greater substance use as well as higher rates of substance dependence (84,85).

Causal Models

Some longitudinal follow-up studies have observed that children with ADHD, compared with controls, have more substance use and related problems later in life, suggesting that ADHD leads to SUD (e.g., Refs. 86, 87). Not all studies, however, have found this relationship. ADHD predicts adolescent cigarette-smoking initiation in some studies (88) but not others (16). In a comparison of hyperactive children and normal controls for alcohol and drug use 15 years after initial contact, no differences between groups were found in substance use frequency or severity (89). Biederman and colleagues (90) reported that

Table 2. Lifetime Mental Disorders in Adolescents with Alcohol Dependence and Community Controls

	Alcohol dependence (%)	Control (%)
Conduct disorder		
Females	75	5
Males	88	14
ODD		
Females	24	5
Males	18	7
ADHD		
Females	16	0
Males	37	12
Major depression		
Females	69	11
Males	37	12
PTSD		
Females	24	0
Males	9	0

Source: Data from Ref. 34.

adolescents with and without ADHD had a similar risk for SUD that was mediated by conduct and bipolar disorders.

Several possible mechanisms for a pathway from ADHD to SUD have been suggested. Particularly since stimulant use improves ADHD symptoms, substance use may be an attempt to self-medicate ADHD symptoms (91). Findings relating ADHD with specific drug use patterns, however, have been inconsistent (77,85). The pathway from ADHD to SUD may also be mediated by CD. Several studies have found that, when correlated CD characteristics are taken into consideration, an independent relationship between ADHD and substance use or SUD is not evident (e.g., Refs. 33, 90). Other studies have found an independent association between ADHD and SUD beyond that explained by CD (77,79,85).

SUD in a parent may predispose a child to ADHD (35,92,93). The transmitted risk may be specific to ADHD or may be more generally representative of a risk for antisocial characteristics. The results of a family genetic study (94) suggested that ADHD, ODD, CD, and ASPD represent a single entity with polygenic etiology and variable severity. Although aggressivity, impulsivity, inattention, and hyperactivity are correlated (93),

ADHD without associated antisocial characteristics may be a distinct diagnostic entity.

In contrast to bidirectional cause and effect postulated for many comorbid mental disorders, SUD probably does not cause ADHD. By definition, ADHD symptoms must be present before an individual is 7 years old, an age at which significant substance use and related problems are rare. While long-standing problematic substance use causes cognitive deficits (95,96), the cognitive problems associated with ADHD and SUD have distinct features (97). The possibility nevertheless exists that SUD effects in some predisposed individuals may influence ADHD persistence.

Treatment Implications

There is a paucity of data on treatment effects in comorbid ADHD in SUD adolescents. SUD adolescents with comorbid ADHD may have increased difficulty with maintaining SUD recovery because of increased cravings and restlessness as well as decreased concentration and compliance with treatment (84). ADHD treatment may improve outcomes in these cases. Stimulant treatment has been shown to be effective in reducing ADHD symptoms in children and adults (98–100). There has been a concern that, among SUD adolescents, stimulants may adversely influence abstinence by leading to abuse of stimulants themselves or other substances (101), although there have been reports to the contrary (102).

Future Directions

The research to date suggests that ADHD may predispose toward SUD, but that other characteristics substantially influence this pathway. Additional family-genetic and longitudinal studies are needed to refine the causal models, particularly to define the genetic and environmental factors that lead ADHD to be associated with SUD and other related disorders. For ADHD, a combination of pharmacotherapy and psychotherapy, including individual, group social skills, parent training, and school-based methods, may be needed. Similar approaches may be effective for cases in which SUD and ADHD are comorbid. Systematic treatment studies are needed to determine the extent to which such comprehensive approaches are effective and, if they are shown to be promising, cost-effectiveness studies are needed to determine efficacy. The use of alternative medications for ADHD with minimal abuse potential, such as antidepressant medication, also needs to be considered in this population.

MOOD DISORDERS

Definitions

The DSM-IV definition of major depression is familiar to most clinicians, and includes either depressed mood or loss of interest or pleasure and five or more symptoms from a list of nine present during the same 2-week period. For children and adolescents, depressed mood or loss of interest are not required if irritable mood is present, and failure to make expected weight gains is an alternative symptom to weight loss. Dysthymia, indicated by at least 2 years of depressed mood in adults, may be diagnosed in children and adolescents if present for at least 1 year and, as with major depression, irritable mood may be considered equivalent to depressed mood. Note that dysthymia should not be diagnosed when criteria for major depression are met. Bipolar disorder is an important comorbid mental disorder in adults with SUD and has been the subject of some clinical observations regarding relationships with adolescent SUD (e.g., Refs. 103, 104). Little systematic information is available on bipolar disorder with SUD adolescents, however, perhaps in part because bipolar disorder is relatively uncommon and difficult to diagnose in children and adolescents (105).

Relationships with Substance Use Disorders

In individuals with a life history including major depression and SUD, most report an onset of one of the involved disorders prior to age 20 (106). In adolescents with SUD, high rates of major depression have been reported (29,107–109), particularly in females (e.g., Refs. 110, 111). Using the PAARC sample, Clark, Pollock, and colleagues (34) reported that adolescents with alcohol dependence were three times more likely than controls to have a major depression history. For major depression symptoms, an interaction was noted between alcohol dependence and gender in which the difference between alcohol dependence and control groups on the mean number of depression symptoms was greater for females (6.2 vs. 1.5) than for males (3.4 vs. 1.2).

Causal Models

The expectation that depression is a risk factor for SUD, especially for alcohol abuse and dependence, is based in part on the assumption that alcohol consumption improves mood. While there is a commonly held belief that alcohol improves mood (see Ref. 22 for review), the acute effects of alcohol on mood have proven complex and difficult to rigorously investigate. Dose effects are evident, as laboratory experiments with humans suggest that low doses of alcohol improve mood whereas high doses cause dysphoric symptoms (112,113). The extent to which such laboratory experiments can be generalized to the naturalistic development of alcohol use disorders is questionable, however, because the stressors and alcohol doses typically utilized in such experiments are necessarily less intense than those that have been experienced by SUD adolescents (114).

In epidemiological and clinical studies, a mixed picture emerges in which both causal directions between major depression and SUD receive some support. Studies in clinical and community samples clearly indicate that alcohol consumption leads to depressive symptoms. In alcohol-dependent individuals, for example, short periods of abstinence lead to substantial declines in depressive symptoms (115–117). The relative etiological influence of depression on alcohol consumption may also differ somewhat by gender. Hartka and colleagues (118) found that depression predicted later alcohol consumption only in women, although alcohol consumption predicted depression in both men and women. Limited prospective data are available for examining adolescent SUD predictions. Rao and colleagues (119) studied the development of SUD in a 6–8-year prospective follow-up of 26 adolescents with major depression and a control group. SUD rates at follow-up were not significantly higher in the major depression group than in the control group. When SUD did develop, however, the age of onset tended to be earlier in the major depression group than in the control group. Similarly, in SUD adolescents, major depression has been reported to be associated with earlier SUD age of onset (120). Examination of the order of onset of major depression and SUD in adolescents has also yielded relevant information. Among SUD adolescents with major depression, the first-occurring disorder has typically been found to be approximately evenly split between these two disorders (34,120), although major depression following SUD was substantially more common in one sample (111). Although it has been established that SUD leads to depression in some individuals, further research is needed to establish whether depression constitutes a risk factor for SUD development. The evidence presented to date suggests a bidirectional relationship in which major depression increases risk for adolescent SUD and SUD precipitates or exacerbates major depression.

Treatment

Clinical evaluation of adolescents with SUD necessarily includes screening for major depression. While this may seem obvious to the experienced clinician, major depression is too frequently missed in the clinical evaluation of SUD adolescents (121). A period of abstinence has traditionally been thought to be crucial in the evaluation process. Alcohol-dependent individuals will typically have improved depression symptoms following abstinence (122). In an unusual experimental treatment program with adults, patients who elected to continue alcohol use while in treatment experienced increasing subjective discomfort, whereas those who abstained experienced improved mood (123).

When diagnoses have been established and major depression and SUD are present, particularly if persistent after a period of abstinence, initiating treatments for both conditions has been advocated (124,125). The relative chronology of onset of SUD and major depression may have prognostic significance and treatment implications. Among adolescents with SUD and major depression, those with primary depression tend to be females with victimization histories, while those with primary SUD are characterized by SUD in first-degree relatives and poor academic performance (120). In adult men, Brown and colleagues (126) found that depressive symptoms remitted more rapidly in men with primary alcoholism than in those with primary mood disorders. In those with primary mood disorders, alcohol dependence did not intensify depressive symptoms or alter the course of symptom resolution. When primary major depression can be identified in SUD adolescents, treatment for major depression may be more readily justified (110). Psychological treatments for major depression have been developed for adolescents (127) and may be less controversial than pharmacological treatments in this population. In adults with alcohol dependence and major depression, Cornelius and colleagues (128) have demonstrated that fluoxetine was effective in reducing depressive symptoms and alcohol consumption. Since fluoxetine has been shown to be effective for depression in adolescents (129), a similar approach may be appropriate for adolescents with comorbid major depression and alcohol dependence.

POSTTRAUMATIC STRESS DISORDER

Definitions

The DSM-IV defines an exposure to a traumatic event as experiencing or witnessing actual or threatened death or serious injury and responding with intense fear, helplessness, or horror. In children, the response may be manifested as disorganized or agitated behavior. A trauma history is a necessary, but not sufficient, condition for the presence of PTSD. PTSD also requires that the traumatic event be persistently experienced through intrusive recollections, dreams or responses to associated cues, persistent avoidance of stimuli associated with the trauma and numbing of general responsiveness, and persistent symptoms of increased arousal, including sleep difficulties, irritability, and exaggerated startle response. While there has been relatively little research to indicate the prevalence of PTSD in adolescents, high rates of victimization (130) and PTSD (2) in community adolescent samples suggest that understanding the relationships with adolescent SUD is an important priority.

Relationships with Substance Use Disorders

Childhood abuse has been found to be common among adults with substance use disorders (see Ref. 131 for review). In community samples, sexual abuse histories have been found to be associated with increased alcohol consumption (132,133) and higher rates of alcohol use disorders (134,135). This literature suggests that childhood abuse is a risk factor for substance use disorders (136).

Among adolescents, a history of childhood abuse has been found to be associated with high levels of alcohol and drug consumption and related disorders. In a survey of 122,824 public school students in grades 6, 9, and 12, Harrison and colleagues (137) found that physical and sexual abuse histories were associated with an increased likelihood of the use of alcohol, marijuana, and other drugs. This association has been found to be particularly evident for sexual abuse (138–142). High rates of childhood abuse have also been reported among adolescents in treatment for substance-related problems (143,144). Deykin and Buka (145) studied 75 female and 222 male substance-dependent adolescents from seven residential treatment centers. Trauma history was reported by 75%. The lifetime prevalence of PTSD was 45% for females and 24% for males.

Among PAARC subjects with alcohol use disorders, trauma history and PTSD are common. Clark, Lesnick, and Hegedus (114) reported trauma rates in adolescents with alcohol dependence ($n = 132$), adolescents with alcohol abuse ($n = 51$), and community control adolescents ($n = 73$). Traumatic events were classified into four groups of interpersonal trauma and a category of miscellaneous traumas. The four interpersonal trauma categories were physical abuse, sexual abuse, other violent victimization, and witnessing of violence. Among females and males, substantially higher rates of traumatization by interpersonal violence were reported for the alcohol-dependence group (66% and 54% for females and males, respectively) and the alcohol abuse group (44% and 58%) than for the control group (8% and 9%). While common, other miscellaneous traumas were not associated with alcohol use disorders. Females more often than males had histories of sexual abuse (e.g., in the alcohol-dependence group, 43% vs. 13% for females and males, respectively), whereas males more often than females had histories of other violent victimization (8% vs. 23% for females and males, respectively). The lifetime prevalence of PTSD among adolescents with alcohol dependence was 24% for females and 9% for males, compared with 0% in control adolescents (34).

Causal Models

Physical and sexual abuse often occurs prior to SUD and is hypothesized to contribute to the development of SUD through the so-called self-medication mechanisms. Physical or sexual abuse during childhood tends to precede problematic alcohol consumption among juvenile detainees (146–148). In PAARC adolescents with childhood abuse history and alcohol use disorders (114), physical abuse precedes the onset of an alcohol use disorder in most cases (90%), and sexual abuse also typically precedes alcohol use disorders (77%). Adults with PTSD have an increased risk for alcohol-related problems (149). Traumatic experiences may increase the risk for SUD through PTSD and other affective symptoms (131). Adolescents may view alcohol consumption as a means of temporarily controlling internal affective states (150). Dembo and colleagues (151) developed and tested a model of the relationships among childhood abuse, alcohol use, and emotional functioning with data from a longitudinal study of adolescents detained in a criminal justice–system facility. The model showed influences of child abuse experiences on alcohol use and emotional functioning. Emotional functioning mediated the effect of physical and sexual abuse during childhood on alcohol use during a 1-year follow-up period.

Substance use disorders may also increase the risk for PTSD in two ways: 1) substance intoxication may increase the risk for traumatic experiences and 2) substance use may exacerbate PTSD symptoms, resulting in individuals developing PTSD only in association with substance use disorders. Alcohol consumption has been specifically linked to violent victimization (152,153). Among PAARC subjects with alcohol use disorders, violent victimization other than sexual abuse tends to follow the onset of alcohol use disorders (114). For violent victimization, only 23% reported that the traumatic event occurred prior to the development of alcohol use disorder.

Treatment Implications

When PTSD is present in SUD adolescents, assessment of PTSD symptoms, other mental disorders, and other functional effects of trauma and PTSD history need to be considered in a comprehensive assessment. An interview screening for specific traumatic experiences and assessment of PTSD symptoms as well as other mental disorders can be accomplished through the most recent version of the Schedule for Affective Disorders and Schizophrenia for School-Age Children—Present and Lifetime Version (K-SADS-PL) (154). A questionnaire assessment of childhood abuse and neglect is available through the Childhood Trauma Questionnaire (155). Information from multiple sources (156), including the adolescent, his or her parents, and medical and judicial records, should be gathered. For adolescents with PTSD and SUD, additional relevant areas include substance use patterns, situational triggers, and motivations (131).

The presence of PTSD in adolescents suggests that assessment of other functional areas is also important. The substantial influence of PTSD on adolescent functioning, relative to major depression and alcohol use disorders, was studied in PAARC participants (157). The individual main effects and relative effect sizes of PTSD on four quality-of-life areas were explored: 1) psychological functioning (i.e., anxiety, depression, and satisfaction with life), 2) physical functioning (i.e., health complaints), 3) social functioning (i.e., social competence and social anxiety), and 4) role functioning (i.e., academic achievement, school adjustment, and highest level of functioning). PTSD, like major depression, showed significant adverse effects on psychological, physical, and social functioning, whereas alcohol use disorder adversely influenced role functioning. For adolescents with comorbid major depression or PTSD with alcohol use disorders, treatment planning may need to include remedial interventions in all these areas.

Adolescents with PTSD may be treatment-resistant and vulnerable to early relapse. During early stages of abstinence, adults with PTSD often have increased PTSD symptomatology (158). Clinical observation suggests that PTSD symptoms are associated with treatment-resistant SUD (159,160). Individuals with PTSD are at higher risk for early relapse, with PTSD associated with more severe SUD and poor compliance with aftercare (161).

Severe psychosocial stressors lead to relapse in vulnerable individuals. Brown and colleagues (126) found that, among male abstinent alcoholics who experienced marked life adversity, those with higher composite psychosocial vulnerability scores were more likely to relapse than those with lower vulnerability scores. Men who had improved psychosocial functioning (i.e., coping, self-efficacy, social support) following treatment had better outcomes than those with increased vulnerability. Because adolescents with SUD are subject to more stressors than control adolescents (114), interventions to reduce stressors following treatment may be relevant.

Mental Disorders in Adolescents

Cognitive-behavior therapy approaches have been developed for treating PTSD in adolescents (162), and such approaches may be relevant for adolescents with comorbid PTSD and SUD. Treatment in these adolescents must, however, address SUD and PTSD simultaneously (131). Specific approaches to treatment of this population have not been empirically examined. A group cognitive-behavior therapy program has been developed for women with PTSD and SUD (163). The program provides education about these disorders, teaches self-control skills focused on managing affect, works on improving functioning, and includes relapse prevention training. Systematic evaluations of this and other treatment programs are needed with adolescent SUD samples.

OTHER ANXIETY DISORDERS

Definitions

The DSM-IV diagnostic system includes the following anxiety disorders: separation anxiety disorder, panic disorder, agoraphobia, specific phobias, social phobia, obsessive-compulsive disorder, and generalized anxiety disorders, as well as the previously considered posttraumatic stress disorder and acute stress disorder (see Ref. 164 for review). Separation anxiety disorder is defined by excessive and developmentally inappropriate anxiety about separation from parents or other primary attachment figures. Typically less common in adolescents than younger children, a relationship between separation anxiety disorder and adolescent SUD has not been established. Panic disorder and agoraphobia are rare in adolescent samples. Specific phobias are relatively common but probably not a factor in SUD development. Social phobia is nearly as common in adolescent as in adult samples and may influence SUD development and course. Obsessive-compulsive disorder often begins during adolescence, but a relationship with adolescent SUD has not been established. Generalized anxiety disorder may be one of the more common anxiety disorders in adolescents. The criteria for generalized anxiety disorder, however, have been substantially changed in DSM-IV so the applicability of studies using prior criteria is uncertain.

Relationships with Substance Use Disorders

Clinical samples of adults with SUD typically show high rates of social phobia, panic disorder, and agoraphobia (165,166; see Ref. 22 for review). Epidemiological data also support an association between anxiety disorders and SUD in adults (167). Among adolescents with SUD, high rates of social phobia have been noted (e.g., Refs. 29, 168). In the PAARC analysis comparing adolescents with alcohol dependence to community control adolescents, anxiety disorders other than PTSD were not found to be significantly associated with alcohol dependence (34). Whether there is an association between anxiety disorders other than PTSD and SUD among adolescents remains to be definitively determined.

Causal Models

The hypothesis that anxiety disorders lead to alcohol dependence through a self-medication mechanism has been repeatedly proposed, particularly for agoraphobia and social phobia (e.g., Refs. 169–171). The data in support of this viewpoint are problematic, as the effects of alcohol on anxiety have depended on dose, individual differences, anxiety type, and use circumstances (22). Childhood anxiety disorders may influence substance use and related problems that vary by developmental stage as well as the nature of anxiety symptoms. For example, while children at high risk for SUD have been found to have elevated rates of anxiety disorders (35), childhood anxiety disorders were found to inhibit the initiation of tobacco use (16). In adolescents and young adults, on the other hand, anxiety disorders are associated with higher rates of regular tobacco use and nicotine dependence (172,173). Further research is needed to determine the relevance of anxiety disorders to substance effects and adolescent SUD development.

Treatment Implications

Screening for anxiety disorders may be useful in evaluating SUD adolescents, particularly since these disorders may be neglected in clinical assessment (121). Structured interview methods developed for children and adolescents (e.g., the K-SADS) (154) typically include assessment of the relevant anxiety disorders. In addition to evaluating diagnoses, questionnaire measures may provide useful information on the severity and course of anxiety and phobia symptoms in SUD adolescents. Measures of social phobia and general anxiety are available and have been validated for adolescents (e.g., Social Phobia and Anxiety Inventory (174), State Trait Anxiety Inventory for Children (175), Hamilton Anxiety Rating Scale (176).

An abstinent period is useful in the evaluation process. Observations concerning the influence of abstinence and substance consumption constitute an important aspect of adolescent SUD assessment. In adults with alcohol use disorders, periods of abstinence have been associated with improvements in anxiety (115,177). Anxiety and phobias may also alter response to treatment. For example, social phobia may lead to less willingness to participate in group interventions. When anxiety symptoms persist, targeting these symptoms with specific interventions is prudent. As with other forms of psychopathology, simultaneous or sequential treatment for anxiety disorders and SUD may be needed.

Psychological treatments are available for most adolescent anxiety disorders (178) and, in most circumstances with SUD adolescents, are preferred over pharmacological interventions for the initial intervention. Pharmacological treatments for many anxiety disorders are available (see Ref. 179 for review) and may also need to be considered, especially in treatment-resistant cases. Benzodiazepines should be avoided due to their potential for abuse in SUD individuals. In SUD patients, targeted treatments for anxiety disorders have been advocated, and cases for which specific treatment has been thought to contribute to relapse prevention have been presented (180). These general guidelines, however apparent, are not currently supported by empirical literature.

Future Directions

Considerable work needs to be done to determine the extent to which anxiety disorders other than PTSD are relevant for adolescent SUD etiology and treatment. Clinical and community studies have indicated that anxiety syndromes lead to SUD and are caused by substance consumption. Progress in this area may be inhibited by the tendency to hypothesize that only one or the other causal direction is true. In fact, a more complex model may be more valid in which SUD and psychopathology contribute to a positive-feedback loop. This loop may have a neurobiological basis, as alcohol consumption has been found to be associated with diminished benzodiazepine receptor binding (181,182). The literature to date suggests that several complexities need to be considered in future studies, including the following: 1) each anxiety disorder may have a unique relationship with SUD; 2) SUD involving specific substances may have unique relationships with each anxiety disorder; and 3) different relationships may be evident for substance initiation, early substance-related problems, and substance dependence. It is unlikely that a single approach to studying these complex relationships will prove sufficient; clinical, community, and laboratory studies are needed to clarify them.

CONCLUSIONS

Substantial challenges remain in understanding the influences of comorbid mental disorders on adolescent SUD. Given that the relationships among the relevant disorders are probably complex, new conceptualizations, assessment methods, analysis approaches, and treatment interventions need to be developed and systematically tested. The concepts emerging in the discipline of developmental psychopathology may be particularly applicable to the problem of understanding these relationships. Developmental psychopathology is a macroparadigm emphasizing the importance of qualitative change over time, particularly with reference to major changes that typically occur across the life cycle (183). Progress has been made in the construction of a developmental conceptualization of substance use disorders (e.g., Ref. 184). While the methodological challenges this conceptualization poses have been considered (185), there has been relatively little application of developmentally informed conceptualizations and relevant statistically techniques to data available to characterize the relationships among alcohol use disorders, other substance use disorders, and other mental disorders. Since SUD and associated mental disorders are complex problems with multiple etiologies, genetic, family, epidemiological, and clinical studies may help define clinically meaningful subgroups that would allow earlier identification of individuals at risk, and could provide more specific treatments.

Assessment

A comprehensive assessment, including systematic evaluation of disruptive behavior disorders, mood disorders, and anxiety disorders, is the basis for effective treatment planning in programs for SUD adolescents. A consensus has been reached regarding the criteria for SUD and other mental disorder diagnoses through the development of the American Psychiatric Association DSM system. Variation in the typically unstructured clinical assessment is a significant source of clinician disagreement and may lead to inaccurate diagnostic formulations, particularly lack of detection of relevant mental disorders (186). In adolescent inpatients identified by semistructured interview as having alcohol abuse or dependence, the results of a systematic assessment and diagnostic formulation process were compared with hospital records (121). Of cases in whom the disorders were indicated by semistructured interview, hospital records detected 74% with alcohol use disorders, 92% with disruptive behavior disorders, 60% with mood disorders, and only 24% with anxiety disorders. Similar results have been reported in other adolescent samples (187). Systematic diagnostic interviewing thus provides a more comprehensive assessment than the typical clinical procedures and has been advocated for clinical evaluations (186). In adolescents suspected as having substance abuse or dependence, the following other mental disorders should be specifically evaluated: ADHD, ODD, CD, major depression, and PTSD. A follow-up assessment after an abstinent period of 4 weeks further refines the psychopathology assessment. In addition to evaluating a limited observation period for immediate clinical decisions, assessing the prior life course of substance use disorders may also be instructive (e.g., Ref. 188).

Extensive and multifaceted problems are often revealed by a comprehensive assessment, as SUD adolescents typically have multiple SUD and other mental disorders. In PAARC adolescents with alcohol dependence (34), cannabis abuse or dependence was present in the majority of females (69%) and males (77%). A configural frequency analysis indicated that conduct disorder and major depression clustered together and that both were present in a majority of females (60%) and a substantial proportion of males (38%) with alcohol dependence. These combinations of disorders may have treatment implications that are distinct from the considerations evident for each independent disorder.

Adolescent substance use disorders have risk factors and consequences that change and interact over time. For example, a childhood history of physical or sexual abuse or other important traumas is present in the majority of adolescents with SUD (e.g., Ref. 114). Childhood abuse may be important in understanding the etiology of SUD in adolescents, and can lead to anxiety and depression in these cases (189). Parent–adolescent relationships, peer relationships, school functioning, and health functioning form a minimum additional assessment domain list. Problems in multiple areas may be briefly and efficiently assessed through the use of questionnaires, such as the Drug Use Screening Inventory (190). PAARC adolescents with alcohol use disorders were found to be impaired, compared with control adolescents, in the 10 areas of functioning assessed by this measure (174). For a more comprehensive assessment, however, multiple informants may be needed. In an examination of family functioning in the PAARC sample, for example, adolescents' and their mothers' views on family functioning differed (191). Problematic family relationships contribute to increased association with antisocial and substance-using peers (192). Adolescent SUD may be associated with impaired school functioning (157). Assessment and intervention in these areas are important for successful adolescent SUD treatment (193). While a comprehensive assessment presents a considerable challenge to the clinician, time spent in the initial assessment may avoid unnecessary evaluations during the course of treatment

(186). While more effective and efficient intervention planning likely results from comprehensive assessment, the specific areas that need to be included and the resulting improvement in management must be determined through clinical research.

Treatment

Empirical studies on the effects of comorbid mental disorders on the course of adolescent SUD treatment are limited, although the observations made to date have apparent implications for optimizing treatment programs. Treatment programs for SUD adolescents need to focus on eliminating substance use, improving psychopathology, and addressing problems with family and social functioning. Achieving reduction in substance use is essential to effective interventions. Psychopathological symptoms increase during periods of alcohol and drug use (194) and improve with abstinence. Brown and colleagues (195,196) have shown that, following SUD treatment, adolescents with less drug and alcohol use show improved emotion and interpersonal functioning in multiple settings including family, school, and work. Successfully achieving reduced substance use or abstinence may, however, require addressing the substantial problems in multiple domains presented by these adolescents.

Treatment programs are needed that address problems in SUD and comorbid mental disorders, as well as family, peer, and school functioning, with systematic methods for coordinating interventions. Multisystemic treatment is such a treatment model—a multidimensional approach devised by Henggeler and colleagues (62,63,193) combining family, peer, school and community interventions with individual treatment. Multisystemic treatment has been demonstrated to improve antisocial behaviors in adolescents (193,197,198), as well as in families with a history of child abuse and neglect (199). When applied to adolescents with SUD, multisystemic treatment has been reported to reduce substance use, criminal offending, and parent-figure alcohol use (193). The rationale for this treatment model is clearly supported by the empirical literature on adolescent SUD, and observations to date suggest that the approach may be effective for SUD and related problems.

Other psychological and pharmacological treatments may also be relevant for this population. Adolescent coping skills may also influence treatment outcome. In adolescents following treatment for SUD, Myers, Brown, and Mott (200) found that wishful thinking and social support predicted total days using substances and the length of initial abstinence. The findings suggest that unrealistically low stress appraisal may decrease active coping efforts, leading to increased relapse risk. Psychopathology has been found to be associated

Mental Disorders in Adolescents

with decreased efficacy to avoid heavy drinking in both alcoholic and non-alcoholic adolescents (55). Interventions focused on teaching accurate stress appraisal, active cognitive coping strategies, and actions to enhance social support may be useful in preventing relapse. The role of pharmacological approaches to adolescent SUD remains controversial. As Kaminer (201) points out, the scope of pharmacological treatment is limited by possible developmental risks, unproven long-term benefits, and social stigma. Pharmacological interventions focused on specific comorbid mental disorders may be more effective and acceptable to parents, practitioners, and adolescents.

While multidimensional treatment programs represent the ideal—and perhaps the most realistic—approach to adolescent SUD, the cost of such comprehensive programs may limit their application. Cost containment through managed health care has had major ramifications on the delivery and availability of programs for SUD adolescents in recent years. Particularly when compensation to the health care provider is at risk with intensive interventions, there is a conflict of interest and an unfortunate incentive to provide less care (202). An empirical basis for specific recommendations will increase the likelihood that increased costs associated with more comprehensive services will be accepted. Further studies to determine the characteristics of effective and efficient treatment for SUD adolescents are urgently needed. While the cost of providing comprehensive interventions for SUD is undoubtedly considerable, the societal cost of neglecting these highly problematic adolescents is even greater.

ACKNOWLEDGMENTS

The preparation of this chapter was supported by grants from NIAAA (P50 AA08746, K02 AA00291) and NIDA (P50 DA05605).

REFERENCES

1. P Cohen, J Cohen, S Kasen, CN Velez, C Hartmark, J Johnson, M Rojas, J Brook, EL Streuning. Age- and gender-specific prevalence. J Child Psychol Psychiatry 34:851–867, 1993.
2. HA Reinhertz, IM Giaconia, ES Lefkowitz, B Pakiz, AK Frost. Prevalence of psychiatric disorders in a community population of older adolescents. J Am Acad Child Adolesc Psychiatry 32: 369–377, 1993.
3. P Rohde, PM Lewinsohn, JR Seeley. Psychiatric comorbidity with problematic

alcohol use in high school students. J Am Acad Child Adolesc Psychiatry 35(1):101–109, 1996.
4. RE Tarter, M Vanyukov. Alcoholism: a developmental disorder. J Consult Clin Psychol 62(6):1096–1107, 1994.
5. RA Zucker. The four alcoholisms: a developmental account of the etiologic process. In: PC Rivers, ed. Alcohol and Addictive Behaviors. Lincoln, NB: University of Nebraska Press, 1987.
6. DB Clark, OG Bukstein. Psychopathology in adolescent alcohol abuse and dependence Alcohol Health Res World. 22:117–126, 1998.
7. TF Babor, M Hofman, FK DelBoca, V Hesselbrock, RE Meyer, ZS Dolinsky, B Rounsaville. Types of alcoholics. I. Evidence for an empirically derived typology based on indicators of vulnerability and severity. Arch Gen Psychiatry 49:599–608, 1992.
8. L Buydens-Branchey, MH Branchey, D Noumair. Age of alcoholism onset. I. Relationship to psychopathology. Arch Gen Psychiatry 46:225–230, 1989.
9. CR Cloninger. Neurogenetic adaptive mechanisms in alcoholism. Science 236:410–416, 1987.
10. M Irwin, M Schuckit, TL Smith. Clinical importance of age at onset in type 1 and type 2 primary alcoholics. Arch Gen Psychiatry 47:320–324, 1990.
11. M McGue, W Slutske, J Taylor, WG Iacono. Personality and substance use disorders. I. Effects of gender and alcoholism subtype. Alcoholism: Clin Exp Res 21:513–520, 1997.
12. LC Morey, HA Skinner, RK Blashfield. A typology of alcohol abusers: correlates and implications. J Abnorm Psychol 93:408–417, 1984.
13. RE Tarter, H McBride, H Buonpane, DU Schneider. Differentiation of alcoholics: childhood history of minimal brain dysfunction, family history, and drinking pattern. Arch Gen Psychiatry 34:761–768, 1977.
14. MA Schuckit, TL Smith, R Anthenelli, M Irwin. Clinical course of alcoholism in 636 male inpatients. Am J Psychiatry 150:786–792, 1993.
15. DB Clark, L Kirisci, RE Tarter. Adolescent versus adult onset and the development of substance use disorders in males. Drug Alcohol Depend 49:115–121, 1998.
16. DB Clark, L Kirisci, HB Moss. Early adolescent gateway drug use in sons of fathers with substance use disorders. Addict Behav 23:561–566, 1998.
17. DB Clark, AM Parker, KG Lynch. Psychopathology, substance use and substance related problems. J Child Clin Psychol. 28:333–341, 1999.
18. RJ Cadoret, E Troughton, J Bagford, G Woodward, MA Steward. Adoption study demonstrating two genetic pathways to drug abuse. Arch Gen Psychiatry 52:42–52, 1995.
19. TE Wilens, J Biederman, E Mick, SV Faraone, T Spencer. Attention deficit hyperactivity disorder (ADHD) is associated with early onset substance use disorders. J Nerv Ment Disord 185:475–482, 1997.
20. RK Brooner, D Temple, DS Svikis. Dimensions of alcoholism: a multivariate analysis. J Stud Alcohol 51:77–81, 1990.

21. PD Farber, KA Kharari, FM Douglass. A factor analytic study of reasons for drinking: empirical validation of positive and negative reinforcement dimensions. J Consult Clin Psychol 48(6):780–781, 1980.
22. DB Clark, MA Sayette. Anxiety and the development of alcoholism: clinical and scientific issues. Am J Addict 2:59–76, 1993.
23. M Cox, E Klinger. A motivational model of alcohol use. J Abnorm Psychol 97:168–180, 1988.
24. ML Cooper. Motivations for alcohol use among adolescents: developments and validation of a four-factor model. Psychol Assess 6:117–128, 1994.
25. LN Robins, J Tipp, T Przydeck. Antisocial personality. In: Psychiatric Disorders in America: The Epidemiologic Catchment Area Study. LN Robins, DA Regier, eds. New York: Free Press division of Macmillan, pp 258–290, 1991.
26. BB Lahey, B Applegate, RA Barkley, B Garfinkel, K McBurnett, L Kerdyk, L Greenhill, GW Hynd, PJ Frick, J Newcorn, J Biederman, T Ollendick, EL Hart, D, Perez, I Waldman, D Schaffer. DSM-IV field trials for oppositional defiant disorder and conduct disorder in children and adolescents. Am J Psychiatry 151:1163–1171, 1994.
27. R Loeber. Development and risk factors of juvenile antisocial behavior and delinquency. Clin Psychol Rev 10:1–41, 1990.
28. DR Lynam. Early identification of chronic offenders: who is the fledgling psychopath? Psychol Bull 126(2):209–234, 1996.
29. JG Hovens, DP Cantwell, R Kiriakos. Psychiatric comorbidity in hospitalized adolescent substance abusers. J Acad Child Adol Psychiatry 33:476–483, 1994.
30. B Neighbors, T Kempton, R Forehand. Co-occurrence of substance abuse with conduct, anxiety, and depression disorders in juvenile delinquents. Addict Behav 17:379–386, 1992.
31. M Zoccolillo, J Meyers, S Assiter. Conduct disorder, substance dependence and adolescent motherhood. Am J Orthopsychiatry 67(1):152–157, 1997.
32. DM Fergusson, MT Lynskey, LJ Horwood. Alcohol misuse and juvenile offending in adolescence. Addict 91(4):483–494, 1996.
33. MT Lynskey, DM Fergusson. Childhood conduct problems, attention deficit behaviors, and adolescent alcohol, tobacco, and illicit drug use. J Abnorm Child Psychol 23(3):281–302, 1995.
34. DB Clark, NK Pollock, OG Bukstein, AC Mezzich, JT Bromberger, JE Donovan. Gender and comorbid psychopathology in adolescents with alcohol dependence. J Am Acad Child Adolesc Psychiatry 36(9):1195–1203, 1997.
35. DB Clark, HB Moss, L Kirisci, AC Mezzich, R Miles, P Ott. Psychopathology in preadolescent sons of substance abusers. J Am Acad Child Adolesc Psychiatry 36:495–502, 1997.
36. SE Young, SK Mikulich, MB Goodwin, J Hardy, CL Martin, MS Zoccolillo, TJ Crowley. Treated delinquent boys' substance use: onset, pattern, relationship to conduct and mood disorders. Drug Alcohol Depend 37:149–162, 1995.
37. MG Myers, SA Brown, MA Mott. Preadolescent conduct disorder and behaviors

predict relapse and progression of addiction for adolescent alcohol and drug abusers. Alcoholism Clin Exp Res 19(6):1528–1536, 1995.
38. E Gorenstein, J Newman. Disinhibitory psychopathology: a new perspective and model for research. Psychol Rev 87:301–315, 1980.
39. CE Lewis, KK Buchholz. Alcoholism, antisocial behavior and family history. Br J Addict 86:177–194, 1991.
40. PE Greenbaum, EC Brown, RM Friedman. Alcohol expectancies among adolescents with conduct disorder: prediction and mediation of drinking. Addict Behav 20(3):321–333, 1995.
41. M Zoccolillo, A Pickles, D Quinton, M Rutter. The outcome of childhood conduct disorder: implications for defining adult personality disorder and conduct disorder. Psychol Med 22:971–986, 1992.
42. P Reebye, MM Moretti, JC Lessard. Conduct disorder and substance use disorder: comorbidity in a clinical sample of preadolescents and adolescents. Can J Psychiatry 40:313–319, 1995.
43. EO Johnson, AM Arria, G Borges, N Ialongo, JC Anthony. The growth of conduct problem behaviors from middle childhood to early adolescence: sex differences and the suspected influence of early alcohol use. J Stud Alcohol 56:661–671, 1995.
44. SA Brown, A Gleghorn MA Schuckit, MG Myers, MA Mott. Conduct disorder among adolescent alcohol and drug abusers. J Stud Alcohol 57:314–324, 1996.
45. M Rutter. Comments on Fergusson et al.'s "Alcohol misuse and juvenile offending in adolescence." Addiction 91(4):495–510, 1996.
46. DP Farrington. Comments on Fergusson et al.'s "Alcohol misuse and juvenile offending in adolescence." Addict 91(4):495–510, 1996.
47. R Jessor, SL Jessor. Problem Behavior and Psychosocial Development: A Longitudinal Study of Youth. New York: Academic Press, 1977.
48. NH DeCourville. Testing the applicability of problem behavior theory to substance use in a longitudinal study. Psychol Addict Behav 9(1):53–66, 1995.
49. JE Donovan, R Jessor. Structure of problem behavior in adolescence and young adulthood. J Consult Clin Psychol 53(6):890–904, 1985.
50. R Jessor. Problem-behavior theory, psychosocial development and adolescent problem drinking. Br J Addict 82:331–342, 1987.
51. R Jessor, JE Donovan, FM Costa. Beyond Adolescence: Problem Behavior and Young Adult Development. Cambridge, England: Cambridge University Press, 1991.
52. R Jessor, J Van Den Bos, J Vanderryn, FM Costa, MS Turbin. Protective factors in adolescent problem behavior: moderator effects and developmental change. Develop Psychol 31(6):923–933, 1995.
53. M Stouthamer-Loeber, R Loeber, DP Farrington, Q Zhang, W van Kammen, E Maguin. The double edge of protective and risk factors for delinquency: interrelations and developmental patterns. Develop Psychopathol 5:683–701, 1993.
54. Y Kaminer, RE Tarter, OG Bukstein, M Kabene. Comparison between treatment

completers and noncompleters among dually diagnosed substance-abusing adolescents. J Am Acad Child Adolesc Psychiatry 31(6):1046–1049, 1992.
55. HB Moss, L Kirisci, AC Mezzich. Psychiatric comorbidity and self-efficacy to resist heavy drinking in alcoholic and nonalcoholic adolescents. Am J Addict 3:204–212, 1994.
56. P Chamberlain, JG Rosicky. Efficacy of family therapy treatment for conduct disorder and delinquency. J Marital Fam Ther 21(4):441–460, 1995.
57. WR Shadish, K Ragsdale, RR Glaser, LM Montgomery. The efficacy and effectiveness of marital and family therapy: a perspective from meta-analysis. J Marital Fam Ther 21(4):345–360, 1995.
58. WM Pinsof, LC Wynne. The efficacy of marital and family therapy: an empirical overview, conclusion, and recommendations. J Marital Fam Ther 21(4):585–613, 1995.
59. AE Kazdin. Parent management training: evidence, outcomes, and issues. J Am Acad Child Adolesc Psychiatry 36(10):1349–1356, 1997.
60. L Bank, JH Marlowe, JB Reid, GR Patterson, MR Weinrott. A comparative evaluation of parent-training interventions for families of chronic delinquents. J Abnorm Child Psychol 19(1):15–33, 1991.
61. DB Clark, BL Baker. Predicting outcome in parent training. J Consult Clin Psychol 51:309–311, 1983.
62. SW Henggeler, CM Bourduin. Family Therapy and Beyond: A Multisystemic Approach to Treating Children and Adolescents. Pacific Grove, CA: Brooks/Cole, 1990.
63. SW Henggeler, GB Melton, LA Smith. Family preservation using multisystemic therapy: an effective alternative to incarcerating serious juvenile offenders. J Consult Clin Psychol 60(6):953–961, 1992.
64. H Joanning, F Thomas, W Quinn, R Mullen. Treating adolescent drug abuse: a comparison of family systems therapy, group therapy, and family drug education. J Marital Fam Ther 18(4):345–356, 1992.
65. GA Figurelli, BW Hartman, FX Kowalski. Assessment of change in scores on personal control orientation and use of drugs and alcohol of adolescents who participate in a cognitively oriented pretreatment intervention. Psychol Report 75:939–944, 1994.
66. N Ralph, C McMenamy. Treatment outcomes in an adolescent chemical dependency program. Adolescence 31(121):91–107, 1996.
67. HA Liddle, GA Dakof. Efficacy of family-based treatment for drug abuse. J Marital Fam Ther 21(4):511–544, 1995.
68. SW Henggeler, CM Borduin, GB Melton, BJ Mann, LA Smith, JA Hall, L Cone, BR Fucci. Effects of multisystemic therapy on drug use and abuse in serious juvenile offenders: a progress report from two outcome studies. Fam Dynam Addict Q 1(3):40–51, 1991.
69. TE Moffitt. Adolescent-limited and life-course-persistent antisocial behavior: a developmental taxonomy. Psychol Rev 100:674–701, 1993.
70. RG Klein, H Abikoff, E Klass, D Ganeles, LM Seese, S Pollack. Clinical efficacy

of methylphenidate in conduct disorder with and without attention deficit hyperactivity disorder. Arch Gen Psychiatry 54:1073–1080, 1997.
71. GR Patterson, CM Narrett. Development of a reliable and valid treatment program for aggressive young children. Int J Ment Health 9(3):19–26, 1990.
72. SW Henggeler, SK Schoenwald, CM Borduin, MD Rowland, PB Cunningham. Multisystemic Treatment of Antisocial Behavior in Children and Adolescents. New York: Guilford Press, 1998.
73. R Loeber, K Keenan. The interaction between conduct disorder and its comorbid condition: effects of age and gender. Clin Psychol Rev 14:497–523, 1994.
74. EH Cook, MA Stein, MD Krasowski, NJ Cox, DM Olkon, JE Kieffer, B Leventhal. Association of attention-deficit disorder and the dopamine transporter gene. Am J Hum Genet 56:993–998, 1995.
75. M Gill, G Daly, S Heron, Z Hawi, M Fitzgerald. Confirmation of association between attention deficit hyperactivity disorder and a dopamine transporter polymorphism. Molec Psychiatry 2:311–313, 1997.
76. J Biederman, SV Farone, T Spencer, T Wilens, D Norman, KA Lapey, E Mick, BK Lehman, A Doyle. Patterns of psychiatric comorbidity, cognition, and psychosocial functioning in adults with attention deficit hyperactivity disorder. Am J Psychiatry 150:1792–1798, 1993.
77. J Biederman, T Wilens, E Mick, S Milberger, TJ Spencer, SV Farone. Psychoactive substance use disorders in adults with attention deficit hyperactivity disorder (ADHD): effects of ADHD and psychiatric comorbidity. Am J Psychiatry 152:1652–1658, 1995.
78. WO Shekim, RF Asarnow, E Hess, K Zaucha, N Wheeler. A clinical and demographic profile of a sample of adults with attention deficit hyperactivity disorder, residual state. Compr Psychiatry 31(5):416–425, 1990.
79. KM Carroll, BJ Rounsaville. History and significance of childhood attention deficit disorder in treatment-seeking cocaine abusers. Compr Psychiatry 34(2):75–82, 1993.
80. DW Goodwin, F Schulsinger, L Hermansen, SB Guze, G Winokur. Alcoholism and the hyperactive child syndrome. J Nerv Ment Disord 160(5):349–353, 1975.
81. SL Eyre, BJ Rounsaville, HD Kleber. History of childhood hyperactivity in a clinic population of opiate addicts. J Nerv Ment Disord 170(9):522–529, 1982.
82. L Demilio. Psychiatric syndromes in adolescent substance abusers. Am J Psychiatry 146:1212–1214, 1989.
83. R Milin, JA Halikas, JE Meller, C Morse. Psychopathology among substance abusing juvenile offenders. J Am Acad Child Adolesc Psychiatry 30(4):569–574, 1991.
84. BR Horner, KE Scheibe. Prevalence and implications of attention-deficit hyperactivity disorder among adolescents in treatment for substance abuse. J Am Acad Child Adolesc Psychiatry 36(1):30–36, 1997.
85. LL Thompson, PD Riggs, SK Mikulich, TJ Crowley. Contribution of ADHD symptoms to substance problems and delinquency in conduct-disordered adolescents. J Abnorm Child Psychol 24(3):325–347, 1996.

86. AGA Blouin, RA Borenstein, RL Trites. Teenage alcohol use among hyperactive children: a five-year follow-up study. J Ped Psychol 3(4):188–194, 1978.
87. S Mannuzza, RG Klein, A Bessler, P Malloy, M LaPadula. Adult outcome of hyperactive boys educational achievement, occupational rank, and psychiatric status. Arch Gen Psychiatry 50:565–576, 1993.
88. S Milberger, J Biederman, SV Faraone, L Chen, J Jones. ADHD is associated with early initiation of cigarette smoking in children and adolescents. J Am Acad Child Adolesc Psychiatry 36:37–44, 1997.
89. L Hechtman, G Weiss. Controlled prospective fifteen-year follow-up of hyperactives as adults: non-medical drug and alcohol use and anti-social behavior. Can J Psychiatry 31:557–567, 1986.
90. J Biederman, T Wilens, E Mick, SV Farone, W Weber, S Curtis, A Thornell, K Pfister, J Jetton, J Soriano. Is ADHD a risk factor for psychoactive substance use disorders? Findings from a four-year prospective follow-up study. J Am Acad Child Adolesc Psychiatry 36:21–29, 1997.
91. EJ Khantzian. The self-medication hypothesis of addictive disorders: focus on heroin and cocaine dependence. Am J Psychiatry 142:1259–1264, 1985.
92. HB Moss, TC Blackson, C Martin, RE Tarter. Heightened motor activity in male offspring of substance abusing fathers: association with temperament, behavior, and psychiatric diagnosis. Biol Psychiatry 32:1135–1147, 1992.
93. CS Martin, M Earlywine, TC Blackson, M Vanyukov, HB Moss, RE Tarter. Aggressivity, inattention, hyperactivity, and impulsivity in boys at high and low risk for substance abuse. J Abnorm Child Psychol 22:177–203, 1994.
94. SV Farone, J Biederman, K Keenan, MT Tsuang. Separation of DSM-III attention deficit disorder and conduct disorder: evidence from a family-genetic study of American child psychiatric patients. Psychol Med 21:109–121, 1991.
95. RE Tarter, HB Moss, A Arria, D Van Thiel. Cognitive impairment in substance abusers. In: The Residual Effects of Drugs on Performance. J Spencer, ed. Washington DC: U.S. Superintendent of Documents, 1991.
96. TH Harrell, LM Honaker, E Davis. Cognitive and behavioral dimensions of dysfunction in alcohol and polydrug abusers. J Subst Abuse 3:415–426, 1991.
97. JM Vaeth, AM Horton, Jr., M Ahadpour. Attention deficit disorder, alcoholism, and drug abuse: MMPI correlates. Int J Neurosci 63:115–124, 1992.
98. TE Wilens, J Biederman. The stimulants. In: Psychiatric Clinics of North America. D Schaffer, ed. Philadelphia: WB Saunders, pp 191–222, 1992.
99. TE Wilens, J Biederman, TJ Spender, J Prince. Pharmacotherapy of adult attention deficit/hyperactivity disorder: a review. J Clin Psychopharmacol 15(4):270–279, 1995.
100. T Spencer, T Wilens, J Biederman, SV Farone, JS Ablon, K Lapey. A double-blind, crossover comparison of methylphenidate and placebo in adults with childhood-onset attention-deficit hyperactivity disorder. Arch Gen Psychiatry 52:434–443, 1995.
101. SL Jaffe. Intranasal abuse of prescribed methylphenidate by an alcohol and

drug abusing adolescent with ADHD. J Am Acad Child Adolesc Psychiatry 30(5):773–775, 1991.
102. DH Langer, KP Sweeney, DE Bartenbach, PM Davis, KB Menander. Evidence of lack of abuse or dependence following pemoline treatment: results of a retrospective study. Drug Alcohol Dep 17:213–227, 1986.
103. R Famularo, K Stone, C Popper. Preadolescent alcohol abuse and dependence. Am J Psychiatry 142:1187–1189, 1985.
104. ND Ryan, J Puig-Antich, P Ambrosini, H Rabinovich, D Robinson, B Nelson, S Iyengar, J Twomey. The clinical picture of major depression in children and adolescents. Arch Gen Psychiatry 44:854–861, 1987.
105. MA Bowring, M Kovacs. Difficulties in diagnosing manic disorders among children and adolescents. J Am Acad Child Adolesc Psychiatry 31:611–614, 1992.
106. KA Christie, JD Burke, DA Regie. Epidemiological evidence for early onset of mental disorders and higher risk of drug abuse in young adults. Am J Psychiatry 145(8):971–975, 1988.
107. L Demilio. Psychiatric syndromes in adolescent substance abusers. Am J Psychiatry 146:1212–1214, 1989.
108. PE Greenbaum, ME Prange, RM Friedman, SE Silver. Substance abuse prevalence and comorbidity with other psychiatric disorders among adolescents with severe emotional disturbances. J Am Acad Child Adolesc Psychiatry 30:575–583, 1991.
109. JH Kashani, MB Keller, N Solomon, JC Reid, D Mazzola. Double depression in adolescent substance users. J Affect Disord 8:153–157, 1985.
110. EY Deykin, JC Levy, V Wells. Adolescent depression alcohol and drug abuse. Am J Pub Health 77:178–182, 1987.
111. OG Bukstein, LJ Glancy, Y Kaminer. Patterns of affective comorbidity in a clinical population of dually diagnosed adolescent substance abusers. J Am Acad Child Adolesc Psychiatry 31(6):1041–1045, 1992.
112. JA Russell, A Mehrabian. The mediating role of emotions in alcohol use. J Stud Alcohol 36:1508–1536, 1975.
113. JA Tucker, RE Vuckinich, MB Sobell. Alcohol's effects on human emotions: a review of the stimulation/depression hypothesis. Int J Addict 17:155–180, 1982.
114. DB Clark, L Lesnick, A Hegedus. Trauma and other stressors in adolescent alcohol dependence and abuse. J Am Acad Child Adolesc Psychiatry 36(12):1744–1751, 1997.
115. SA Brown, M Irwin, MA Schuckit. Changes in anxiety among abstinent male alcoholics. J Stud Alcohol 52:55–61, 1991.
116. SA Brown, RK Inaba, JC Gillin, MA Schuckit, MA Stewart. Alcoholism and affective disorder: clinical course of depressive symptoms. Am J Psychiatry 152:45–52, 1995.
117. CA Dackis, MS Gold, ALC Pottash, DR Sweeney. Evaluating depression in alcoholics. Psychiatry Res 17:105–109, 1986.
118. E Hartka, B Johnstone, EV Leino, M Motoyoshi, MT Temple, KM Fillmore. A

meta-analysis of depressive symptomatology and alcohol consumption over time. Br J Addict 86:1283–1298, 1991.
119. U Rao, ND Ryan, B Birmaher, RE Dahl, DE Williamson, J Kaufman, R Rao, B Nelson. Unipolar depression in adolescents: clinical outcome in adulthood. J Am Acad Child Adolesc Psychiatry 34:566–578, 1995.
120. EY Deykin, SL Buka, TH Zeena. Depressive illness among chemically dependent adolescents. Am J Psychiatry 149:1341–1347, 1992.
121. DB Clark, OG Bukstein, MG Smith, NA Kaczynski, A Mezzich, JE Donovan. Identifying anxiety disorders in adolescents hospitalized for alcohol abuse or dependence. Psychiatr Serv 46:618–620, 1995.
122. SA Brown, MA Schuckit. Changes in depression among abstinent alcoholics. J Stud Alcohol 49:412–417, 1988.
123. AI Alterman, E Gottheil, HD Crawford. Mood changes in an alcoholism treatment program based on drinking decisions. Am J Psychiatry 132:1032–1037, 1975.
124. DS Elliot, D Huizinga, S Menard. Multiple Problem Youth: Delinquency, Substance Use, and Mental Health Problems. New York: Springer-Verlag, 1989.
125. F Osher, LL Kofoed. Treatment of patients with psychiatric and psychoactive substance abuse disorders. Hosp Commun Psychiatry 40:1025–1030, 1989.
126. SA Brown, PW Vik, TL Patterson, I Grant, MA Schuckit. Stress, vulnerability and adult alcohol relapse. J Stud Alcohol 56:538–545, 1995.
127. WD Holmes, KD Wagner. Psychotherapy treatments for depression in children and adolescents. J Psychother Prac Res 1(4):313–323, 1992.
128. JR Cornelius, IM Salloum, JG Ehler, PJ Jarrett, MD Cornelius, MJ Perel, ME Thase, AE Black. Fluoxetine in depressed alcoholics: a double-blind, placebo-controlled trial. Arch Gen Psychiatry 54:700–705, 1997.
129. GJ Emslie, AJ Rush, WA Weinberg, RA Kowatch, CW Hughes, T Carmody, J Rintelmann. A double-blind, randomized, placebo-controlled trial of fluoxetine in children and adolescents with depression. Arch Gen Psychiatry 54:1031–1037, 1997.
130. D Finkelhor, J Dziuba-Leatherman. Children as victims of violence: a national survey. Pediatrics 94(4):413–420, 1994.
131. SH Stewart. Alcohol abuse in individuals exposed to trauma: a critical review. Psychol Bull 120:83–112, 1996.
132. AD Klassen, SC Wilsnack. Sexual experiences and drinking among women in a U.S. national survey. Arch Sex Behav 15:363–392, 1986.
133. SC Wilsnack. Sexuality and women's drinking: findings from a U.S. national study. Alcohol Health Res World 15:147–150, 1991.
134. CS Widom, T Ireland, PJ Glynn. Alcohol abuse in abused and neglected children followed-up: are they at increased risk? J Stud Alcohol 56:207–217, 1995.
135. I Winfield, LK George, M Swartz, DG Blazer. Sexual assault and psychiatric disorders among a community sample of women. Am J Psychiatry 147:335–341, 1990.
136. KJ Sher, BS Gershuny, L Peterson, G Raskin. The role of childhood stressors in

the intergenerational transmission of alcohol use disorders. J Stud Alcohol 58:414–427, 1997.
137. PA Harrison, JA Fulkerson, TJ Beebe. Multiple substance use among adolescent physical and sexual abuse victims. Child Abuse Neglect 21:529–539, 1997.
138. BJ Flanigan, PA Potrykus, D Marti. Alcohol and marijuana use among female adolescent incest victims. Alcoholism Treat Q 5:231–248, 1988.
139. JT Hernandez. Substance abuse among sexually abused adolescents and their families. J Adolesc Health 13:658–662, 1992.
140. JT Hernandez, M Lodico, RJ DiClemente. The effects of child abuse and race on risk-taking in male adolescents. J Nat Med Assoc 85:593–597, 1993.
141. DL Hussey, M Singer. Psychological distress, problem behaviors, and family functioning of sexually abused adolescent inpatients. J Am Acad Child Adolesc Psychiatry 32:954–961, 1993.
142. MI Singer, ML Petchers, D Hussey. The relationship between sexual abuse and substance abuse among psychiatrically hospitalized adolescents. Child Abuse Negl 13:319–325, 1989.
143. GE Edwall, NG Hoffmann, PA Harrison. Psychological correlates of sexual abuse in adolescent girls in chemical dependency treatment. Adolescence 24(94):279–288, 1989.
144. VB Van Hasselt, RT Ammerman, LJ Glancy, OG Bukstein. Maltreatment in psychiatrically hospitalized dually diagnosed adolescent substance abusers. J Am Acad Child Adol Psychiatry 31(5):868–874, 1992.
145. EY Deykin, SL Buka. Prevalence and risk factors for posttraumatic stress disorder among chemically dependent adolescents. Am J Psychiatry 154:752–757, 1997.
146. R Dembo, M Dertke, S Borders, M Washburn, J Schmeidler. The relationship between physical and sexual abuse and tobacco, alcohol, and illicit drug use among youths in a juvenile detention center. Int J Addict 23:351–378, 1988.
147. R Dembo, L Williams, W Wothke, J Schmeidler, CH Brown. The role of family factors, physical abuse and sexual victimization experiences in high-risk youths' alcohol and other drug use and delinquency: a longitudinal model. Violence Victims 7:245–266, 1992.
148. WD Watts, AM Ellis. Sexual abuse and drinking and drug use: implications for prevention. J Drug Educ 23:183–200, 1993.
149. JE Helzer, LN Robins, L McEvoy. Posttraumatic stress disorder in the general population: findings of the Epidemiologic Catchment Area survey. N Engl J Med 317:1630–1634, 1987.
150. EW Labouvie. Alcohol and marijuana use in relation to adolescent stress. Int J Addict 21:333–345, 1986.
151. R Dembo, L Williams, L La Voie, J Schmeidler, J Kern, A Getreu, E Berry, L Genung, ED Wish. A longitudinal study of the relationships among alcohol use, marijuana/hashish use, cocaine use, and emotional/psychological functioning problems in a cohort of high-risk youths. Int J Addict 25(11):1341–1382, 1990.
152. MP Koss, TE Dinero. Discriminant analysis of risk factors for sexual victimiza-

tion among a national sample of college women. J Consult Clin Psychol 57:242–250, 1989.
153. K Pernanen. Alcohol in Human Violence. New York: Guilford Press, 1991.
154. J Kaufman, B Birmaher, D Brent, U Rao, C Flynn, P Moreci, D Williamson, N Ryan. Schedule for Affective Disorders and Schizophrenia for School-Age Children—Present and Lifetime Version (K-SADS-PL): initial reliability and validity data. J Am Acad Child Adolesc Psychiatry 36:980–988, 1997.
155. DP Bernstein, L Fink, L Handelsman, J Foote, M Lovejoy, K Wenzel, E Sapareto, J Ruggiero. Initial reliability and validity of a new retrospective measure of child abuse and neglect. Am J Psychiatry 151:1132–1136, 1994.
156. J Kaufman, B Jones, E Stieglitz, L Vitulano. The use of multiple informants to assess children's maltreatment experiences. J Fam Viol 9:227–248, 1994.
157. DB Clark, L Kirisci. PTSD, depression, alcohol use disorders, and quality of life in adolescents. Anxiety 2:226–233, 1996.
158. JA Kovach. Incest as a treatment issue for alcoholic women. Alcohol Treat Q 3:1–15, 1986.
159. MP Root. Treatment failures: the role of sexual victimization in women's addictive behavior. Am J Orthopsychiatry 59:542–549, 1989.
160. K Bollerud. A model for the treatment of trauma-related syndromes among chemically dependent inpatient women. J Subst Abuse 7:83–87, 1990.
161. KT Brady, T Killeen, ME Saladin, B Dansky, S Becker. Comorbid substance abuse and posttraumatic stress disorder. Clin Res Rep 3:160–164, 1994.
162. P Saigh. The behavioral treatment of child and adolescent posttraumatic stress disorder. Advances Behav Res Ther 14:247–275, 1992.
163. LM Najavits, RD Weiss, BS Liese. Group cognitive-behavioral therapy for women with PTSD and substance use disorder. J Subst Abuse Treatment 13:13–22, 1996.
164. DB Clark, MG Smith, BD Neighbors, LM Skerlec, J Randall. Anxiety disorders in adolescence: characteristics, prevalence, and comorbidities. Clin Psychol Rev 14(2):113–137, 1994.
165. DL Chambless, J Cherney, C Caputo. Anxiety disorders and alcoholism: a study with inpatient alcoholics. J Anx Disord 1:29–40, 1987.
166. HE Ross, FB Glaser, T Germanson. The prevalence of psychiatric disorders in patients with alcohol and other drug problems. Arch Gen Psychiatry 45:1023–1031, 1988.
167. JE Helzer, A Burnam, LT McEvoy. Alcohol abuse and dependence. In: Psychiatric Disorders in America. LN Robins, DA Regier, eds. New York: Free Press, pp 81–115, 1991.
168. D Deas-Nesmith, K Brady, M Wagner, S Campbell. Substance use and psychiatric disorders in adolescents [abstr]. Proceedings of the Annual Meeting of the American Psychiatric Association 650:54, 1994.
169. MG Kushner, KJ Sher, BD Beitman. The relation between alcohol problems and anxiety disorders. Am J Psychiatry 147(6):685–695, 1990.

170. C Westphal. Die agoraphobia: eine neuropathische erscheinung. Archiv fur Psychiatrie and Nervenkrankheiten, 3:138–161, 1871.
171. GT Wilson. Alcohol and anxiety. Behav Res Ther 26(5):369–381, 1988.
172. N Breslau. Psychiatric comorbidity of smoking and nicotine dependence. Behav Genet 25:95–101, 1995.
173. LL Pederson, JJ Koval, K O'Connor. Are psychosocial factors related to smoking in grade 6 students? Addict Behav 22:169–181, 1997.
174. DB Clark, S Turner, D Beidel, J Donovan, L Kirisci, RG Jacob. Reliability and validity of the Social Phobia and Anxiety Inventory for Adolescents. Psychol Assess 6:135–140, 1994.
175. L Kirisci, DB Clark, HB Moss. Reliability and validity of the State-Trait Anxiety Inventory for Children in an adolescent sample: confirmatory factor analysis and item response theory. J Child Adol Subst Abuse 5:57–69, 1996.
176. DB Clark, J Donovan. Reliability and validity of the Hamilton Anxiety Rating Scale in an adolescent sample. J Am Acad Child Adolesc Psychiatry 33:354–360, 1994.
177. K Ludenia, GW Donham, PD Holzer. Anxiety in an alcoholic population: a normative study. J Clin Psychol 40(1):356–358, 1984.
178. GA Bernstein, J Kinlan. Summary of the practice parameters for the assessment and treatment of children and adolescents with anxiety disorders. J Am Acad Child Adolesc Psychiatry 36:1639–1641, 1997.
179. AJ Allen, HL Leonard, SE Swedo. Current knowledge of medications for the treatment of childhood anxiety disorders. J Am Acad Child Adolesc Psychiatry 34:976–986, 1995.
180. FM Quitkin, A Rifkin, J Kaplan. Phobic anxiety syndrome complicated by drug dependence and addiction. Arch Gen Psychiatry 27:159–162, 1972.
181. A Abi-Dargham, J Krystal, E Webb. SPECT imaging of benzodiazepine receptors in alcoholics and healthy controls [abst]. Alcoholism Clin Exp Res 19:10A, 1995.
182. KM Adams, S Gilman, R Koeppe. Decreased benzodiazepine receptor binding in the cingulate cortex of chronic alcoholic patients measured with (11C) flumazenil and PET [abstr]. Alcoholism Clin Exp Res 19:10A, 1995.
183. D Cicchetti. A historical perspective on the discipline of developmental psychopathology. In: Risk and Protective Factors in the Development of Psychopathology. J Rolf, A Masten, D Cicchetti, K Nuechterlein, S Weintraub, eds. New York: Cambridge University Press, 1990.
184. RA Zucker, HE Fitzgerald, HD Moses. Emergence of alcohol problems and the several alcoholisms: a developmental perspective on etiologic and life course trajectory. In: Developmental Psychopathology. Vol 2. Risk, Disorder and Adaptation. D Cicchetti, DJ Cohen, eds. New York: John Wiley & Sons, pp 677–711, 1995.
185. JE Richters. The Hubble hypothesis and the developmentalist's dilemma. Develop Psychopathol 9:193–229, 1997.
186. DB Clark. Psychiatric assessment. In: Sourcebook on Substance Abuse: Etiol-

ogy, Methodology, and Intervention. PJ Ott, RE Tarter, RT Ammerman, eds. Needham Heights, MA: Allyn & Bacon, 1999.
187. ET Aronen, GG Noam, SR Weinstein. Structured diagnostic interviews and clinicians' discharge diagnosis in hospitalized adolescents. J Am Acad Child Adolesc Psychiatry 32:674–781, 1993.
188. RA Zucker, WH Davies, SB Kincaid, HE Fitzgerald, EE Reider. Conceptualization and scaling the developmental structure of behavior disorder: the Lifetime Alcohol Problems Score as an example. Develop Psychopathol 9:453–471, 1997.
189. DB Clark, SL Bailey, KG Lynch. The effects of childhood abuse on adolescents with alcohol use disorders [abstr]. Alcoholism Clin Exper Res 22:72A, 1998.
190. RE Tarter. Evaluation and treatment of adolescent substance abuse: a decision tree model. Am J Drug Alcohol Abuse 16:1–46, 1990.
191. DB Clark, BD Neighbors, LA Lesnick, KG Lynch, JE Donovan. Family functioning and adolescent alcohol use disorders. J Fam Psychol 12(1):81–92, 1998.
192. TJ Dishion, JB Reid, GR Patterson. Empirical guidelines for a family intervention for adolescent drug use. J Chem Depend 2:189, 1988.
193. SG Pickrel, SW Henggeler. Multisystemic therapy for adolescent substance abuse and dependence. Child Adolesc Psychiatr Clin N Am 5:201–211, 1996.
194. LE O'Connor, JW Berry, A Morrison, S Brown. Retrospective reports of psychiatric symptoms before, during, and after drug use in a recovering population. J Psychoact Drugs 24(1):65–68, 1992.
195. SA Brown, MG Myers, MA Mott, PW Vik. Correlates of success following treatment for adolescent substance abuse. Applied Prevent Psychol 3:61–73, 1994.
196. MA Stewart, SA Brown. Family functioning following adolescent substance abuse treatment. J Subst Abuse 5:327–339, 1993.
197. CM Borduin, BJ Mann, LT Cone. Multisystemic treatment of serious juvenile offenders: long-term prevention of criminality and violence. J Consult Clin Psychol 63:569–578, 1995.
198. SW Henggeler, GB Melton, LA Smith. Family preservation using multisystemic treatment: long-term follow-up to a clinical trial with serious juvenile offenders. J Child Fam Stud 2:283, 1993.
199. M Brunk, SW Henggeler, JP Whelen. A comparison of multisystemic therapy and parent training in the brief treatment of child abuse and neglect. J Consult Clin Psychol 55:311, 1987.
200. MG Myers, SA Brown, MA Mott. Coping as a predictor of adolescent substance abuse treatment outcome. J Subst Abuse 5:15–29, 1993.
201. Y Kaminer. Issues in the pharmacological treatment of adolescent substance abuse. J Child Adol Psychopharmacol 5:93–106, 1995.
202. L Semlitz. Adolescent substance abuse treatment and managed care. Child Adol Psychiatric Clin N Am 5:221–241, 1996.

8
Comments on the Psychoanalytically Informed Treatment of Alcoholism

Pietro Castelnuovo-Tedesco[†]
Vanderbilt University School of Medicine
Nashville, Tennessee

INTRODUCTION

Alcoholism is a very complex clinical entity with major parameters that are biological, psychological, and social. The psychoanalytical treatment of this condition is more difficult and complex than had been imagined early in this century, in part because of the problem of identifying the truly significant factors to be addressed with each individual patient. Terms such as "alcoholic" or "substance abuser" are shorthand descriptors of individuals who chronically ingest substances that alter their mood but are toxic to them, especially over time. Unfortunately, however, these terms imply far greater homogeneity and similarity among those so afflicted than is the case. The reverse, in fact, is true: there is *always* a diagnostic problem. The range of psychopathology found in these conditions is considerable, and planning treatment appropriate for the individual must take this into account. The treatment also varies considerably. Terms such as "alcoholism" and "alcoholic" are used in this chapter only because they are quick referents to complex and, in many ways, diverse problems. It is also fitting to mention here that the colloquially used "drinking problem" and its more technical-sounding equivalent "substance abuse" are

---

[†]Deceased.

not only attempts to avoid the stigma attached to the term alcoholism; they also strive to convey that this is not a unitary, easily describable entity.

The purpose of this chapter is to review the changes that have occurred in the psychoanalytical treatment of alcoholics as advances in psychoanalytical theory have contributed to modifications in approach and technique. My purpose is also to highlight some clinical issues that, in my experience, warrant special attention.

THE "CLASSICAL" PSYCHOANALYTICAL LITERATURE

The psychoanalytical literature on the treatment of alcoholism, although not large, is indicative of the important changes that have taken place over time.

In the early decades of psychoanalysis, several papers appeared that explored the personality structure of the alcoholic and the potential benefits of the recently introduced psychoanalytical approach (1–3). The emphasis at that time was on the drive disturbances in alcoholism, particularly on the significance of the oral drives, on the relationship to homosexuality, and on the capacity of alcohol to alter both mood and drive expression and to modulate the emotional status of the drinker.

These contributions were of great significance because they helped to identify key personality characteristics and the role of conflict in the alcoholic disorder, but they did not yet provide a sufficient picture of the personality as a whole, particularly of the subtler aspects of ego functioning that concern the maintenance of internal homeostasis and self-esteem. Most of all, they did not convey an adequate sense of the fragility of the alcoholic patient. The tone of these early contributions, rather, was positive and confident, taking the position that the new treatment—psychoanalysis—which could clarify the typically occurring conflicts, offered a major advance in the management and treatment of the patient. These papers upheld the fundamental psychoanalytical strategy—that a neutral, passive stance could be applied to the treatment of this condition, just as it was already being applied to other disorders.

MODIFICATION OF PSYCHOANALYTICAL METHODS FOR TREATMENT OF ALCOHOLISM AND THE EMERGENCE OF ALCOHOLICS ANONYMOUS

Initially, little consideration was given to the possibility that *unmodified* psychoanalytical treatment might be unsuitable for most alcoholic patients. By

Psychoanalytically Informed Alcoholism Treatment

the late 1930s, however, experience with "classical" psychoanalytical treatment of alcoholics had proven less than consistently encouraging and there was increasing realization—mainly through the work of Robert Knight (4,5), who contributed so much to our understanding of borderline patients—that most alcoholics required a special and modified psychoanalytical approach, with emphasis on supportive and interactive maneuvers. In the 1950s a new approach to treatment, that of Alcoholics Anonymous (AA), came to the fore and quickly asserted itself by its capacity to provide sustained help to many patients who had failed to benefit from other methods. This approach, which stressed the achievement of abstinence and a radical change in the alcoholic's *behavior* through group participation, was very different from the one offered by psychoanalysis, which emphasized instead the resolution of distressed *feelings* and unresolved conflicts in the context of individual therapy. At first these two approaches, psychoanalysis and AA, largely ignored each other and went their separate ways. During subsequent decades, however, an effort was made to study whether the two methods might in some way be integrated. It also became apparent that the results of even modified psychoanalytical treatment were quite variable and that significant complications (particularly, these patients' proneness to serious regressions) were not infrequent. This led Vaillant (6), for example, to raise the question whether psychoanalytical treatment might actually be contraindicated. In the debate that followed (6–8), some took the view that psychoanalytical treatment might disclose the essential psychopathology, making it more evident by unraveling fragile defenses instead of helping to resolve it.

Concurrently, psychoanalytical writings began to reflect increasing awareness of the other method of treatment, AA. AA, coming from a very different direction, was based on the empirical finding that the successful treatment of alcoholism depended on the achievement of sobriety. By means of group membership and peer pressure, positive encouragement, attention to spiritual values, and the establishment of strict expectations of abstinence, the alcoholic was helped to gradually free himself of his dependence on alcohol. The specific goal of this approach was continued abstinence. Yet, at the same time, AA also acknowledged that the alcoholic was prone to relapses and that indeed these were to be expected and anticipated as a characteristic—and in many cases inevitable—part of the disorder. Whereas the psychoanalytical approach looked on alcoholism as a symptomatic expression of intrapsychic conflict, AA was based on the view that alcoholism is a disease. As is true of many other diseases (diabetes, for example), the only possible goal of treatment for alcoholism, given the current state of knowledge, was to contain its symptomatic expressions rather than "cure" its root cause. From the AA perspective, an alcoholic will always be an alcoholic, although it is hoped an abstinent and sober one (most of the time). The question whether alcoholism really fits the "disease" label also was addressed (9), but this is of less importance than more practical issues. As Mack (7) and others have pointed out, the "disease concept" of alcoholism—regardless of its scientific merit—helps to alleviate the alcoholic's sense of failure and his guilt over his addiction. The patient is not held responsible for his addiction, only for his efforts to control it (just as the diabetic is made responsible for taking insulin). On the other hand, a complaint against the psychoanalytical approach is that it may increase the burden on the patient. Through its emphasis on conflicts, it may increase the patient's responsibility for trying to resolve these conflicts before he is ready. Responsibility, in short, may be given too soon and sometimes a "moment" is all it takes to unravel the patient.

For this reason, the analytically oriented therapist must at all times pay close attention to the tasks the patient is currently facing in treatment and consider whether those demands may be too difficult for the patient, especially given his habitual resorting to evasion of feelings and responsibilities by numbing out in drink. For example, a patient who felt trapped and frustrated in a miserable marriage wished to seek a divorce but was unable to act on this because of his own enormous dependency and his wife's insistence that the marriage be "saved." The conflict remained very active and unresolved, creating barely disguised rage and a serious impasse in treatment. Finally, the patient achieved a reprieve from this increasingly untenable situation by going on an alcoholic binge that resulted in his being hospitalized in another city. In this way, the patient achieved a long-term, *de facto* separation from his wife. He also effectively interrupted his psychotherapy, postponing it till a later date.

Today there is wide recognition of the merits of the AA approach, even among psychoanalytical psychotherapists. It has proved effective for many alcoholics and, being free of charge, it has also been applicable to those who otherwise would not be able to afford adequate treatment for their addiction. AA's 12 Steps program has offered clear rules and procedures for the management of this disorder (10).

THE THERAPEUTIC RELATIONSHIP DURING ALCOHOLISM TREATMENT

I now highlight some characteristics of alcoholic patients that are in one sense well known, but that probably have not been sufficiently emphasized in discussions of how these individuals perform in analytically oriented psychotherapy. I am referring to their tendency to alcoholic relapses and to evoking

Psychoanalytically Informed Alcoholism Treatment

disappointment in those (including physicians) who care about them and are trying to be helpful to them. In working with alcoholic patients, one learns how fragile the therapeutic relationship is and how it remains vulnerable to sudden episodes of regression. This tendency to abrupt disruption is true even in those who have been in treatment for an extended period of time and appear to be doing well.

A striking clinical pattern presents itself again and again: the patient unexpectedly misses appointments or even withdraws from treatment because of an alcoholic episode, perhaps to return weeks or months later. During the patient's extended absences the therapist often will not hear a word from the patient, although occasionally he may receive a brief phone call. Superficially, the call may deal with a peripheral matter (e.g., the refilling of a prescription), but its main purpose is to renew contact. Even when there are no phone calls, the therapist often has the sense that the therapeutic relationship has been put "on hold" but not severed. The therapist's countertransference tells him that a part of the patient remains attached to him, that the work of therapy is unfinished, and that sooner or later he will see the patient again—of course, he does not know when that will be. In time this surmise often proves correct. Without notice, the patient phones and, often without explanation, asks for an appointment. The patient takes for granted that the therapist will understand and make time for him. The patient keeps this appointment and typically dives into his current problems but gives little information about what has taken place in the intervening period, almost as if there had been no interruption. Soon it becomes apparent whether the patient has come simply to "check out" the therapist (to see if the latter is in good health and well disposed toward the patient) or whether the patient consciously plans to resume treatment on a regular basis. In either case, this is a moment when the relationship is reaffirmed and consolidated.

This phenomenon of unexpected disappearance and return is one that we have also commonly heard about in the analysis of patients who have alcoholic relatives. For example, patients who had an alcoholic father often recall how the latter suddenly left the family when the children were small and did not reappear until years later. Another frequently described manifestation is the atmosphere of unreliability that surrounds the alcoholic parent; this in turn creates in the children a state of suspense and anxiety. What would happen next? When would father/mother "go off"? Would there be dire consequences (such as physical abuse, severe disappointments, or embarrassments)? What would one do then? Would there be money to live on? A common finding, in short, is a palpable deficit in the alcoholic's capacity to invest himself in his family and act consistently toward them. Even in cases where the alcoholic parent did not actually absent himself, his alcoholism inevitably created a barrier between child and parent that evoked in the child significant feelings of abandonment. Moreover, often the child is thrust into a premature caretaking role and must put aside his own needs to attend to those of the parent. In short, the constant uncertainty of the relationship with an alcoholic relative is something that is described over and over again and may appear so commonplace (and be so regarded by the patient who tells the story) that its special significance is often missed. These patients *expect* to be let down and have difficulty believing in the consistency of a good analytical therapist.

PSYCHODYNAMIC SIGNIFICANCE OF "ACTING OUT"

Associated with these "disappearances" are outbursts of rage and other manifestations of regression that prompt the alcoholic to engage in behavior that is simultaneously damaging to his own social standing and reputation and very painful to those who care about him and his well-being. What stands out about these episodes is the intensity of the alcoholic's rage and rebelliousness, which during periods of sobriety are usually disguised by a façade of blandness or bonhomie. The alcoholic plainly has no adequate way of expressing anger except through profound periodic explosion-like regressions which take the form of intense and destructive acting out. Although some alcoholics appear voluble and gregarious, these characteristics are defensive. Alcoholics typically have great difficulty expressing their emotions in words. The term alexithymia has been applied by some to this phenomenon (11,12). A patient of mine, for example, related circumstances that must have been painful, distressing, and anxiety-provoking in a bland and offhand way. When I tried to bring this to his attention, he sometimes responded with a slightly contemptuous half-smile and almost a shrug.

The difficulty with emotional expression, however, is not limited to simple verbal communication. Often one becomes aware of the alcoholic's tendency to prevaricate, to hide crucial information, and to misrepresent the actual status of a situation or relationship. This is particularly true concerning the extent of his drinking—a circumstance frequently referred to as alcoholic denial. This may occur in such a subtle way that it takes a while for the therapist to reach the conclusion that things have become as serious as indeed they are. These trends enormously complicate treatment; ultimately it becomes apparent, through the transference, that the patient treats the analyst in the same way that he has treated others. There are, in short, pervasive difficulties in the realm of object relations which, together with the patient's proneness to drastic regressions, form the core of the alcoholic's difficulties.

This is a brief sketch of a problem that stands out as a special challenge to treatment. The personal and social pathology that affects the alcoholic is much broader than one might at first imagine, as Blum (13) has demonstrated in her thorough and detailed review of the psychoanalytical literature on alcoholism.

COUNTERTRANSFERENCE, OR THE CASE OF THE DISAPPEARING PATIENT

The reason for dwelling on these characteristics of alcohol-dependent patients is that during psychoanalytical treatment they inevitably manifest themselves as important facets of the transference. The transference of the alcoholic patient is complex, often opaque, and consistently marked by latently hostile thoughts and feelings that are not easily identified or accessible to interpretation. Even if they are correctly identified and skillfully and compassionately interpreted, the patient may have difficulty in connecting emotionally with the meaning of these interpretations. The patient's behavior is also punctuated from time to time by frank alcoholic outbursts that express great rage, impatience, and despair. The patient demonstrates (as an expression of his anal struggles) a wish to "mess up," both literally and metaphorically, and to injure, provoke, and disappoint the therapist, among others. The therapist, in his countertransference, senses that he is being attacked and may, in turn, feel inclined to respond punitively or, at least, defensively. In this context, he may discharge the patient as incapable of responding to treatment. The patient may also create a situation that is so extreme (involving, for example, prolonged hospitalization or incarceration) that, even when the therapist makes exceptional efforts, a consistent program of psychotherapy becomes impossible. The opacity and diffuseness of the patient's reactions—which severely challenge the therapist's wish to be helpful—stimulate his disappointment (in a setting that calls instead for understanding and forbearance) and make it difficult for therapy to continue. These problems pervade the treatment of the alcoholic patient. This instability of key object relationships is a characteristic that alcoholics share with those with some severe personality disorders, particularly borderlines, who likewise have special difficulty containing their anger. Other similarities to borderline personality disorder are the self-destructive and suicidal aspects of chronic alcoholism and in the patients' being prone to violent eruptions. These manifestations, however, cannot be explained simply as an expression of severe psychopathology. Other very troubled individuals (e.g., chronic schizophrenics, passive-dependent or schizoid personalities, severe neurotics, and those with psychosomatic disorders) become very attached to their therapists, often in a stable and seemingly permanent way.

My purpose is to highlight the features that I consider central to the pathology of alcoholic patients and then return to the question of how to maximize the utility of psychoanalytical understanding and psychoanalytically informed treatment. It is important that the therapist be especially aware that the therapeutic relationship is remarkably fragile and that exceptional care must be taken not to disturb the delicate alliance with comments or other behavior that the patient may perceive as unempathic, rejecting, or critical. As a general rule, I believe it is desirable to deal interpretatively with the hostile elements of the transference insofar as this is possible. Yet one must also keep in mind that, given the vagaries of the negative transference in very disturbed personalities, rageful and intransigent feelings will often flood the therapeutic relationship and make the situation very difficult and occasionally unmanageable. In this group of patients, these episodes usually take the form of alcoholic acting out. The fact that this happens, despite the analyst's best efforts, tends to increase his sense of futility and discouragement. One must be prepared for this, to the extent that one can, by understanding this problem and recognizing how likely it is to arise.

PSYCHOANALYTICAL APPROACHES AND ALCOHOLICS ANONYMOUS MAY BE COMPLEMENTARY

Another question that for some is still unresolved is whether treatment by the methods of AA can be combined with analytical psychotherapy or whether the two are mutually exclusive. Experience over the past two decades has reaffirmed that the two modalities can be successfully combined (8,9), each making a special contribution. Participation in AA is especially helpful during the early phases of treatment when the achievement of sobriety is a primary goal. Throughout the course of treatment, AA is of assistance by helping the alcoholic to confront the denial of his disturbance and to recognize the need for sustained efforts at abstinence. Depending on the nature of the case, analytical psychotherapy can be usefully introduced either from the very beginning of treatment or later, when the patient's recovery has stabilized somewhat. It is important to keep in mind the central truth that analytical psychotherapy is the modality most likely to help resolve the patient's internal conflicts and severe life dilemmas. In the milder cases—classified by Knight (5) as "reactive" alcoholics, in whom the ego is reasonably strong and not excessively warped—analytical psychotherapy may function effectively as the only treatment. On the other hand, the most severe cases—those whom Knight (5) called "essential" alcoholics, characterized by predominant oral-level fixations and a striking lack of real-life accomplishments—may be best treated by AA methods alone. In psychotherapy, these patients' egos may not be strong enough to deal with the conflicts that are inevitably mobilized.

Clearly, then, choice of treatment is not a matter that can be decided casually; it depends on careful assessment of the patient's psychological strengths and vulnerabilities. For example, psychotherapy, in contrast to AA with its strong inspirational/suppressive/supportive components, may not be able to provide a structure that sufficiently contains the patient. Nonetheless, in persons who have been effectively treated with AA methods alone (i.e., without formal psychotherapy), one often finds that a distinct rigidity of personality has settled in. The patient has successfully remained abstinent, but significant emotional problems are still evident and have not been addressed. There is often a phobic avoidance of alcohol and an obsessive investment of great time and energy in the affairs of AA. Sometimes this is the best that one can hope for, and it should be accepted as a very satisfactory outcome in these cases of severe disturbance. In the less severe cases, it is possible to strive for personal growth and for something more profound than sustained abstinence. One may be able to achieve through analytical psychotherapy a significant modification of the alcoholic's conflicts and struggles and the restoration of greater plasticity and flexibility to his personality.

In short, AA and analytical psychotherapy are not mutually exclusive but can be complementary. Each therapeutic approach, at its best, has contributions to make. AA offers the achievement of sustained sobriety, a reduction in the individual's often profound guilt over his drinking and tendency to "mess up," a place of refuge, and a sense of communion, encouragement, and support in the context of a group of individuals who are similarly afflicted; this can lead to a softening of the harshness of the superego as a consequence of a benign identification with the group. All these factors help to contain and diminish feelings of loneliness, isolation, rage, and despair. By helping the alcoholic accept his limitations in his capacity to handle alcohol, AA offers him a life that is safer and more protected than what otherwise would be his lot.

Psychoanalytical therapy of the alcoholic patient helps to promote self-understanding, strengthening of the ego's coping capacities, amelioration of pathogenic and cruelly destructive wishes, the development of innate talents and abilities, and the pursuit of relationships that are both more stable and more fulfilling. These may permit the alcoholic to enjoy a degree of happiness and achievement previously denied to him.

REFERENCES

1. Abraham K. The psychological relation between sexuality and alcoholism [1908]. In: Selected Papers of Karl Abraham. New York: Basic Books, 1960.
2. Brill, AA. Alcohol and the individual. NY Med J 109:928–930, 1919.
3. Radó S. The psychoanalysis of pharmacothymia (drug addiction). Psychoanal Q 2:1–23, 1933.
4. Knight RP. The dynamics and treatment of chronic alcoholic addiction. Bull Menninger Clin 1:233–250, 1937.
5. Knight RP. The psychodynamics of chronic alcoholism. J Nerv Ment Disord 86:538–548, 1937.
6. Vaillant GE. Dangers of psychotherapy in the treatment of alcoholism. In: Dynamic Approaches to the Understanding and Treatment of Alcoholism. MH Bean, NE Zinberg, eds. New York: Free Press, 1981.
7. Mack JE. Alcoholism, A.A., and the governance of the self. In: Dynamic Approaches to the Understanding and Treatment of Alcoholism. MH Bean, NE Zinberg, eds. New York: Free Press, pp 128–162, 1981.
8. Dodes LM. The psychology of combining dynamic psychotherapy and Alcoholics Anonymous. Bull Menninger Clin 52:283–293, 1988.
9. Fingarette H. Heavy Drinking. The Myth of Alcoholism as a Disease. Berkeley, CA: University of California Press, 1988.
10. Alcoholics Anonymous World Services. Twelve Steps and Twelve Traditions. New York: Alcoholics Anonymous World Services, 1952.
11. Krystal H. Alexithymia and psychotherapy. Am J Psychother 33:17–31, 1979.
12. Krystal H. Alexithymia and the effectiveness of psychoanalytic treatment. Int J Psychoanal Psychother 9:353–388, 1982–1983.
13. Blum EA. Psychoanalytic views of alcoholism: a review. Q J Stud Alcohol 27:297–299, 1966.

9
Cardiovascular Disease and Substance Use Disorders

Robert P. Albanese, Jr., and W. Blake Haren
*Medical University of South Carolina
and Ralph H. Johnson VA Medical Center
Charleston, South Carolina*

John R. Hubbard*
*Vanderbilt University Medical School
and Nashville VA Medical Center
Nashville, Tennessee*

INTRODUCTION

Coronary artery disease is the leading cause of death in Western societies, and its prevalence in rural/agrarian cultures is increasing rapidly as sedentary lifestyles and other Western influences grow. In the United States, about one-third of individuals who have a heart attack do not make complete recovery, and coronary heart disease is the number 1 cause of disability in the U.S. labor force. Stroke is the third leading cause of death in America, behind heart disease and cancer (1). Because substance-related disorders are 1) also very common and debilitating and 2) believed to be associated with cardiovascular disease, it is worthwhile to review the influence of alcohol and drugs of abuse on cardiovascular health.

---

*Currently in private practice.

Substances with abuse potential are quite numerous and a single drug may appear in various forms. Therefore, we limit our discussion to four of the most important substances of abuse in social and economic terms: ethanol, cocaine, cannabis, and opiates (2).

ETHANOL

Alcohol is the most widely abused substance in the United States and in the world. In 1997, about 32 million Americans engaged in binge drinking, and approximately 11 million Americans (over 5% of the population) were heavy drinkers (2). Ethanol is rather unique among substances of abuse in that it is legal to consume in most countries, and also because there is evidence that it can have a positive *or* a negative effect on cardiovascular health, depending on the dose and the physiology of the person consuming it. A U- or J-shaped curve has been observed as the relationship between alcohol intake and the incidence of cardiovascular disease. In other words, those who abstain from alcohol have higher rates of coronary artery disease than do those who use "moderate" amounts of alcohol. Those who use alcohol heavily have significant increases in cardiovascular diseases (3).

Quantifying the cardioprotective dose of alcoholic beverages with great precision is nearly impossible because most studies are based on the subjects' estimates on dietary recall questionnaires. Therefore, the term "moderate" may not represent the same amount of alcohol in every study, may differ between genders (and other variables), and thus may be different from person to person.

Benefit of Alcohol in Cardiovascular Disease

In an early study on alcohol and coronary artery disease, Marmot et al. (3) screened 1422 middle-aged, male civil servants in and around London between 1967 and 1969 using a 3-day dietary recall format. Ten years later the investigators compared mortality rates of those who used various amounts of alcohol. Even correcting for smoking, systolic blood pressure, and serum cholesterol, the authors found the now-famous U-shaped curve. They grouped the men according to consumption of no alcohol per day, up to 9 g (approximately one alcoholic beverage) per day, 34 g (three to four beverages) per day, and over 34 g per day. Of note, the U-shaped curve was seen for all-cause mortality, with the cardiovascular death curve assigned a relative risk of 1.0 for the 0.1–9 g/day group. They found a relative risk of 1.5 for the 9.1–34-g/day group, and 0.9 for the over-34-g/day group. The abstainer group had a relative risk of death due to coronary artery disease of 2.1.

The London group, however, was not the first to publish the observation that alcohol may have a cardioprotective effect. In 1974, Klatsky, Friedman, and Siegelaub (4) published the first relatively large-scale (464 patients) epidemiological study that demonstrated a cardioprotective effect of moderate drinking (defining moderate drinking as two or fewer alcoholic beverages per day). Yano et al. (5) published in 1977 that beer (up to 60 ml per day) had a protective effect in a cohort of 7705 Japanese men living in Hawaii against death due to coronary artery disease and also nonfatal myocardial infarction.

In 1979, St. Leger (6) looked at a number of different factors with the potential to influence risk of cardiovascular disease. The most significant finding was a strong negative association between deaths due to cardiovascular disease and alcohol consumption; St. Leger and his coauthors felt that this effect was attributable entirely to the drinking of wine.

Kozararevic et al. (7), in a cohort of 11,121 men, found that alcohol consumption was inversely related to risk of death from coronary artery disease, but increased the risk of trauma and stroke in Yugoslav men aged 35–62. Their 1980 study used a complex system of estimating alcohol intake, as they were trying to equalize a number of kinds of beverages with different alcohol contents. Briefly, they found that the death rate due to heart disease among those who consumed two or more drinks per day was about half that of infrequent drinkers (less than once per week).

Most recent studies have continued to support the hypothesis that moderate consumption of alcohol reduces the risk of coronary disease. Analyzing data from the Physician's Health Study, Camargo et al. (8) examined data obtained from 21,530 male physicians between the ages of 40 and 84. While they found that drinking two or more alcohol-containing drinks per day increased the risk of death from cancer, two to six drinks per day resulted in decreased total mortality. Men who consumed two or more drinks per day had a 56% lower risk of angina and 47% lower risk for myocardial infarction. They concluded that "alcohol consumption had strong, independent, inverse associations with the risk for angina pectoris and myocardial infarction."

The salutary effects of moderate intake of red wine may explain what has been called the "French paradox," the low rates of death due to coronary artery disease among French people, who have a diet high in saturated fat (9). Only Japan has lower male cardiac death rates than France (225 per 100,000 versus 201 per 100,000), and French women have lower risk (84 per 100,000) than women of all other nationalities (10).

Still other studies suggest that it is the ethanol itself that exerts the salutary effect, and therefore any alcoholic beverage could confer benefits. Rimm (11) reviewed a number of studies in 1996 demonstrating cardiac benefit in moderate drinking. Of 12 studies looking at one or more kinds of alcoholic beverages, seven demonstrated benefits from wine drinking, seven from beer, and six showed a positive effect from consumption of "spirits."

It should be noted that there are other cardioprotective agents, such as aspirin, that may negate relative protective effect of alcohol. The interaction of other medications and/or natural agents with alcohol in cardioprotection is not well known.

Mechanism of Cardioprotection by Ethanol

As shown in Table 1, the proposed mechanisms for the cardioprotective effect of moderate alcohol consumption include decreased plasma fibrinogen, increased serum high-density lipoprotein (HDL), decreased oxidation of low-density lipoprotein (LDL), decreased platelet activity, and stress reduction (12–22).

The cardioprotective effects of alcohol may be mediated through increased antioxidant levels (15). It has been established that phenolic flavinoids, which are found in the skin of the grape (and therefore are much more plentiful in red wine), are antioxidants that inhibit the oxidation of LDL (13). LDL, in its oxidized form, is believed to be much more atherogenic. The most important flavinols in red wine are thought to be quercetin, myricetin, catechin, and epi(gallo)catechin (13).

Alcohol intake, in any form, has the effect of raising HDL levels (16). The degree to which alcohol raises HDL is not precisely known, but in one study of five nonsmoking men, HDL increased by 12.4% after 4 weeks of 50 g of alcohol per day (17). This increase in the favorable form of cholesterol is thought to appear within as little as 3 weeks, as a rule, and in general it appears in individuals who do not have hepatic damage. By damaging the liver's ability to synthesize HDL, alcoholic hepatitis would appear to negate this effect. Also, the effect does not appear to rely on the HDL subfraction.

Other possible mechanisms of reduction of coronary artery disease in the moderate or light alcohol user include antithrombotic actions and stress reduction. With regard to the former, fibrinogen levels are lowered in alco-

Table 1. Mechanisms of Cardiovascular Benefit in Moderate Alcohol Consumption

Inhibition of oxidation of low-density lipoprotein (LDL)
Increasing levels of high-density lipoprotein (HDL)
Decreasing levels of fibrinogen
Decreased platelet activity
Stress reduction

hol users (18,19), and platelets are less adherent as there is a decreased thromboxane to prostacyclin (20,21). This phenomenon is similar to the action of aspirin, which inhibits the action of thromboxane relative to prostacyclin, the former being an agent of platelet thrombus formation and the latter inhibitory (22).

Deleterious Cardiovascular Effects of Alcohol

Acute ingestion of alcohol can have many deleterious effects on the cardiovascular system and can cause noncompliance with medications. Tachycardia and elevated blood pressure are common effects of alcohol, perhaps due to vagal withdrawal. For example, Rossinen et al. (23) had 20 patients with stable exertional angina Holter-monitored while given either juice alone or juice mixed with 1.25 g of ethanol. The mean heart rate increased from 57 to 64 beats per minute, while the mean systolic blood pressures increased from 132 to 141 mm Hg.

Alcohol can also cause nonsinus arrhythmias (24). In a study by Greenspon and Schaal (25), 14 patients with a history of alcohol consumption and rhythm disturbance were given 90 ml of 80-proof whiskey. Ten of the 14 patients developed sustained or nonsustained atrial or ventricular tachydysrhythmias.

Chronic alcohol intake can lead to cardiomyopathy, leading to heart failure (26). In 1981, Matthews et al. (27) reported that of 22 asymptomatic chronic alcoholics, 15 (68%) had echocardiographic changes consistent with alcoholic cardiomyopathy.

Heart failure in the alcoholic is thought to happen in many distinct ways. Arrhythmias may precipitate heart failure, particularly atrial fibrillation, after an acute episode of alcohol ingestion. Atrial fibrillation deprives the left ventricle of the left atrial contribution to cardiac output, which can be significant in individuals who are barely compensated. Second, there is the alcoholic cardiomyopathy, the mechanism of which remains to some extent obscure. Third, nutritional deficiencies can result in conditions such as beriberi, which can have important cardiac manifestations. Fourth, contaminants can occasionally be cardiotoxic, as in the case of the outbreak of cardiomyopathy in Canada as a consequence of excessive cobalt in beer (28). Chronic hypertension, which may be related to alcohol use, leads to left ventricular hypertrophy, which can proceed to congestive heart failure. Finally, the drinker may develop "cirrhotic" cardiomyopathy. The proposed mechanisms of heart failure due to alcohol are shown in Table 2.

Alcoholic cardiomyopathy is a *dilated* cardiomyopathy and is not uncommon. Alcoholic cardiomyopathy in the absence of vascular disease and

Table 2. Mechanisms of Alcohol-Associated Heart Failure

Type of heart failure in alcoholism	Mechanism
1. Alcohol heart muscle disease	Decreased myocardial protein synthesis, free radical damage to myocardium
2. Atrial fibrillation	Decreased contribution to cardiac output from atrial contractions
3. "Wet" beriberi (thiamine deficiency)	"High-output" state with decreased systemic vascular resistance
4. Contaminant cardipmyopathy	Contaminants in alcoholic beverage directly toxic to myocardium
5. Cirrhotic cardiomyopathy	A "high-output" state similar to thiamine deficiency, featuring decreased systemic vascular resistance
6. Hypertrophic cardiomyopathy	Chronic hypertension causing left ventricular hypertrophy and diastolic dysfunction

malnutrition has been called alcohol heart-muscle disease (AHMD) (29). It is thought that ethanol exerts a dose-related toxic effect on cardiac muscle, and, as with alcoholic liver disease, women are perhaps more susceptible to this effect than men (30). There are probably a number of factors that may contribute to individual susceptibility to this phenomenon, including hypertension, smoking, established cardiac disease, disorders of the immune system, and genetic differences in alcohol metabolism (29).

The toxic effect of alcohol on the myocardium may be direct or indirect. Alcohol is metabolized to acetaldehyde, and acetaldehyde is in turn metabolized to acetate. These metabolites are thought to be cardiotoxic in their own right; for example, it has been demonstrated that both alcohol and acetaldehyde reduce the Na+,K+ -activated ATPase activities of the myocardial plasma membranes in vitro (31). They also damage other organs and cause metabolic disarray. Preedy et al. (29) demonstrated that alcohol ingestion reduces the rate of synthesis of cardiac mixed and myofibrillary proteins. They measured myocardial protein synthesis in rats 2–5 hours after intraperitoneal injections of ethanol and found a decrease of 22%.

Beriberi, or thiamine deficiency, is unusual because the vitamin is present in so many foods. It is possible in alcoholic patients, however, because alcoholism can lead to decreased dietary intake and defective absorption of the thiamine. The two disease states, thiamine deficiency and AHMD, are not identical, however. They both feature chamber dilation, tachycardia, elevated

Cardiovascular Disease

venous pressure, and peripheral edema; it is important to note, however, that the alcoholic cardiomyopathy is a low-output state, whereas beriberi is a high-output state (32). The cardiac output (stroke volume × heart rate) is elevated in beriberi because peripheral vascular dilation is prominent in the disorder, resulting in tachycardia; in alcoholic cardiomyopathy, there is depressed cardiac output due to decreased myocardial contractility (33). When thiamine deficiency occurs, there is usually a mixed clinical picture, featuring Wernicke-Korsakoff's, "wet" beriberi (congestive heart failure), and "dry" beriberi (peripheral neuropathy) (34).

There is yet another entity in the cardiomyopathy encountered in alcoholics: the so-called "cirrhotic cardiomyopathy." Like beriberi, cirrhotic cardiomyopathy is a high-output cardiac state, with increased heart rate and decreased systemic vascular resistance. It is not seen exclusively in alcoholic cirrhosis. The mechanism of this entity has not been fully elucidated, but impairment of the beta-adrenergic receptor has been proposed (35).

An ethanol intake of as little as 30–40 g/day (approximately two to four beers) can have a pressor effect. The effect abates within several days of achieving abstinence. The manner in which this effect is mediated remains obscure. Acute ingestion does not alter plasma concentrations of renin, adrenaline, noradrenalin, aldosterone, or cortisol, and there is no evidence of activation of the sympathetic nervous system (36). It is possible that in some heavy drinkers who are chronically hypertensive, the hypertrophic, less compliant left ventricle could evidence diastolic dysfunction, indirectly leading to yet another type of heart failure.

Excessive alcohol intake can, as noted, precipitate atrial arrhythmias—*holiday heart syndrome*, a syndrome of supraventricular tachydysrhythmias classically caused by a period of heavy alcohol use, usually manifests itself as an acute-onset episode of atrial fibrillation (38). Typically the atrial fibrillation reverts spontaneously to sinus rhythm within 24 hours. Other rhythm disturbances seen in this setting include atrial flutter, premature atrial contractions, and junctional tachycardia.

Ethanol is a common cause of secondary hypertriglyceridemia, usually a Type IV or V hyperlipidemia. It is second only to diabetes mellitus as a cause of hypertriglyceridemia (16). Moderate users usually have significantly higher triglyceride levels than abstainers. Withdrawal of alcohol leads to a rapid decrease in triglyceride levels. HDL levels are also elevated in ethanol users, such that elevations in HDL, triglycerides, and GGT are virtually diagnostic for alcohol use (39).

In drinkers, partial sleep apnea may be converted to total sleep apnea, especially if they consume alcohol in the evening hours. Sleep apnea can result in chronic hypoxemia and hypercapnea, with respiratory acidosis and polycythemia. These conditions can in turn lead to pulmonary vasoconstriction and pulmonary hypertension (40). Pulmonary hypertension can in time lead to right-heart failure with hepatic congestion and lower-extremity edema.

There is evidence that long-term exposure to alcohol can result in a Cushingoid appearance with central obesity, plethora, striae, and hypertension. It has been called "alcohol-induced pseudo-Cushing's syndrome" (41). Hypertension, no matter what the cause, is one of the most important risk factors for coronary artery disease.

The question of whether alcohol is contributory or causative in cerebral infraction is complicated by the fact that a high percentage of heavy drinkers are also smokers. The evidence that alcohol alone may precipitate stroke is overwhelming, but evidence exists for alcohol acting in combination with other factors to cause cerebral infarction (42). You et al. (43) found the odds ratios for cerebral infarction to be 11.6 for diabetes, 6.8 for hypertension, 2.7 for heart disease, 2.5 for smoking, 15.3 for long-term heavy drinking (greater than or equal to 60 g ethanol or four to five beers per day). These findings were in 201 first-stroke patients aged 15–55 years. For ischemic stroke, alcohol appears to demonstrate the J-shaped curve, indicating that moderate users have lower risk of stroke than abstainers and heavy users. By contrast, the influence on risk of hemorrhagic stroke is an increase with increasing consumption throughout the spectrum of usage patterns (44). In 1996 Camargo (45) published a review of the epidemiological data, concluding that while alcohol exhibited a J-shaped curve with respect to effect on ischemic stroke, and increased the risk of hemorrhagic stroke at all usage levels, the overall effect is to inhibit stroke, since 80% of strokes are ischemic.

Alcohol may contribute to the risk of stroke by several mechanisms. First is the well-known pressor effect of alcohol. Alcoholics may also develop deep venous thromboses (prolonged stasis), which may embolize to the brain if the patient has a communicating defect of the heart, especially ventricular septal defect (VSD). Alcohol has been demonstrated to activate the clotting cascade in vitro (42), although in vivo the effect is likely to be invisible to lower dosages. We have already noted that alcoholic cardiomyopathy is a *dilated* cardiomyopathy, and in such patients mural thrombi are not uncommon. "Holiday heart" dysrhythmias include atrial fibrillation, usually transient; such patients may form small atrial thrombi while their atria are fibrillating, and when the dysrhythmia resolves the thrombi are embolized (46).

Other possible mechanisms of brain infarction include infectious vasculopathies associated with alcohol use, obstructive sleep apnea caused by or worsened by alcohol, and hypoxia due to alcohol-induced vasoconstriction.

Table 3. Mechanisms of Stroke Due to Alcohol

Alcohol-induced hypertension
Embolic phenomena
Alcohol-induced coagulopathy
Dysrhythmias
Infectious vasculopathies
Trauma to vascular structures

Finally, trauma is common in intoxicated individuals; according to U.S. Department of Justice statistics, 40.9% of traffic fatalities are alcohol-related and 40% of violent offenders report drinking at the time of the offense (47). Physical assaults and motor vehicle accidents may result in direct damage to arteries, provoking arterial dissection, including of the carotids. Such injuries reduce flow and may have thrombosis and/or embolus as a result of intimal injury (42,46,48). Trauma to the cranium may also result in intracranial hemorrhage as a result of shear injury on intracranial vascular structures. Mechanisms of stroke due to alcohol are shown in Table 3.

Alcohol, especially red wine, has been suspected to be a causative agent in dietary migraine (49). Littlewood et al. (50) disguised red wine and vodka in appearance and taste, and challenged red-wine-sensitive migraineurs (keeping alcohol content equal); they found that nine of 11 of those who received red wine developed migraines but none of the eight vodka recipients did. Proposed mechanisms include stimulation of this release of serotonin (51), which is thought to be a precipitator of migraines, and inhibition of monoamine oxidase, which would increase 5-HT levels. Of note, in Littlewood's study, the diluted red wine had "negligible tyramine content." Jarman, Glover and Sandler (52) demonstrated that serotonin was released from platelets exposed to red wine, but not those exposed to white wines or beer.

Overall, the cardioprotective effect of alcohol at certain doses must be put into context of the general risk/benefit to patients. Alcohol is the most common substance of abuse dependence, causes many accidents, and has direct deleterious effects such as CNS toxicity.

COCAINE

Cocaine, or benzoylmethylecgonine [$C_{17}H_{21}NO_4$], is an alkaloid extract from the leaves of the coca plant (*Erythroxylon coca*). Cocaine has been associated with myocardial infarction, cardiac dysrhythmia, and cerebrovascular disease, including intracranial hemorrhage. The drug has two forms: cocaine HCl, which is water-soluble and used intranasally and intravenously, and the "freebase" form, also known as "crack." In 1997, an estimated 1.5 million Americans were current cocaine users (2).

The most common cocaine-associated complaint among patients who present to emergency rooms is chest pain (53). In a study by Counselman et al. (54), 24 of 40 patients presenting to the emergency room with cocaine-related complaints had chest pain; the primary finding of the study was that a majority (53%) of those patients had an elevated CPK, although none of the patients had a myocardial infarction. Although most cocaine-associated chest pain does not usually appear to be ischemic (55), myocardial infarction is not an uncommon cardiac consequence of cocaine abuse. The mechanism of cocaine-induced cardiac disease is not completely understood.

Cocaine blocks the reuptake of norepinephrine and dopamine by presynaptic adrenergic neurons. It is therefore a sympathomimetic and is dopaminergic in the CNS (56). Dopaminergic activity is centrally augmented by enhanced release of dopamine (57), and cocaine increases the central stimulation of the adrenal medulla, increasing the release of sympathetic amines (58). Elevated levels of circulating catecholamines are thought to contribute to medial thickening and intimal hyperplasia of arteries throughout the body and also to cause premature atherosclerosis (59). Case reports support this observation (60,64,68). Many of the case reports of sudden cardiac death are in young patients who have few, if any, risk factors for coronary artery disease. This observation supports the hypothesis that cocaine adversely affects the myocardial oxygen supply/demand ratio or could possibly be arrhythmogenic per se (61).

The central dopaminergic effects of cocaine probably explain the psychosis so frequently associated with ongoing abuse of the drug. Paranoia is typical (62). The paranoid psychological state is an anxious or agitated one; psychological anxiety coupled with the sympathomimetic autonomic (increase in rate pressure product) action of cocaine would account for a significant increase in myocardial oxygen demand. In an individual with compromised myocardial blood supply, because of either cocaine itself or underlying coronary artery disease, a high level of anxiety or agitation could provoke ischemia and infarction.

Intimal hyperplasia, thrombus formation, and premature coronary atherosclerosis have been demonstrated in postmortem examinations and case reports (63–65). Cocaine may be thrombogenic by way of increasing circulating levels of epinephrine and serotonin, and also by increasing the release of thromboxane A2 (66). Some scientists have proposed that still another mechanism of diminished coronary artery perfusion could be vasospasm, and it has been demonstrated in vitro and in vivo that cocaine increases the endothelial cell release of endothelin (a vasoconstrictor) in arterial tissue (67). Vasospasm appears to be the primary action of cocaine in the approximately 18 case reports of mesenteric ischemia due to the drug (68). Sullivan et al. (69) demonstrated decreased digital blood flow in cocaine-exposed white males, the duration of the effect being dose-dependent. The mechanisms of cardiac ischemia in cocaine users are shown in Table 4.

Because of a number of case reports of cocaine in relation to sudden cardiac death, many believe that cocaine is intrinsically arrhythmogenic. The evidence is mostly from case reports and animal models. Kanani et al. (70) showed that in dogs cocaine infusions widened the QRS complex and lowered the ventricular fibrillation threshold, and that the effect was inhibited by a dopamine antagonist; these results could imply that the effect is dopamine-mediated (70). In dogs cocaine actually *increased* the ventricular fibrillation threshold, but found delayed conduction (70,71). Perera, Kraebber, and Schwartz (72) reported the case of a 17-year-old girl who, in the setting of a binge on cocaine, developed a prolonged QT interval that subsequently normalized. It is not absolutely necessary to invoke a special arrhythmogenicity to explain dysrhythmias in the cocaine user, however, because ischemia is in itself arrhythmogenic.

Although the relationship between cocaine and stroke has not been conclusively proven, there are numerous case reports in the literature, and some retrospective studies indicate that there is a correlation (73). Herning et al. (74) measured cerebral blood flow in cocaine users and found that, in middle and anterior cerebral arteries, flow was significantly decreased in the cocaine users compared to controls; there was only partial normalization with abstinence. As with other cocaine-associated ischemic phenomena, vasospasm appears to be the most important mechanism (75,76). Intracranial hemorrhage

Table 4. Mechanisms of Cardiac Ischemia in Cocaine Users

Decreased supply	Increased demand
Intimal proliferation of arterial walls	Noradrenergic increase in blood pressure
Medial thickening of arterial walls	
Cocaine-induced arterial thrombus formation	Noradrenergic increase in heart rate
Cocaine-induced arrhythmia	Dopaminergic psychological agitation

is also a consequence of cocaine use, apparently occurring most often in individuals with occult vascular abnormalities (77,78).

CANNABIS

Marijuana, a substance prepared from the *Cannabis sativa* plant, is by far the most commonly used illicit drug in the United States. In 1997, approximately 11 million Americans were current marijuana/hashish users (about 5% of the population) (2).

Many individuals, including some healthcare professionals, have come to regard cannabis as being rather benign among the substances of abuse. Aggression, disinhibition, or other problematic effects of alcohol and other drugs do not typically characterize the intoxicated state of marijuana. Furthermore, cannabinoids are increasingly perceived as having possible uses in medicine, for example, as an antinauseant, appetite stimulant (in patients with HIV), and antiglaucoma drug (79). However cannabis, particularly when smoked, has harmful effects.

Cannabis can induce significant sinus tachycardia, with resting heart rates up to and beyond 160 beats per minutes (80). The tachycardiac effect appears to be dose-related (81), and due at least in part to an increased sympathoadrenal discharge. Gash et al. (82) found elevated sympathetic neurotransmitter levels in 14 healthy men 30 minutes after smoking marijuana cigarettes; these elevations persisted for at least 2 hours. Smoking marijuana does not appear to provoke ventricular dysrhythmias, but the increased oxygen consumption can at least occasionally lead to ischemia and infarction, as noted in case reports (83–85). In fact, the influence of marijuana smoking on myocardial oxygen supply and demand my be even more deleterious than that of a similar amount of high-nicotine tobacco. Aronow and Cassidy (86) found that among habitual cigarette, but not cannabis smokers, exercise tolerance to angina was decreased more by smoking one marijuana cigarette (50%) than by smoking one high-nicotine tobacco cigarette (23%).

The action of cannabis on the heart is more complex, however. Smoking marijuana has been demonstrated not only to increase the heart rate but also to increase levels of carboxyhemoglobin. Blood-pressure responses are variable, with the typical experience being no change or a slight decrease, with orthostatic hypotension appearing at high doses (87). It is therefore not surprising that in another study of cannabis and exercise tolerance, Aronow and Cassidy (88) found that smoking cannabis decreased the anginal exercise threshold by 48%, compared with 8.6% with placebo marijuana cigarettes. Furthermore, Prakash et al. (89), in a double-blind crossover study of 10 men

Cardiovascular Disease

with stable angina pectoris, demonstrated that smoking marijuana can decrease stroke index and ejection fraction. The decrease in ejected fraction 15 minutes after smoking was approximately 18% compared with 7.5% after placebo marijuana, whereas the decreases in stroke index were approximately 29% with marijuana compared with approximately 12% with placebo marijuana.

The psychiatric effects of cannabis can also, under certain circumstances, place patients at increased risk for cardiac events. Common psychological phenomena produced by the drug include panic reactions, toxic delirium, acute paranoia, and psychosis in general (87). Individuals with compromised myocardial oxygen supply at baseline, such as those who have significant coronary artery disease, could go into negative balance in an excited state and experience the symptoms of ischemia or infarction.

Because the cardiac and pulmonary systems are so intimately associated, factors that negatively affect pulmonary oxygen delivery will have adverse consequences for the heart. Since marijuana smoke contains three times more tar than cigarette smoke and raises carboxyhemoglobin levels fivefold greater than tobacco, it is surprising that more marijuana-associated lung disease is not seen (90). Nevertheless, these phenomena could be dangerous in an individual with compromised coronary perfusion or who suffers from congestive heart failure. Patients who smoke marijuana but not tobacco probably smoke far fewer cigarettes than tobacco smokers, and patients who use cannabis tend to be younger; perhaps this is why we do not encounter more cannabis-induced myocardial infarction.

There is at least one case report in the literature of an apparent cannabis-induced dilated cardiomyopathy (91). In this case report, certain other possible causes of the cardiac disease were not definitively ruled out, as there was no biopsy or postmortem. The condition is apparently not encountered in the United States, or, if it is, it is obscured by other factors. The actions of cannabis on myocardial oxygen supply and demand are shown in Table 5.

Table 5. Actions of Cannabis on Myocardial Oxygen Supply and Demand

Supply	Demand
Increased carboxyhemoglobin	Tachycardia
Decreased ejection fraction	Agitated psychological state (panic, paranoia)
Decreased stroke index	

OPIATES AND OPIOIDS

Opiates (extracts of the opium poppy, or *Papaver somniferum*, plant such as codeine or morphine) and opioids (artificially synthesized compounds such as meperidine) are popular substances of abuse that can be found in a number of different forms. Many opiates/opioids are important pain medications, that can be used for appropriate purposes, but can also be abused. Others, such as heroin, are currently used in the United States for recreational use only. Opiates and opioids vary considerably in anesthetic effectiveness, duration, and risk of abuse/dependence. Heroin has been called "semisynthetic" because it is a chemically altered form of a natural opiate; it is an acetylated morphine molecule. In 1997, there were 325,000 reported heroin users in the United States, but the National Household Survey on Drug Abuse (NHDSA) has estimated the true number to be closer to 400,000 (2).

Heterogeneity in route of administration is even more characteristic of this group of drugs than it is of cocaine. They can be consumed orally (prescription pain relievers), smoked (opium), or injected, sniffed, and snorted (heroin).

As may be the case with alcohol, there is a therapeutic role for the opiate in the area of cardiac disease. Patients who present to emergency departments with chest pain are typically treated with morphine, which decreases pain and anxiety. For patients with congestive heart failure, it is particularly helpful in decreasing air hunger and increasing venous capacitance, lessening the load on the overburdened left ventricle.

In a study designed to discern the mechanism of opiate-mediated venodilation in humans, Grossman et al. (92) constricted the hand veins of their subjects with infusions of phenylephrine. Then they infused morphine, which stimulates histamine release from mast cells, and fentanyl, which does not stimulate histamine release but does have affinity for μ-opiate receptors. They found that morphine precipitated venodilation but fentanyl did not. Furthermore, they found that the effect was negated by coinfusion of histamine-blocking agents, and only partially antagonized by coinfusion of naloxone (92).

The *direct* cardiac effects of heroin have been studied in vitro. In 1991, Peterna et al. (93) perfused rabbit hearts with heroin or morphine and compared them with controls. They found no changes in creatine phosphokinase, lactate dehydrogenase, heart rate, systolic ventricular pressure, or diastolic ventricular pressure. There were also no changes in coronary blood flow (93). These findings were similar to those of Nawrath et al. (94), who found that morphine and ethylketocyclazocine did not affect excitation and contraction

Cardiovascular Disease

in isolated ventricular heart muscle from guinea pigs, rabbits, and humans. Pons-Llado et al. (95) performed echocardiographic examinations on 68 asymptomatic heroin users and compared them with 41 normal controls. Of the heroin users, none had had an episode of clinical endocarditis. They found more valvular abnormalities in the heroin group, but no changes in morphological or functional parameters of myocardium.

Heroin overdose has been associated with abnormal electrocardiograms. In a study of 25 acutely overdosed heroin addicts, Glauser, Downie, and Smith (96) observed nonspecific ST-T changes, sinus tachycardia, and left and right atrial enlargement. Less common were atrial fibrillation and ventricular tachycardia. Predictably hypoxemia was common among the patients studied, and may therefore have been causative.

There are case reports and series of myocardial damage associated with rhabdomyolysis in patients who overdosed on heroin and had hypoxic coma, but the mechanism of this phenomenon is unknown. It could be due to an as yet unrecognized effect of the drug itself, or perhaps a consequence of the cellular components released in rhabdomyolysis (97,98). The evidence suggests that the cardiac effects per se of such drugs as morphine and heroin are much more likely to be indirect.

One well-known and dangerous consequence of intravenous drug use is bacterial endocarditis; what is not well known is the level of risk for this disorder in intravenous drug users. In Holland, Spijkerman et al. (99) examined data on intravenous drug users from 1986 to 1994 and found an incidence of 1.3/100 person-years of bacterial endocarditis. In these data it appeared that HIV infection and previous history of endocarditis were independent risk factors for endocarditis (99). Dressler and Roberts (100) examined hearts from necropsy in 168 opiate addicts; 40% had active endocarditis and another 8% had evidence of prior disease. These figures may be biased, however, as most of these patients died from cardiac disorders. Endocarditis in this setting is much more likely to be right-sided than in nonusers of intravenous drugs, and the organism is usually *Staphylococcus aureus* (101). The clinical picture is an abrupt-onset febrile illness, which may be accompanied by a tricuspid murmur. Pulmonary manifestations are predictably common. Fortunately it is the tricuspid valve that is most often affected; because it is the valve with the lowest pressure gradient, localized disease is unlikely to be hemodynamically significant. The prognosis is usually good (102). Left-sided endocarditis occasionally occurs in injection-drug users, and carries a worse prognosis.

Other infectious agents can be introduced via injection-drug use, such as viral hepatitides. As discussed in the section on alcohol, any cause of cirrhosis can produce cirrhotic cardiomyopathy, including viral hepatitis. Injection-drug use is one of the major routes of transmission of HIV, and cardiomyopathy has been recognized as one of the characteristics of advanced disease. Barbaro et al. (103) evaluated 952 HIV-positive patients, of whom 8% had a dilated cardiomyopathy. Sixty-three of those patients had biopsy-proven myocarditis, with the rest evidencing fibrosis. The incidence was greatest in patient with CD4 counts less than 300 and in those receiving AZT (103).

Yet another vascular complication of heroin use in noncardiogenic pulmonary edema was first described by William Osler in 1880. The exact mechanism is unknown, but apparently the use of heroin, naloxone, and even oral agents can produce this phenomenon (104). It appears to be due to changes in permeability of the pulmonary capillary bed. Since opiates and opioids decrease the sensitivity to carbon dioxide of the respiratory center of the CNS, respiratory depression is a common consequence of the use of drugs such as heroin. The "heroin overdose syndrome" consists of the triad of abnormal mental status, decreased respiration, and miotic pupils (105). In view of the respiratory depression and the fact that the noncardiogenic pulmonary edema occurs independent of route of administration, the most likely cause seems to be hypoxemia.

Among drugs of abuse, heroin is the most likely to be injected. Much of the vascular disease associated with heroin use is related to the process of injection itself. There are approximately 10 case reports of needle embolization with intravenous drug use; in one case there was a sequel of endocarditis (106). Other direct damage to blood vessels caused by injection-drug use includes septic emboli (107), mycotic aneurysms (108), microangiopathic hemolytic anemia (109), arterial embolization with tissue necrosis and gangrene (110,111), and necrotizing angiitis, a disorder with characteristics of periarteritis nodosa (112). There are case reports of pulmonary hypertension in injection-drug users, which could be due to talc microemboli (113) or multiple thromboemboli (114). Cardiac and vascular effects of opiates and opioids are listed in Table 6.

Table 6. Cardiac and Vascular Effects of Opiates and Opioids

Cardiac effects	Vascular effects
Rhabdomyolysis-associated cardiomyopathy	Histamine mediated vasodilation
	Talc emboli
Bacterial endocarditis	Thromboemboli
HIV cardiomyopathy	Septic emboli
	Noncardiogenic pulmonary edema
	Necrotizing angitis

CONCLUSIONS

Alcohol is the most commonly abused substance in the world, and in the Unites States the three most commonly encountered illegal drugs are cannabis, cocaine, and heroin. The detrimental effects of these drugs on cardiovascular and neurovascular health are only partially understood; there is reason to be concerned that their effects could be synergistic. It is known, for example, that in the presence of ethanolemia, cocaine is metabolized to cocaethylene, a metabolite that is more potent and longer-acting than the parent substance (115). It has also been suggested that the tachycardiac effects of cocaine and cannabis are additive (47). Chambers et al. (116) found that there seemed to be an especially increased risk of endocarditis in patients who injected cocaine—most of those patients "speedball," that is, inject cocaine and heroin simultaneously. There could therefore be a synergy of risk for the infection when cocaine and heroin are used together. In clinical experience we frequently encounter patients who use various combinations of these agents simultaneously.

It is intuitive that a measurable economic impact could be discerned in the relationship between cardiac diseases and substance use disorders. Examining Medicare data, Ingster and Cartwright (117) found that among patients hospitalized with cardiac conditions, comorbid substance use disorders increased hospital length of stay. They noted that the time of hospitalization was increased by 51% for the elderly and 61% for the disabled, represented by an increase in cost of $174,498,071 in 1987 (117).

We do not fully understand the interactions between substance abuse and cardiovascular disease. It is possible that where one exists, the other is frequently present but not diagnosed. A generation of Americans who established new limits in recreational substance abuse is reaching late middle age; if their use patterns follow them, we would do well to know how they interact with established risk factors for various types of cardiovascular disease.

REFERENCES

1. American Heart Association. 1999 Heart and Stroke Statistical Update.
2. Department of Health and Human Services. Preliminary Results from the 1997 National Household Survey on Drug Abuse.
3. Marmot MG, Rose G, Shipley MJ, Thomas BJ. Alcohol and mortality: a U-shaped curve. Lancet i(8220 Pt 1):580–583, 1981.
4. Klatsky AL, Friedman GD, Siegelaub AB. Alcohol consumption before myo-

cardial infarction: results from the Kaiser-Permanente epidemiologic study of myocardial infarction. Ann Intern Med 81:294–301, 1974.
5. Yano K, Rhoads GG, Kagan A. Coffee, alcohol and risk of coronary heart disease among Japanese men living in Hawaii. N Engl J Med 267(8):405–409, 1977.
6. St Leger AS, Cochrane AL, Moore F. Factors associated with cardiac mortality in developed countries with particular reference to the consumption of wine. Lancet i(8124):1017–1020, 1979.
7. Kozararevic D, McGee D, Vojvodic N, Racic Z, Dawber T, Gordon T, Zukel W. Frequency of alcohol consumption and morbidity and mortality: the Yugoslavia Cardiovascular Disease Study. Lancet i(8169):613–616, 1980.
8. Camargo CA, Stampfer MJ, Glynn RJ, Grodstein F, Graziano JM, Manson JE, Buring JE, Hennekens CH. Moderate alcohol consumption and risk for angina pectoris or myocardial infarction in us male physicians. Ann Intern Med 126:364–371, 1997.
9. Klatsky AL. Epidemiology of coronary heart disease: influence of alcohol. Alcohol Clin Exp Res 18(1):88–96, 1994.
10. 1998 World Health Organization Statistics Manual. Geneva: World Health Organization, 1998.
11. Rimm EB. Invited commentary—alcohol consumption and coronary artery disease: good habits may be more important than just good wine. Am J Epidemiol 143(11):1094–1098, 1996.
12. Ridker PM, Vaughan DE, Stampfer MJ, Glynn RJ, Hennekens CH. Association of moderate alcohol consumption and plasma concentration of endogenous tissue-type plasminogen activator. JAMA 272(12):929–933, 1994.
13. Aviram M, Hayek T, Fuhrman B. Red Wine Consumption Inhibits LDL Oxidation and Aggregation in Humans and in Atherosclerotic Mice. Amsterdam: IOS Press, 1997.
14. Fenn CG, Littleton JM. Inhibition of platelet aggregation by ethanol in vitro shows specificity for aggregating agent used and is influenced by platelet lipid composition. Thromb Haemost 48(1):49–52, 1982.
15. Wilhelmsen L, Marmot M. Ischaemic Heart Disease: Risk Factors and Prevention. In: Diseases of the Heart. Julian DG, ed. London: WB Saunders, p 921, 1996.
16. Steinberg D, Pearson TA, Kuller LH. Alcohol and atherosclerosis (Davis Conference). Ann Intern Med 114:967–976, 1991.
17. Gottrand F, Beghin L, Duhal N, Lacroix B, Bonte JP, Fruchart JC, Luc G. Moderate red wine consumption in healthy volunteers reduced plasma clearance of apolipoprotein AII. Eur J Clin Invest 29(5):387–394, 1999.
18. Ridker PM, Vaughan De, Stampfer MJ, Glynn RJ, Hennekenes CH. Association of moderate alcohol consumption and plasma concentration of endogenous tissue-type plasminogen activator. JAMA 272(12):929–933, 1994.
19. Meade TW, et al. Characteristics affecting fibrinolytic activity and plasma fibrinogen concentrations. Br Med J 1(6157):153–156, 1979.

20. Landolfi R, Steiner M. Ethanol raises prostacyclin in vivo and in vitro. Blood 64(3):679–682, 1984.
21. Mehta P, Mehta J, Lawson D, Patel S. Ethanol stimulates prostacyclin biosynthesis by human neutrophils and potentiates antiplatelet aggregatory effects of prostacyclin. Thromb Res 48(6):653–661, 1987.
22. Easton JD, Hauser SL, Martin JB. Cerebrovascular diseases. In: Harrison's Textbook of Internal Medicine [online]. McGraw-Hill, 1999.
23. Rossinen J, Partanen J, Koskinen P, Toivonen L, Kupari M, Nieminen MS. Acute heavy alcohol intake increases silent myocardial ischaemia in patients with stable angina pectoris. Heart 75(6):563–567, 1996.
24. Robertson JIS, Ball SG. Hypertension. In: Diseases of the Heart. Julian DG, ed. London: WB Saunders, p 1162, 1996.
25. Greenpon AJ, Schaal SF. The "holiday heart": electrophysiologic studies of alcohol effects in alcoholics. Ann Intern Med 98(2):135–139, 1983.
26. Sleight P. Short term and long term effects of alcohol on blood pressure, cardiovascular risk and all cause mortality. Blood Pressure 5:201–205, 1996.
27. Mathews EC Jr, Gardin JM, Henry WL, Del Negro AA, Fletcher RD, Snow JA, Esptein SE. Echocardiographic abnormalities in chronic alcoholics with and without heart failure. Am Cardiology 47(3):570–578, 1981.
28. Poole-Wilson PA. Dilated and restrictive cardiomyopathy. In: Diseases of the Heart. Julian DG, ed. London: WB Saunders, p 485, 1996.
29. Preedy V, Atkinson L, Richardson P, Peters T. Mechanisms of ethanol-induced cardiac damage. Br Heart J 69:197–200, 1993.
30. Urbano-Marquez A, Estruch R, Fernandez-Sola J, Nicolas JM, Pare JC, Rubin E. The greater risk of alcoholic cardiomyopathy and myopathy in women compared with men. JAMA 274(2):149–154, 1995.
31. Williams JW, Tada M, Katz AM, Rubin E. Effect of ethanol and acetaldehyde on the (Na+, K+)-activated adenosine triphosphatase activity of cardiac plasma membranes. Biochem Pharmacol 24:27–32, 1975.
32. Poole-Wilson PA. Chronic heart failure. In: Diseases of the Heart. Julian DG, ed. London: WB Saunders, 1996.
33. Moushmoush B, Abi-Mansour P. Alcohol and the heart. Arch Intern Med 151:36–42, 1991.
34. Wilson JD. Vitamin deficiency and excess: thiamine (beriberi). Chapter 79. In: Harrison's Textbook of Internal Medicine [online]. McGraw-Hill, 1999.
35. Ma Z, Lee SS. Cirrhotic cardiomyopathy: getting to the heart of the matter. Hepatology 24(2):451–459, 1996.
36. Robertson JIS, Ball SG. Hypertension. In: Diseases of the Heart. Julian DG, ed. London: WB Saunders, p 1144, 1996.
37. Dargie HJ, McMurray J. Heart failure: management, drug treatment and prevention. In: Diseases of the Heart. Julian DG, ed. London: WB Saunders, p 550, 1996.
38. Menz V, Grimm W, Hoffman J, Maisch B. Alcohol and rhythm disturbance: the holiday heart syndrome. Hertz 21(4):227–231, 1996.

39. Thompson GR. Pathophysiology of blood lipids. In: Diseases of the Heart. Julian DG, ed. London: WB Saunders, p 84, 1996.
40. Lipkin DP. Miscellaneous disorders and agents affecting the heart. In: Diseases of the Heart. Julian DG, ed. London: WB Saunders, p 1339, 1996.
41. Robertson JIS, Ball SG. Hypertension. In: Diseases of the Heart. Julian DG, ed. London: WB Saunders, p 1201, 1996.
42. Hillbom M, Kaste M. Alcohol abuse and brain infarction. Ann Med 22(5):347–352, 1990.
43. You RX, McNeil JJ, O'Malley HM, Davis SM, Thrift AG, Donnan GA. Risk factors for stroke due to cerebral infarction in young adults. Stroke 28(10):1913–1918, 1997.
44. Rehm J, Bondy S. Alcohol and all-cause mortality: an overview. Novartis Foundation Symposium 216:223–232; discussion 232–236, 1998.
45. Camargo CA. Case-control and cohort studies of moderate alcohol consumption and stroke. Clinica Chimica Acta 246: 107–119, 1996.
46. Hillbom M, Juvela S, Karttunen V. Mechanisms of alcohol-related strokes. Novartis Foundation Symposium 216:193–204, 1998.
47. Greenfield LA. Office of Justice Programs. Bureau of Justice Statistics. US Department of Justice, 1998.
48. Lucas C, Moulin T, Deplanque D, Tatu L, Chavot D. Stroke patterns of internal carotid artery dissection in 40 patients. Stroke 29(12):2646–2648, 1988.
49. Sandler M, Li NY, Jarrett N, Glover V. Dietary migraine: recent progress in the red (and white) wine story. Cephalagia 15(2):101–103, 1995.
50. Littlewood JT, Gibb C, Glover V, Sandler M, Davies PT, Rose FC. Red wine as a cause of migraine. Lancet i(8585):558–559, 1988.
51. Pattichis K, Louca LL, Jarman J, Sandler M, Glover V. 5-Hydroxytryptamne release from platelets by different red wines: implications for migraine. Eur J Pharmacol 292(2):173–177, 1995.
52. Jarman J, Glover V, Sandler M. Release of (14C) 5-hydroxytryptamine from human platelets by red wine. Life Sci 48(24):2297–2300, 1991.
53. Hoffman RS, Hollander JE. Evaluation of patients with chest pain after cocaine use. Crit Care Clin 12(4):809–828, 1997.
54. Counselman F, McLaughlin E, Kardon E, Bhambani-Bhavnani A. Creatine phosphokinase evaluation in patients presenting to the emergency department with cocaine-related complaints. Am J Emerg Med 15(3):221–223, 1997.
55. Feldman JA, Bui LD, Mitchell PM, Perera TB, Lee VW, Bernard SA, Fish SS. The evaluation of cocaine-induced chest pain with acute myocardial perfusion imaging. Acad Emerg Med 6(2):103–109, 1999.
56. Ritchie JM, Greene NM. Local Anesthetics. In: The Pharmacologic Basis of Therapeutics. 5th ed. Gilman AG, Goodman LS, Rall TW, et al. New York: Macmillan, pp 309–310, 1985.
57. Moore KE, Chiueh CC, Zeldes G. Release of neurotransmitters from the brain in vivo by amphetamine, methylphenidate and cocaine. In: Cocaine and Other

Stimulants. Ellinwood EH, Kilbey MM, eds. New York: Plenum, pp 143–160, 1977.
58. Chiueh CC, Kopin IJ. Centrally mediated release by cocaine of endogenous epinephrine and norepinephrine from the sympathoadrenal medullary system of the unanesthetized rats. J Pharmacol Exp Ther 205:148–154.
59. Karch SB. Cocaine toxicity by organ system. In: Pathology of Drug Abuse. 2nd ed. Karch SB, ed. Boca Raton, FL: CRC Press, 1993.
60. Wilson LD. Rapid progression of coronary artery disease in the setting of chronic cocaine abuse. J Emerg Med 16(4) 631–634, 1998.
61. Kerns W, Garvery L, Owens J. Cocaine-induced wide complex dysrhythmia. J Emerg Med 15(3):321–329, 1997.
62. Rosse RB, Collins JP Jr, Fay-McCarthy, Alim TN, Wyatt RJ, Deutsch SI. Phenomenologic comparison of the idiopathic psychosis of schizophrenia and drug-induced cocaine and phencyclidine psychoses: a retrospective study. Clin Neuropharmacol 17(4):359–369, 1994.
63. Wilson LD. Rapid progression of coronary artery disease in the setting of chronic cocaine abuse. J Emerg Med 16(4):631–634, 1998.
64. Roh LS, Hamele-Bena D. Cocaine-induced ischemic myocardial disease. Am J Forensic Med Pathol 11(2):130–135, 1990.
65. Mirzayan R, Hanks SE, Weaver FA. Cocaine-induced thrombosis of common iliac and popliteal arteries. Ann Vasc Surg 12:476–481, 1998.
66. Ellenhorn MJ, Schonwald S, Ordog G, Wassberger J, Ellenhorn S. Cocaine abuse. In: Ellenhorn's Medical Toxicology. 2nd ed. New York: Williams and Wilkins, 1997.
67. Wilbert-Lampen U, Seliger C, Zilker T, Rainer MA. Cocaine increases the endothelial release of immunoreactive endothelin and its concentrations in human plasma and urine: reversal by coincubation with sigma-receptor antagonists. Circulation 98(5):385–390, 1998.
68. Hoang MP, Lee EL, Anand A. Histological spectrum of arterial and arteriolar lesions in acute and chronic cocaine-induced mesenteric ischemia. Am J Surg Pathol 22(11):1404–1410, 1988.
69. Sullivan JT, Becker PM, Preston KL, Wise RA, Wigely FM, Testa MP, Jasinski DR. Cocaine effects on digital blood flow and diffusing capacity for carbon monoxide among chronic cocaine users. Am J Med 102:232–238, 1997.
70. Kanani PM, Guse PA, Smith WM, Barnett A, Ellinwood EH. Acute deleterious effects of cocaine on cardiac conduction, hemodynamics, and ventricular fibrillation threshold: effects on interaction with a selective dopamine d1 antagonist SCH 39166. J Cardiovasc Pharmacol 32(1)42–48, 1998.
71. Tisdale JE, Shimoyama H, Sabbah HN, Webb CR. The effect of cocaine on ventricular fibrillation threshold in the normal canine heart. Pharmacotherapy 16(3):429–437, 1996.
72. Perera R, Kraebber A, Schwartz MJ. Prolonged QT interval and cocaine use. J Electrocardiol 30(4):337–339, 1997.

73. Petitti DB, Sidney S, Quesenberry C, Berstein A. Stroke and cocaine or amphetamine use. Epidemiology 9(6):596–600, 1998.
74. Herning RI, King DE, Better W, Cadet JL. Cocaine dependence: a clinical syndrome requiring neuroprotection. Ann NY Acad Sci 825:323–327, 1997.
75. Kaufman MJ, Levin JM, Ross HM, Lange N, Rose SL, Kukes TH, Mendelson JH, Lukas SE, Cohen BM, Renshaw PF. Cocaine-induced cerebral vasoconstriction detected in humans with magnetic resonance angiography. JAMA 279(5):376–380, 1998.
76. Wallace EA, Wisniewski G, Zubal G, vanDyck GH, Pfau SE, Smith EO, Rosen MI, Sullivan MC, Woods SW, Kosten TR. Acute cocaine effects on absolute cerebral blood flow. Psychopharmacology (Berl) 128(2):17–20, 1996.
77. Fessler RD, Esshaki CM, Stankewitz RC, Johnson RR, Diaz FG. The neurovascular complications of cocaine. Surg Neurol 47(4):339–345, 1997.
78. Green RM, Kelly KM, Gabrielssen T, Levine S, Vanderzant D. Multiple intracerebral hemorrhages after smoking "crack" cocaine. Stroke 21(6):957–962, 1990.
79. Voth EA, Schwartz RH. Medicinal applications of delta-9-tetrahydrocannabinol and marijuana. Ann Intern Med 126:791–798, 1997.
80. Hanna JM, Strauss RH, Itagaki B, Kwon WJ, Stanyon R, Bindon J, Hong SK. Marijuana smoking and cold tolerance in man. Aviat Space Environ Med 47(6):634–639, 1976.
81. Johnson S, Domino EF. Some cardiovascular effects of marijuana smoking in normal volunteers. Clin Pharmacol Therapeutics 12(5):762–768, 1971.
82. Gash A, et al. Effects of smoking marijuana on left ventricular performance and plasma norepinephrine: studies in normal men. Ann Intern Med 89(4):448–452, 1978.
83. Roth WT, Tinkleinberg JR, Kopell BS, Hollister LE. Continuous electrocardiographic monitoring during marihuana intoxication. Clin Pharmacol Therap 14(4):553–540, 1973.
84. Charles R, Holt S, Kirkham N. Myocardial infarction and marijuana. Clin Toxicol 14(4):433–438, 1979.
85. MacInnes DC, Miller KM. Fatal coronary thrombosis associated with cannabis smoking. Royal Coll Gen Pract 34:575–576, 1986.
86. Aronow WS, Cassidy J. Effect of smoking marijuana and of a high-nicotine cigarette on angina pectoris. Clin Pharmacol Ther (17)5:549–554, 1975.
87. Hollister LE. Health aspects of cannabis. Pharmacol Rev 38(1):1–20, 1986.
88. Aronow WS, Cassidy J. The effect of marijuana and placebo marijuana on angina pectoris. N Engl J Med 291:65–67, 1974.
89. Prakash R, et al. Effects of marijuana and placebo marijuana smoking on hemodynamics in coronary disease. Clin Pharmacol Ther 18:90–95, 1975.
90. Wu TC, et al. Pulmonary hazards of smoking marijuana as compared with tobacco. N Engl J Med 318(6):347–351, 1988.
91. Ghalat PS, Kalra ML. Charas (cannabis) cardiomyopathy. J Indian Med Assoc 83(5):158–159, 1985.

92. Grossman M, Aboise A, Tangphao O, Blaschke T, Hoffman B. Morphine-induced venodilation in humans. Clin Pharmacol Ther 60(5):554–559, 1996.
93. Paterna S, Di Pasquale P, Montaina G, Procaccianti P, Antona A, Scaglione R, Parrinello G, Martino S, Licata G. Effect of heroin and morphine on cardiac performance in isolated and perfused rabbit heart: evaluation of cardiac hemodynamics, myocardial enzyme activity and ultrastructure features. Cardiologia 36(10):811–815, 1991.
94. Nawrath H, Rupp J, Jakob H, Sack U, Mertzlufft F, Dick W. Failure of opioids to affect excitation and contraction in isolated ventricular heart muscle. Experientia 45:337–339, 1989.
95. Pons-Llado G, Carreras F, Borras X, Cadafalch J, Fuster M, Guardia J, Casas M. Findings on Doppler echocardiography in asymptomatic intravenous heroin users. Am J Cardiol 69(3):238–241, 1992.
96. Glauser FL, Downie RL, Smith WR. Electrocardiographic abnormalities in acute heroin overdosage. Bull Narc 29(1):85–89, 1977.
97. Scherrer P, Delaloye-Bischof A, Turini G, Perret C. Participation myocardique à la rhabdomyolyse non traumatique après surdosage aux opiaces. Schwiez Med Wschr 115:1166–1170, 1985.
98. Melandri R, Re G, Lanzarini C, Rapezzi C, Leonoe O, Zele I, Rocchi G. Myocardial damage and rhabdomylosis associate with prolonged hypoxic coma following opiate overdose. Clin Toxicol 34(2):199–203, 1996.
99. Spijkerman IJ, van Ameijden EJ, Mientjes GH, Coutinho RA, van den Hoek A. Human inmunodeficiency virus infection and other risk factors for skin abscesses and endocarditis among injection drug users. J Clin Epidemiol 49(10):1149–1154, 1996.
100. Dressler FA, Roberts WC. Modes of death and types of cardiac disease in opiate addicts: analysis of 168 necropsy cases. Am J Cardiol 64:909–920, 1989.
101. Friedland GH, Selwyn PA. Infections (excluding AIDS) in injection drug users. In: Harrison's Textbook of Internal Medicine [online]. McGraw-Hill, 1999.
102. Hoechst SR, Berber M. Right-sided endocarditis in intravenous drug users. Ann Intern Med 117:560–566, 1992.
103. Barbaro G, Di Lorenzo G, Grisorio B, Barbarini G for the Gruppo Italiano per lo Studio Cardiologico dei Pazienti Affetti da AIDS. N Engl J Med 339:1093–1099, 1998.
104. Ingram RH, Braunwald E. Dyspnea and pulmonary edema. In: Harrison's Textbook of Internal Medicine [online]. McGraw-Hill, 1999.
105. Sporer K. Acute heroin overdose. Ann Intern Med 130(7):584–590, 1999.
106. Thorne LB, Collins KA. Speedballing with needle embolization: case study and review of the literature. J Forensic Sci 43(5):1074–1076, 1998.
107. Yeager RA, Hobson RW, Padberg FT, Lynch TG, Chakravarty M. Vascular complications related to drug abuse. J Trauma 27(3):305–308, 1987.
108. Morgan JM, Morgan AD, Addis B, Bradley GW, Spiro SG. Fatal hemorrhage from mycotic aneurysm of the pulmonary artery. Thorax 41:71, 1986.

109. Schofferman J, Billesdon J, Hall R. Microangiopathic hemolytic anemia: another complication of drug abuse. JAMA 230(5):721, 1974.
110. Silverman SH, Turner WW Jr. Intraarterial drug abuse: new treatment options. J Vasc Surg 14:111–116, 1991.
111. Somers WJ, Lowe FC. Localized gangrene of the scrotum and penis: a complication of heroin injection into the femoral vessels. J Urol 136(1):111–113, 1986.
112. Halpern M, Citron BP. Necrotizing angiitis associated with drug abuse. Am J Roentgenol Radium Ther Nucl Med 111(4):663–671, 1971.
113. Saadjian A, Gueunoun M, Philip-Joet F, Magnan A, Ebagosti A, Garbe L, Araud A, Levy S. Hypertension arterielle pulmonaire secondaire à des micro-emboles de talc chez une heroinomane seropositive au virus immunodepresseur humain. Archives des maladies du coeur 84:1369–1373, 1991.
114. Talebzadeh VC, Chevrolet JC, Chatelain P, Helfer C, Cox JN. Myocardite à eosinophiles et hypertension pulmonaire chez une toxicomane. Ann Pathol 10(1):40–46, 1990.
115. Gatley JS, Gifford AN, Volkow ND, Fowler JS. Cocaine. In: Handbook of Substance Abuse. Tarter RE, Ammerman RT, Ott PJ, eds. New York: Plenum, 1998.
116. Chambers H, Morris DL, Tauber MG, Modin G. Cocaine use and the risk for endocarditis in intravenous drug users. Ann Intern Med 106:833–836, 1987.
117. Ingster LM, Cartwright WS. Drug disorders and cardiovascular disease: the impact on annual hospital length of stay for the Medicare population. Am J Drug Alcohol Abuse 21(1):93–110, 1998.

10
The Relationship of Substance Abuse to the Human Immunodeficiency Virus

Background to Management

Stephen A. Wyatt* and Richard S. Schottenfeld
Yale University
New Haven, Connecticut

INTRODUCTION

Infection with the human immunodeficiency virus (HIV) profoundly complicates treatment of patients with substance use disorders. One particularly troubling issue, experienced by both patients and treatment providers, is that this grievous situation could have been avoided with appropriate prevention and substance abuse treatment. A primary goal in working with these patients is to improve their well-being through a reduction of their substance abuse problems, which can result in improvement in self-care and compliance with HIV treatment protocols. It often takes significant motivating efforts by the treatment team for these complex patients to be consistent in their participation in treatment. The intent of this chapter is to contribute to the clinician's understanding of these comorbid conditions and improve their effectiveness in motivating and treating the patient. Upon gaining a better understanding of the

---

Current affiliation: Stonington Institute, North Stonington, Connecticut.

relationship of these two illnesses the clinician may be in the position of improving not only the patient's longevity but his or her quality of life as well.

In this chapter we present a brief review of the history of HIV and the acquired immunodeficiency syndrome (AIDS), followed by a discussion of the epidemiology of two intersecting conditions: HIV infection and substance use disorders. The discussion focuses on rates of HIV infection in different geographic and demographic groups of patients with substance use disorders and on rates of drug and alcohol problems in HIV-infected patients. We then review key issues that arise in clinical work with HIV-infected patients with addictive disorders and in addicted patients at risk for HIV infection. These issues include assessment of HIV risk in addicted patients; prevention of risk, diagnosis, and management of psychiatric comorbidity in these patients; and, finally, diagnosis and management of substance use disorders in HIV-infected patients. Important common clinical management issues are discussed, including management of compliance and adherence to medical care in HIV-infected patients with substance use disorders. We conclude with a discussion of the drug interactions one might encounter in patients with these complex medical and psychiatric problems.

HISTORY

In 1981, the first reported case studies of what was later identified as AIDS described five male homosexuals with pneumocystis pneumonia, acute cytomegalovirus infections, and mucosal candidiasis (1). All five men had a history of inhalant-drug use, and one had concurrent intravenous drug use. By 1983 it was clear that certain behaviors put people at a significant risk of infection, and people with identified risk factors (injection drug use, homosexual activity) were asked to refrain from donating blood or plasma (2). Also in 1983, patients with lymphadenopathy and AIDS were found to be carriers of a previously unidentified cytopathic retrovirus (3,4). The year ended with a recommendation that AIDS be added to the list of conditions reportable to health departments (5). In 1985 a serological assay became available to detect HIV antibodies in the serum (6). As a result of the assay it was determined that a greater number of people were infected with the virus than were diagnosed with AIDS. It was also clear that the period between onset of infection and the development of opportunistic infections (OIs) or AIDS had great variability (6).

The definition of AIDS has also evolved over the years. The surveillance case definition was first published in 1984 (7) and revised in 1985, 1987, and most recently in 1993. Until 1993, the surveillance criteria were rare opportunistic infections along with non-Hodgkin's lymphoma, wasting syndrome, HIV encephalopathy, disseminated mycobacterial disease, and evidence of HIV infection (4,8). The 1993 revision was expanded to include persons with evidence of severe HIV-related immunosuppression with or without evidence of an opportunistic infection. This criterion is a CD4+ T-lymphocyte count of fewer than 200 cells/µl or a total lymphocyte count <14% (9). Also added to the criteria in 1993 were pulmonary tuberculosis, recurrent pneumonia, and invasive cervical cancers in persons with HIV-seropositive status. This resulted in a large increase in the incidence that year and should be kept in mind during any evaluation of this data. In 1996, a recommendation was made that clinicians include in their monitoring of HIV-infected patients the rate of HIV replication as indicated by viral load (10). New, more effective antiviral treatments have clearly been shown to reduce viral loads and thus the onset of AIDS-related illnesses. This has brought about a whole new way of thinking about this disease, and the diagnostic criteria may once again need revision.

EPIDEMIOLOGY

As of 1997, approximately 11 million people worldwide had died from AIDS. That same year approximately 22 million people worldwide were living with the infection (11). In the United States, as reported to the CDC through June 1997, 641,086 men, women, and children have been diagnosed with AIDS and less than half of them were still alive (12). By the end of 1996, 290,000 people were *reported* to be HIV-seropositive in the United States (13). The true number has been estimated to be greater than three times that. The back-estimation of those living with the virus in the United States in 1992 is between 600,000 and 900,000 persons, and the prevalence of the virus has risen since then (14). There are difficulties in the reporting of HIV infections because of the social stigma of the disease and the consideration that reporting will lead to a decrease in testing and counseling of high-risk individuals. In the United States only 29 states mandate confidential HIV reporting and three of those report only pediatric cases (13).

The Centers for Disease Control and Prevention (CDC) reported the first cases of AIDS in gay men. In fact, 95% of the initial cases in the United States were gay or bisexual men. By 1987 17% of cases were associated with intravenous drug use. Drug use has remained a primary risk for infection; injection drug use now accounts for about one-third of the existing cases and about one-half of all new infections (15,16). Injection drug use is involved in the transmission of the virus directly, through sharing of contaminated needles and syringes, and indirectly, through sexual partners and maternal transmission in birth. A variety of factors—including frequency of sharing injection equipment with other persons, the number of needle-sharing partners, and the use of "shooting galleries" where the sharing of equipment is common—affect the rate of HIV infection in injection drug users (IDUs) (17). Heroin and cocaine are the drugs most closely associated with HIV infections (18). From 1990 to 1995 the estimated AIDS-OI incidence increased 44% for IDUs. This increase has been less than 5% annually since 1993, reflecting a slowing in the growth of the injection-drug-use-related AIDS incidence in the United States (15).

In the northeastern United States and along the Atlantic coast, AIDS became a part of the IDU community in the early 1980s and has remained prevalent in the region (19,20). Serologic surveys taken of individuals entering drug treatment in 1991–92 revealed an average prevalence of 7% (21). In 1992, the highest seroprevalence was in New York City, where the rate reached 40%, and in New Jersey, at 33%. In the South and Midwest, the seroprevalence was a more modest 12% and 7%, respectively (21). The seroprevalence was only 3% for those entering drug treatment in the West. The reasons for these differences are unclear and not entirely explained by differences in rates of injection drug use in these communities. It may reflect differences in the culture of IDUs along with more progressive HIV-prevention programs seen in some areas of the country (22).

Of the 126 countries reporting injection drug use in 1997, 98 detected HIV among the IDUs. There are approximately 3.4 to 5.5 million IDUs in the world (23), out of the 8–10 million heroin, 30–40 million cocaine, and 30 million amphetamine users. Injection drug use accounts for approximately 5–10% of adult HIV infections worldwide (24). Poverty, social dislocation, and political instability are associated with the prevalence of injection drug use and the risk of HIV transmission. Drug traffickers also contribute to this by the destabilization of governments and their public health programs established to address these problems.

In Europe, injection drug use plays a role in 40% of adult and adolescent AIDS cases. This is due in part to the rapid rise of injection drug use in Spain, Portugal, and Italy (25). In Romania and Russia, where as late as the early 1990s there had been no clear evidence of the AIDS epidemic, there has now been a significant increase in reported AIDS. The escalating incidence is thought to be related to increasing injection drug use in these countries (26). Injection drug use is also the predominant mode of transmission in North Africa, the Middle East, some regions of Southeast Asia, China, and the southern cone of South America (Uruguay, Paraguay, Argentina, and Chile) (23). In some areas of the Far East and South America, where there has been opposition to harm-reduction efforts (i.e., no education or prevention programs), up to 70% of the IDU population is believed to carry the virus (23,26). A characteristic of the HIV epidemic among IDUs is its rapid spread. Upon reaching a threshold of approximately 10% infected individuals in the IDU community, it can rise to 40 or 50% within a 1–4-year period (27).

In 1996, a greater percentage of Americans with AIDS were African-American than Caucasian: 41% to 38%, respectively (15). Compared to Caucasians, African-Americans have a six times greater rate of AIDS OIs (15). African-American men have a greater rate of infection through injection drug use in the Northeast and along the Atlantic coast than through male-to-male sex (28). In all other areas of the United States, the primary mode of transmission for African-American men is through male-to-male sex (28). In the Hispanic population, there is a difference of primary mode of transmission depending on the country of origin (29,30). Injection drug use is the primary mode of transmission in Puerto Rican Americans, while individuals originating from Mexico and Cuba are more likely to have been infected by male-to-male sexual transmission (15). The prevalence rate in 1991–92 of HIV-seropositive status in a cohort of Puerto Ricans entering drug treatment in the Northeast was reported at 40% (31). The greater prevalence of HIV/AIDS for African-Americans and some Hispanic IDUs is thought to be associated with certain HIV risk behaviors more common in these populations, such as injection of cocaine or heroin–cocaine "speedball" combinations, and the more frequent use of "shooting galleries," where groups of people gather to use drugs by injection (32–34).

There has been a change in the sexual demographics in the rates of HIV infections in the United States. Male patients accounted for 85% of the 573,800 patients reported with AIDS by late 1996. However, the incidence of HIV is now rising more rapidly among women. Between 1990 and 1995, the incidence increased 103% in women and 27% in men (15). Of the 13,105 women reported to have received the diagnosis of AIDS-OIs in 1997, 79.8% were African-American or Hispanic (35). In 1997, the annual rate of AIDS reported for black women was 19.8 times higher than for white women (35).

In 1996, the CDC reported that 26% of persons with AIDS were IDUs practicing heterosexual sex, and 4% of cases were their sexual partners (13,15). There is also an increased rate of HIV seen in STD clinics for IDUs compared to other heterosexual men and women. The higher seroprevalence rates for younger female IDUs compared with those for men also suggest that many of these women were infected heterosexually (13). There were close to 7000 children reported living with AIDS by the end of 1996; 55% of these neonatal infections were associated with maternal IDU (15).

Most HIV infections are acquired by people 13–25 years old, and the median age for AIDS is 35 years old (13,15,36). Heterosexual transmission accounted for one-third of the reported AIDS cases of 13–25-year-olds in 1995. Traditionally there has been a higher incidence of seroconversion among the group just starting the use of intravenous drugs, but this trend is changing (37). This may indicate the effectiveness of education and risk-reduction efforts.

HIV, SUBSTANCE ABUSE AND THE IMPACT ON INFANTS

An assessment of HIV risk in mothers of 6750 children with perinatally acquired AIDS in the United States revealed: 41% with history of injection drug use, 34% had had sexual contact with a partner with or at risk for HIV/AIDS, 2% were recipients of contaminated blood or blood products, and in 13% no risk was specified (38). Not only are infants born to drug-dependent HIV-seropositive women at significant risk of becoming HIV-seropositive themselves, they are also at higher risk for a variety of other adverse outcomes (39). There is a rising incidence of mothers infected with HIV secondary to drug use. The association between cocaine use and high-risk sexual activity, including sex for drugs and multiple sexual partners, has led to a rising incidence of HIV infection in cocaine-using mothers. Sex with multiple partners increases the chances of reinfection with multiple HIV serotypes and greater virulence of infection. These features may be responsible for the higher rates of persistent infant seropositive status at 6 months in this population (40). Additionally, maternal drug use during pregnancy may also adversely affect the mother's immune system, placing her at a higher risk of OIs. Intrauterine effects of cocaine include vasculitis and inflammation, which can result in increased likelihood of fetal transmission (41).

Connor et al., in 1994, reported evidence of reduced fetal transmission through the administration of zidovudine during pregnancy (42). This has now been well established as a powerful aid in reducing the risk of infant transmission (38). Persistent compliance with the medication regimen is needed to benefit from the treatment, a behavior not normally associated with the substance-abusing pregnant population and often difficult to accomplish (43). Perinatal infection can also be reduced through expedient delivery following the rupture of membranes. In some cases this may be an indication for cesarean section (44). This is further evidence of the need for a thorough assessment of drug dependence during prenatal assessment and appropriate follow-up during pregnancy.

RISK ASSESSMENT

The first step in the evaluation of any patient for the risk of HIV infection is to assess risk behaviors. Commonly used assessments all include an evaluation of the patient's substance use patterns and sexual activity. It is clear that injection drug use, especially if coupled with sharing of injection equipment (i.e., needles, syringe, or "cookers"), puts an individual at increased risk for infection. There is mounting evidence that other forms of drug use are also associated with increased risk, particularly through their association with high-risk sexual activity. Consequently, the assessment should include potential for exposure to contaminated injection equipment, and participation in high-risk sexual activity, defined as unprotected intercourse, multiple partners, partners with a history of injection drug use, sex for money or drugs, and male-to-male sex. In addition to these specific high-risk behaviors, other factors associated with risk include knowledge of risk behaviors, ability to control impulses, and history of other related infections such as tuberculosis, hepatitis, and sexually transmitted diseases (45).

Standardized risk assessments have generally been developed for research and survey purposes but may be helpful in clinical identification of high risk in patients who may initially underreport their behavior due to social stigma. Structured assessment in clinical practice may also reduce risk behavior by providing an opportunity to educate patients about high-risk behavior. Direct and indirect questions can be used to make their risks more clear. Four assessment instruments are in common use in clinical and research practice: the NIDA-developed AIDS Initial Assessment Questionnaire (AIA), the HIV Risk-Taking Behaviour Scale (HRBS) (46), the RISK for AIDS Behavior Scale (RAB) (47), and the AIDS Risk Inventory (ARI-I) (45).

The AIA was developed for NIDA-funded AIDS research on risk assessment and risk-reduction projects. The final version, published in 1991, includes a demographic section; histories of remote, recent, and current drug use; previous treatment; sexual activity; association between sex, money, and drugs; health; legal status; work and income; and, finally, a section allowing for the interviewer's feedback on the validity of the answers. This assessment is long and cumbersome and may be difficult to use clinically. The RAB Scale, the most widely used scale at this time, is a revised and shortened version of the AIA. This questionnaire was developed for the Risk Assessment Project, which followed the serologic status of a cohort of IDUs in Philadelphia, and it has been shown to be both valid and reliable (48,49). It is a self-assessment instrument consisting of 38 closed-ended questions and takes about 15 minutes to complete. Scores on the RAB correlate with those on the AIA and are good predictors of HIV seroconversion (47). A potential drawback of the RAB may be a lack of sensitivity to changes in sexual risk behaviors (45). The HRBS is a brief, 11-item interviewer-administered scale that examines the behavior of IDUs in relation to both injecting and sexual behavior. Reliability studies on this scale have been favorable, and initial analyses indicate that the scale has satisfactory psychometric properties (46). The ARI was developed for use in clinical trials in an attempt to detect quantitative differences in risk of HIV infection using an instrument sensitive enough to identify changes in risk during treatment. Its tree-like structure enables the interviewer to move quickly over areas that are not applicable to a particular patient, allowing for more in-depth interviewing in specific areas of importance to the individual patient. In initial tests, the broad distribution of scores on the ARI suggests that it may be sufficiently sensitive to select clinically meaningful changes in risk behavior (50).

BARRIERS TO EARLY IDENTIFICATION OF HIV INFECTION

IDUs are less likely to seek early HIV counseling, testing, or treatment (51). This is partly because of the marginalization of these patients and their lack of access to primary healthcare services. The reluctance of this population to seek healthcare may also be related to the negative attitudes of healthcare providers about treating IDUs. These patients are often viewed as manipulative, unmotivated, and undeserving of care. In one survey of physicians, only 28% reported feeling comfortable caring for them (52). The high frequency of HIV testing without follow-up seen in the substance abuse population is another indication of the problem. When healthcare/HIV care is delivered in a drug treatment program, compliance is improved (53).

Delays in seeking healthcare worsen the IDUs' prognosis (10) and potentially increase their chances of transmitting infection. Delays in establishing seropositive status are associated with higher initial viral loads, lower CD4+ cell counts, and a worse prognosis (54–58). The same indices can predict response to treatment and death, and are therefore useful in the evaluation of individual injection drug use patients prior to the onset of antiviral therapy (59).

COMORBID MENTAL HEALTH PROBLEMS IN HIV-INFECTED SUBSTANCE ABUSERS

Rates of psychiatric comorbidity and psychopathology are high among patients with HIV (60), ranging from 50 to 80% in some studies (61). As noted, substance use disorders are critical risk factors for HIV infection, and there is a strong relationship between substance use disorders and other mental illnesses (62–64). The high rates of psychiatric and substance abuse comorbidity in patients with HIV infection complicate the diagnosis and management of these patients (65,66). In this section we review disorders of cognition, personality, affect, and anxiety as they relate to the HIV-infected substance abuser.

Cognitive Impairments

Neurological defects secondary to HIV infection may be due to the direct effects of the retroviruses on the nervous system or to secondary infections after significant immune-system compromise. The dementias are often classified in two ways: according to the underlying pathophysiology and according to the neurological location of injury. HIV-1 passes the blood–brain barrier easily, resulting in a greater concentration of the virus in the brain than in other organs of the body (67). It is replicated in the monocytes and multinucleated macrophages within the brain (68). The primary site of destruction is in the subcortical regions of the brain. There is now evidence that the excitatory N-methyl D-aspartate (NMDA) receptors may be sensitized by the HIV-1 coat protein gp120, resulting in neurotoxic elevations of calcium (69). A great deal of work is being carried out in an attempt at retarding this neurotoxicity, but to date there are no clearly effective clinical treatments.

Minor cognitive impairment not meeting the criteria for a diagnosis of dementia is detectable in 0.4% of patients in the asymptomatic period (70). Rarely, there may be an early-phase dementia, which occurs soon after infection with HIV and reflects an encephalopathy (70). There may also be an uncommonly reported middle-phase dementia, which presents similarly to multiple sclerosis after what appears to be an autoimmune reaction affecting the white matter of the brain (71).

The third phase of HIV-associated dementia, initially classified as AIDS dementia complex, is now referred to as HIV-1-associated cognitive/motor complex. The etiology of this disorder is associated with either diffuse HIV pathology or focal lesions secondary to OIs. This complex was once thought to involve approximately 40% of AIDS patients, but this is now thought to have been an overestimate. One study by the World Health Organization

(WHO) showed a point prevalence of between 8 and 16% of patients with AIDS. Estimates of annual incidence have approximated 7.0% (72,73). In patients in the late stage of disease, it has been estimated that 27% may have diagnosable dementia (74). The true incidence secondary to cerebral HIV infections is difficult to determine. It may be overestimated secondary to the high prevalence of pre-existing cognitive difficulties seen in many patients at risk for HIV-1 infection, and the uncertainty in determining the related contributions of AIDS-related secondary encephalopathies and chronic substance abuse (75).

A decline in the CD4 cell count is associated with a dramatic increase in the prevalence of neurological involvement, including dementia (76). Of note, dementia is associated with poor prognosis (75). The Multicenter AIDS Cohort Study (72) demonstrated a median survival of 6 months after diagnosis, although the potential impact of combination antiretroviral therapy has yet to be assessed.

Neurocognitively, the HIV dementia complex has many similarities to that seen with chronic substance abuse, including problems with attention, concentration, cognitive flexibility, verbal memory, and psychomotor speed (77,78). There is also evidence of an escalation in appearance of symptoms of cognitive decline in the chronic substance-abusing HIV-positive patient over that seen in non-substance-abusing HIV-positive patients (79). In this and other studies there is generally, although not invariably, evidence that substance abuse patients with concurrent HIV-seropositive status have a more prominent decline in neurocognitive abilities than those who are seronegative (80). Age and educational background are also important factors in the decline of cognitive abilities in these patients (81,82). Clearly, continued substance dependence negatively effects the status of the already cognitively impaired HIV-positive patient.

Assessment of cognitive impairments in HIV-infected patients is critical both to initiate treatments for the underlying cause of the neurological decline and because cognitive impairments may adversely affect compliance with complicated medication regimens. The Mini Mental Status Exam is a rapid, easily preformed assessment tool to evaluate for possible dementia or evidence of a variety of neurological deficits. However, it may not be sufficiently sensitive to pick up subtle early changes, especially in patients with premorbid levels of functioning. The Neuropsychological Impairment Scale (NIS) is a self-assessment scale that has shown greater sensitivity in evaluating these patients. It can assist the clinician in following the potential development of cognitive difficulties during the course of a patient's illness (83). More complete neuropsychological testing, including the Rey Verbal Memory Task for detection of cortical abnormalities, and Trailmaking B, symbol digit, and nonverbal memory tests may be needed for identification of subcortical dementias (84,85).

Specialized approaches may be beneficial in improving compliance with complex medication schedules in patients with cognitive impairments. Information can be presented in simple language and repeated format, making use of written, verbal, and illustrated materials. One multimodal approach incorporating cognitive remediation strategies such as behavioral games, role playing, quizzes, memory books, large-format presentations, and frequent feedback has been found effective in reducing high-risk behavior in a small sample of opiate- and cocaine-dependent, HIV-seropositive patients (86).

Zidovudine (AZT) may be helpful in the treatment of HIV dementia. A randomized, double-blind, placebo-controlled study provided evidence that HIV dementia patients have improvement of neuropsychological performance following administration of high-dose (2000 mg/day) of AZT (87). There is evidence that the incidence of HIV dementia and opportunistic brain disease can be reduced after the administration of AZT if started not only before but also after the onset of AIDS dementia (88). Unfortunately, there was no evidence that AZT was protective against HIV dementia complex when a large cohort of these patients were followed over time (72). No clear evidence exists that other antiviral therapies effectively reduce the incidence of brain disease in the HIV-positive patient (89). However, an open-label trial of the nonnucleoside reverse transcriptase inhibitor atevirdine has shown preliminary favorable results (90). Unfortunately, it is lack of compliance with difficult drug regimens in the substance-use-disordered population that remains the barrier to their benefiting from effective preventive treatment for HIV-related dementia.

Personality Disorders

The estimated prevalence of personality disorders in HIV-positive patients varies from 16% to 30% (91). Borderline personality disorder was found to account for 73% of all personality diagnoses made in HIV-positive individuals in one retrospective study (92). Characteristic hallmarks of borderline personality disorder, including impulsivity and unstable relationships, are also risk factors for HIV transmission and complicate diagnosis and management. HIV-positive homosexual men with personality disorder have been shown to have more psychiatric symptoms associated with their illness (93). However, in a systematic study performed by Johnson et al., although there was a high prevalence of personality disorders among a homosexual population at risk, there was no excess of personality disorders in the infected cohort.

Personality-disordered patients can be very difficult to treat. Sometimes the complexities encountered in attempting to treat these patients' symptoms can actually signal the presence of a personality disorder. "Splitting" is a characteristic defense used by borderline patients, who have a tendency to see others, including caregivers, as either all good or all bad. These distortions may cause disruption among members of the treatment team if distrust or negative attitudes about one another arise from the patient's distorted reports. The use of dialectic behavioral treatment (DBT), as described by Linehan, has been quite effective in the treatment of these patients (94). Important aspects of the treatment include consistent limit setting and frequent, direct communication among members of the treatment team to prevent disruptions. Medication management of these patients often leads to polypsychopharmacotherapy in an attempt to ameliorate anxious, depressive, impulsive, and self-destructive behavior. While polypharmacy should be avoided, there is a high prevalence in personality-disordered patients of co-occurring Axis I disorders in which pharmacological interventions are indicated.

Depression, Mania, and Suicide

Depression and suicide in the HIV-positive population have a higher prevalence than in the general population, at a rate similar to other populations with chronic illness (95–97). The increased rates of affective disorders may be associated with the co-occurrence of a substance use disorder or chronic illness (64,97).

Isolation, lack of social support, bereavement, and the marginalization and stigma associated with AIDS may also contribute to depression (98–101). Fukunishi et al., in Japan, have shown that the lack of social supports provided to HIV-positive patients has a significant effect on the reporting of depressive symptoms and may be associated with avoidant coping behaviors, which may lead to further isolation and delay in effective medical care (98,102).

Suicidal ideation and behavior are frequently encountered problems. The relative risk of suicide in men with AIDS varies from 7 to 36 times that of age-matched controls (103). The times of greatest vulnerability are upon notification of seropositive status, development of an AIDS-defining illness, and death of a partner or close friend (104). Homosexuals and IDUs, independent of HIV status, have a greater prevalence of affective disorders than the general population (105) and a markedly elevated risk of suicide compared with the general population (106). Thus, it is important that clinicians maintain a heightened awareness of the potential for suicide in these patients.

There is conflicting evidence about whether depression increases the progression of the HIV illness. HIV-seropositive homosexual men without AIDS who entered the Multicenter AIDS Cohort Study in 1984 or 1985 were followed for a total of 8 years. Data from this study yielded no evidence that depressive symptoms predicted worsening of HIV disease (107). Burack et al., in a study controlled for drug and alcohol use, found evidence favoring a correlation between the rate at which CD4 levels decline and severity of depression (108), but this association was not supported in a significantly larger study (107). There is evidence that the level of depression is more closely associated with psychosocial problems than with the severity of HIV infection (109), and a greater severity of psychosocial problems is seen frequently in the depressed substance-abusing population. The involvement of alcohol and substance abuse can hasten progressive physical deterioration and also worsen the depression, hopelessness, and despair.

Patients with moderate levels of depression—as detected by a score of 14–21 on the Beck Depression Inventory (BDI)—on intake into a general medical clinic are more likely to show improvement in their depressive symptoms with an improvement in their HIV disease—as determined by the Karnofsky Scale of Physical Performance—than are those who enter treatment with severe depression (BDI >22). Differentiation between secondary depressive symptoms, which will improve slightly with treatment of HIV, and major depression is thus important to prevent adding an unnecessary medication to an often already complicated pharmacological regimen (110). However, missing a diagnosis of treatable depression is more often the problem in HIV medical clinics (99). A WHO study showed that only 9% of patients meeting criteria of depression were receiving antidepressant therapy at the time of assessment (95). Use of simple general screening procedures for depression would improve identification of patients who could benefit from treatment (99,104).

Dementia is often associated with depression in the HIV/AIDS population, and this combination is associated with a particularly poor prognosis (95). Concurrent substance abuse only compounds this problem. Depressed HIV-infected patients may report an increased number of somatic symptoms that are not necessarily indicative of HIV disease progression (109,111,112) or related to HIV pathophysiology (113). These symptoms include poor appetite and sleep, weight loss, and increased fatigability (111,112). Differentiation of the origin of these other symptoms can be particularly difficult in the drug-dependent HIV depressed patient, especially shortly after initiation of abstinence.

Depression is treatable in HIV-infected patients. In a four-cell, double-blind study utilizing interpersonal psychotherapy, cognitive-behavioral therapy, supportive psychotherapy, and supportive psychotherapy with imipramine, interpersonal psychotherapy was shown to be the most effective psychotherapy for patients who have experienced the significant life events associated with HIV infection (114). Grassi et al. were able to demonstrate significant improvement in depressive symptoms in patients treated with paroxetine (115). Because of the similar clinical efficacy of medications in this class, there is reason to believe that the use of other serotonin-reuptake inhibitors would have a similar response. Amitriptyline may help not only with depressive symptoms but also with pain associated with peripheral neuropathies, diarrhea and associated abdominal discomfort, and prolonged sleep latency, all problems more frequently encountered in this population. The psychostimulants methylphenidate and dextroamphetamine can also be very effective in treating the depressed HIV-positive patient (116). This is particularly true in the acutely depressed patient with significant loss of appetite, anergy, and wasting. Standard effective doses of methylphenidate range from as low as 5.0 mg once a day to 20 mg twice a day, with reports of using as much as 80 mg per day. In patients with a substance abuse history, it is recommended that this treatment be either reserved for those who are morbidly depressed with physical deterioration or as a short-term treatment during the initial phase of treatment with a more typical antidepressive. Methylphenidate is a controlled substance and should be used judiciously in this population.

Mania is also seen in greater frequency in the HIV-seropositive population (117), even in patients with no family history of this disorder or prior occurrence. The occurrence of manic symptoms in the HIV-infected patient may be an adverse effect of medications or result from systemic illness or HIV-related brain damage (118). Mania is often a late and ominous sign appearing within months of death (119). A heightened awareness of the mania as an indication of worsening systemic illness may lead to the earlier detection of a treatable complication. Regardless of etiology, mania may need primary treatment. In the patient with no renal or hepatic complications, lithium and valproic acid may be the medications of choice. Gabapentin, because of its low potential for drug interactions and use in chronic pain management, could be an important pharmacological addition to the management of these patients. To date, gabapentin does not appear to be as effective as the other, more established medications in primary management of mania (120).

Anxiety Disorders

There is no evidence that HIV infection alone results in neurobiological changes increasing the prevalence of anxiety. However, symptoms of anxiety have had a significantly greater prevalence in HIV-positive men with major depression and/or adjustment disorders than in a comparable sample of HIV-negative controls. There was also a significant increase in prevalence of adjustment disorder with anxiety in the HIV-positive population over a control group of high-risk patients (121). In this same study, the rates of generalized anxiety disorder (GAD) were relatively low. This is consistent with the low rate of GAD seen in the general population and the large spread of prevalence rates—0%–28%—seen in studies of the chronically ill (122). When coping styles are examined, it is quite clear that feelings of a loss of mastery or control over one's life is an important predictor of anxiety associated with an adjustment disorder in the chronically ill (123,124). The powerful emotional response associated with the fact that one is infected with what until recently was a uniformly lethal illness, and remains an illness fraught with complications, leaves many with a level of stress not previously encountered. Substance-dependent patients are especially notorious for their inability to adequately cope with life stresses.

Evaluation and treatment of anxiety symptoms in the HIV-seronegative patient may play a role in the prevention of transmission of the disease and improve management of HIV-infected patients. Psychiatric symptoms, including various measures of anxiety, are predictive of greater risk behavior in opiate-dependent individuals (125), and reducing anxiety may also reduce high-risk behaviors and improve patient adherence to treatment.

The use of benzodiazepines in this patient population is problematic. In patients with substance use disorders, the abuse liability of benzodiazepines may be quite high. Excessive doses may lead to worsening of cognitive functioning and increased risk-taking behavior. Withdrawal symptoms following abrupt discontinuation, including increased anxiety, irritability, and seizure, may further complicate treatment. Because of these problems, use of alternative treatment for anxiety symptoms may be indicated. The selective serotonin-reuptake inhibitors (SSRIs) have really become a mainstay in the treatment of anxiety. They have significant effects on the relief of anxiety and associated dysphoria. Their low side-effect profile often makes them easily tolerated in a population notoriously sensitive to medications. Tricyclic antidepressants (TCAs) can also be effective in relieving not only the physical symtoms of anxiety but also the frequently associated depressed mood. Sleep latency may also be improved with bedtime dosing of TCA medications, particularly those with greater anticholinergic properties. The sleep problems are often associated with the aggressive irritable mood seen in these patients. Trazodone is a sedative that appears to protect normal sleep cycles and may also have limited beneficial effects on concurrent depressed irritable mood. Finally, propranolol in nonhypotensive, nonasthmatic patients with significant autonomic symptomatology surrounding their anxiety may also be helpful (126). When using propranolol, one should keep in mind that depression is a potential side effect.

It is often difficult to get these patients to take medications other then benzodiazepines long enough to get the targeted result. Patients with a history of substance abuse may expect immediate relief from the medication. A strong alliance between the physician and patient can be most helpful in encouraging the patient to continue the treatment. Patients may also benefit from behavioral and cognitive approaches to relieve anxiety, including relaxation techniques. With the combination of good medical management, psychopharmacological treatment, case management, and at least a modicum of interpersonal/cognitive-behavioral therapy, these patients can have a consistent and lasting improvement in their level of anxiety.

SPECIFIC DRUGS OF ABUSE AND HIV: DIAGNOSIS AND MANAGEMENT

Opiates

An association between heroin dependence and impaired immune system functioning was noted prior to the onset of the AIDS epidemic (127,128). Opioids, including heroin and morphine, affect T-lymphocyte functioning both by brain-mediated pathways (129) and by direct actions on the lymphocytes themselves (130). The most severe adverse effects of opioid dependence on immune system functioning, however, are related to use of contaminated injection equipment, adulterants in street drugs, malnutrition, and other correlates of addiction. IDUs are at high risk for infection with a variety of pathogens associated with immunosuppression, including cytomegalovirus, Epstein-Barr virus, and hepatitis B and C. Malnutrition may also contribute to immunosuppression in heroin addicts (131). Alterations in immune system parameters observed in heroin addicts include elevations of T-lymphocyte counts, reduced proliferative response of peripheral blood lymphocytes to mitogens, and suppressed natural-killer-cell activity (132). Of note, immune system functioning is improved substantially during methadone maintenance treatment, compared to that in heroin addicts, supporting the safety of prescribed opioid use and the effectiveness of methadone maintenance tre/atment for improving health status (133).

Over the past three decades, the effectiveness of methadone maintenance treatment has been repeatedly demonstrated in controlled clinical trials, quasi-experimental studies (e.g., evaluation of the effects of program closure), and clinical practice. Methadone maintenance leads to substantial reductions in the use of injection drugs and illicit opioids. Notably, the incidence of new HIV infection in methadone-maintained patients is substantially lower than in untreated heroin addicts in the same geographical area (134). Provision of methadone maintenance is one of the most important means of reducing HIV transmission among opioid-dependent IDUs (135). Additionally, provision of medical care in association with methadone maintenance treatment improves adherence to medical care recommendations as well as the health status of HIV-infected patients (136). Despite the overall effectiveness of methadone maintenance treatment, limited access to this treatment, inadequate dosing, medically unwarranted restrictions on the length of time patients may remain in treatment, and inadequate funding for necessary counseling and other services continue to limit its beneficial impact. An additional problem is that many patients continue to abuse cocaine and other drugs during maintenance treatment.

Alternatives to methadone maintenance for heroin-dependent patients include long-term residential treatment in a therapeutic community (e.g., Daytop, Phoenix House) or medically supervised withdrawal followed by outpatient treatment. Naltrexone may help prevent relapse in detoxified patients, but adherence and retention rates with naltrexone treatment are typically low. HIV-infected patients with pain syndromes requiring occasional or continued opioid analgesia also cannot be treated with naltrexone. These patients can be treated with methadone maintenance, in which case it is important to recognize that the daily maintenance dose does not provide pain relief. Methadone-maintained patients with severe pain may require adjunctive treatment with a different opioid analgesic. Care should be taken to avoid use of partial opioid agonists or mixed agonist/antagonists (e.g., buprenorphine, pentazocine) so as not to precipitate withdrawal. Because of tolerance to the effects of opioids, methadone-maintained patients might also require higher doses or more frequent administration of opioid analgesics.

Cocaine

Heroin has been the drug most closely associated with transmission of HIV infections through injection drug use (18), but in some regions, particularly the

South and Southwest, transmission is currently most associated with injection use of cocaine and amphetamine (18). The increased prevalence of HIV-seropositive status among cocaine users is apparently linked to two sets of associated behaviors: sexuality and injection drug use (33,137). Sexually transmitted disease related to cocaine use appears to be partially dependent on the route of administration of the cocaine. A survey conducted in 1991 showed evidence of higher-risk sexual practices in those who use a "freebased," or smokeable, form of cocaine. These individuals reported not only more frequent sex partners but also more drug use surrounding individual sexual acts, and, what might seem intuitive, more frequent unprotected sex. This population also had higher rates of drugs for sex activity than the cocaine hydrochloride group, those primarily using intranasally (138). Similar results were found in a study of inner-city young adult crack cocaine smokers in which high-risk sexual activity, sex for drugs, and male-to-male sex were associated with crack cocaine use, which was thus found to be a powerful risk for HIV transmission (139). Schwarcz et al. found similar rates of HIV-seropositive status in those smoking cocaine and IDUs in a group of African-American youths in San Francisco (140)

During 1993–1994, individuals using injection cocaine and heroin in combination accounted for a major new group of HIV-seropositive people, as a result of both needle sharing and the potential combined immunosuppressive effects of heroin and cocaine (33,34,141,142).

There are both biological and behavioral associations between cocaine and HIV infection. Cocaine has well documented adverse pathophysiological effects on the brain, and can result in vasculitis, vasospasm, and hemorrhage. Cocaine can adversely alter the endothelium of cerebral blood vessels and the blood–brain barrier, potentially influencing the progression to AIDS in HIV-seropositive patients (143). Cocaine use by seropositive patients is associated with increased progression of the illness (144).

There is no clearly effective pharmacological treatment for cocaine dependence. Cognitive-behavioral and other psychotherapies have shown some, but limited, efficacy. There has been evidence in controlled studies of improvement of depression in HIV-positive patients after the administration of a variety of antidepressant agents (145). Batki et al. showed reductions in depressive symptoms and cocaine use in a cohort of cocaine-dependent HIV-seropositive depressed patients treated with fluoxetine (146). There is evidence that the SSRI medications have fewer side effects than the TCAs, particularly in individuals with advanced HIV disease (145).

Alcohol

Alcohol use has often been reported as a risk factor in the transmission of HIV (147,148). Although there is some difficulty separating out the effects of alcohol when used in combination with other drugs of abuse, there does appear to be an identifiable risk in the use of alcohol alone (149). The prevalence of HIV infection among patients entering alcohol treatment programs ranges from 1–13% of patients unscreened for male-to-male sexual behavior on the East Coast (150–152) to 3–5% in a sample screened for homosexual activity in San Francisco (148,153).

Expectancies of the effects of alcohol are often associated with disinhibited behaviors and emotions. These alcohol-associated behaviors reinforce drinking, and often result in increased consumption and high-risk sexual activity (154). There is evidence that male-to-male sexual behavior coupled with alcohol intoxication increases the risk for HIV transmission until the level of "alcohol impairment" moves into the high range where the risk begins to fall (155). However, when these highly impaired individuals had a strong sense that alcohol improved their socialization skills and sexual attractiveness, they remained at high risk. Men with a stronger expectancy that intoxication leads to sexual activity are more likely to drink at the time of sexual activity (156). Both heterosexual and homosexual individuals are at greater risk of HIV transmission if sexual activities occur with someone other than their primary sexual partner. Homosexual men are at greater risk of transmission if they socialize in bars (155). Overall, there is a stronger association between intoxication during a sexual encounter and transmission of the virus than there is with the severity of dependence on alcohol (157). Increasing awareness of the association between intoxication and sexual behavior may help individuals take steps to reduce their HIV risk.

In addition to raising the risk of HIV transmission by increasing high-risk sexual activity, alcohol intoxication may be associated with increased HIV disease progression. Alcohol-dependent individuals often delay seeking medical advice, resulting in a late diagnosis of AIDS and a worse prognosis (158). Alcohol dependence may also increase the risk of infection secondary to greater exposure to IDUs (150). Finally, the biological effects of alcohol may increase susceptibility to infection.

Currently there are conflicting data about the direct effect of alcohol on HIV disease progression. Length of delay in seeking treatment after identification of seropositive status has been shown to be partially dependent on the presence of alcohol problems—men who have alcohol problems delay treatment for 1.3 years more than men without alcohol problems. There were no differences, however, between women with and without alcohol problems. Women on the whole were much better about seeking care, entering into treatment 28.5 months sooner than men after the determination of seropositive status (159).

Since alcohol problems are highly prevalent and may complicate treatment of HIV-infected patients, screening for alcohol problems should be a routine component of the initial evaluation of patients. The four-question CAGE (has tried to **C**ut back, is **A**nnoyed by criticism of drinking, feels **G**uilty about drinking behavior, and feels the need for an **E**ye-opener drink) assessment can facilitate detection. Assessment and management issues for patients with alcohol problems have recently been reviewed (160).

Alcoholics Anonymous remains a strong force in helping people through recovery. Physicians working with HIV patients can have a very positive effect on their patients by encouraging participation in 12-Step programs. Naltrexone or disulfiram can also be important adjuncts in the care of these patients. Contraindications to the use of these medications in this patient population are no different from those in the general population of alcohol-dependent patients, but patients should be clinically evaluated for hepatotoxicity and neuropathies; treatment with disulfiram and naltrexone would not be suitable for patients requiring opioids for pain relief. The potentially harmful interaction of these medications is discussed below.

PREVENTION OF HIV ASSOCIATED WITH SUBSTANCE ABUSE

Although newer combination therapies have the potential to lower the viral load, which may also reduce the likelihood of contagion, reducing risk behaviors remains the most important strategy for preventing the spread of HIV (162). Among drug abusers, behaviors associated with sharing injection equipment and high-risk sexual activities are fundamental in the transmission of HIV. Consequently, prevention efforts must target these behaviors.

Despite initial skepticism about the likelihood of producing behavioral change in drug abusers, HIV-prevention efforts have been successful in this population. Because of stigmatization and the marginalized status of drug abusers, initial prevention efforts were directed at outreach and counseling about risk reduction. The results of NIDA's National AIDS Demonstration Research Projects provide compelling evidence that even relatively limited educational counseling about risk reduction can have beneficial effects. Many early attempts at risk reduction attempted to teach addicts to clean needles and injection equipment using bleach. While this approach helped to raise awareness of the problem and was a first attempt at peer-led outreach and counseling (162), its effectiveness was limited because of underestimation of the difficulties of implementation and inadequate understanding of the circumstances in which injection drug use occurs (163). Outreach has also been remarkably effective in encouraging out-of-treatment drug users to enter drug abuse treatment and to reduce injection drug use and sharing of equipment. In recent years, many sites have reported a decline in rates of injection drug use among treatment-seeking opiate addicts (164,165), attributable in part to HIV-prevention efforts and increased awareness of risk.

Increasing the availability of sterile injection equipment has been identified as another option in preventing HIV transmission. State and local laws in many areas of the country prohibiting dispensing of injection equipment without a prescription have limited the accessibility of sterile injection equipment. With repeal of these laws (and of drug paraphernalia laws, which also encourage addicts to discard their own injection equipment and then use whatever is available at the time), addicts may purchase sterile needles and syringes inexpensively at local pharmacies, many of which are open 24 hours a day, 7 days a week. Needle exchange remains another, somewhat more controversial, option. Objections to needle-exchange programs typically center on concerns that the programs will market needles and syringes to drug users, lower the threshold for injection drug use, convey that injection drug use is safe and "clean," and utilize public funds to support drug use. Proponents of needle and syringe exchange programs (NSEPs) counter that the typical NSEP provides, in addition to sterile injection equipment, a number of other risk-reduction and beneficial services, such as counseling about risk reduction, including reducing risk from sexual activities as well as drug use, and referral to medical, legal, and social services and drug abuse treatment (166). In a recent review of 12 NSEPs, beneficial effects were found in six programs, four reported neither beneficial nor adverse effects, and two reported possible adverse effects (increased prevalence of HIV). Regarding the last two programs, supporters contend that rates would have been even higher in the absence of the NSEP and that adverse selection accounted for adverse findings (i.e., drug users with the most severe injection drug use behaviors were most likely to use the program).

The use of inhaled nitrate drugs, most often reported in the homosexual population, is associated with increased prevalence of HIV-seropositive status in the male-to-male-sex group (167). These drugs can increase muscle relaxation and are reported to heighten sexual response. Questions about the use of these drugs, especially in the homosexual population, can be of significant importance in assessing risk of HIV transmission and should be included in any through clinical interview.

Risk-reduction counseling for patients in drug abuse treatment also remains an important priority. While drug abuse treatment substantially reduces drug abuse and HIV risk directly related to drug use, in the absence of specific interventions, other high-risk activities may be unaffected by drug abuse treatment (168). The effectiveness and cost-effectiveness of intensive counseling directed at very high-risk groups (e.g., patients in STD clinics) have been supported in recent studies (169). Similar high-intensity risk-reduction counseling for patients in drug abuse treatment may also be effective. Modifications of the counseling procedures for cognitively impaired patients and HIV-infected patients are currently being investigated (86).

GENERAL TREATMENT ISSUES

In recent years many important advances in treating HIV-seropositive patients have established the potential for both increased quality and duration of life with early presentation and management (10,12). The impact of these treatments on drug-dependent patients, however, has been far less than on other groups. HIV-infected active IDUs and those not in drug treatment are less likely to have sought out or be receiving treatment for their infection. Part of the problem is the lack of a consistent source of healthcare or health insurance (170,171). Even when free potent antiviral treatment was offered in a Vancouver study, only 17% of the eligible cohort received maximum treatment. Older male patients in drug treatment were most likely, and HIV-seropositive females and IDUs least likely, to take advantage of potent HIV regimens (171). In the United States, IDUs experience greater morbidity and mortality than non-IDUs and male homosexuals when similar opportunities for potent HIV regimens are made available. These findings suggest that simply increasing availability of antiviral medications is not sufficient. Continued outreach is needed to encourage HIV-infected drug users to begin retroviral treatment. Additionally, engagement in drug abuse treatment will also improve adherence to medical treatment.

Contributing to the lack of consistent healthcare provided to IDUs is that many physicians lack the training to adequately care for IDUs, and drug-dependent patients in general. Many physicians also have negative attitudes concerning these patients (136). The comorbid neuropsychiatric problems and other drug-related general medical problems (61), along with frequent and profoundly difficult social issues, make these patients very difficult to treat.

Substance Abuse and HIV

The medical complexity of these patients combined with behavioral challenges such as their being demanding, overly dependent, self-destructive, and often involved in criminal activity may also contribute to negative attitudes of healthcare professionals and reluctance to treat them. These factors, however, clearly point to the importance of developing an orderly, well-established, and comprehensive treatment plan that addresses behavioral and social issues as well as the patient's medical needs. When engaged in stable primary care with an experienced physician and adequate support services, individuals with a history of injection drug use have clinical outcomes equal to those without this history (172).

Cultural factors—including ethnic, racial, or language differences—may also make treatment difficult for the drug-dependent patient. A physician may have trouble understanding the level of stress experienced by a patient because of such cultural differences. Establishing trust may also be difficult. Disease and "wellness" may have a different meaning to the patient. Patients may not attribute the importance to HIV status that the physician would expect. Addressing these issues requires patience, the ability to build rapport, and an understanding of the principles of building motivation.

A major advance in the treatment of HIV is the use of highly active antiviral therapy (HAART), which has well-documented efficacy in reducing the rates of progression to AIDS or death (173,174). These regimens, although effective, are costly and require close adherence to complex medication schedules. Because intermittent therapy can result in a proliferation of resistant viral strains and reduced efficacy of other antivirals of the same class (175), deferring treatment with HAART in patients who cannot adhere to the treatment protocols may be appropriate (176). Nonadherence also complicates evaluation of the reasons for persistent viremia (e.g., medication resistance or inadequate dose secondary to noncompliance). These considerations make it advisable to encourage active drug users to participate in drug abuse treatment prior to undertaking a complex medical regimen. Stabilization in drug abuse treatment also provides an opportunity to address other psychosocial issues that might interfere with adherence (e.g., cognitive deficits or homelessness) (177). Prophylactic treatment of OIs can be initiated during the stabilization period. The primary physician may also elect to initiate single or double antiviral treatments at some point along this continuum of care.

The initial comprehensive assessment at the entry point into drug abuse treatment or medical care for HIV provides an important opportunity to begin building a therapeutic alliance with the patient. During the evaluation process, the patient has an opportunity to review his life history and current medical, emotional, and social condition in ways that may improve his awareness of the impact of drug abuse and HIV on his life and encourage treatment engagement. The initial evaluation also provides an opportunity to begin to educate the patient about the treatments that will be prescribed. Evaluation of the viral load can provide important information about prognosis and can be used to assess response to treatment. Patients need to be educated about the importance of this index and about the medications prescribed to treat HIV.

DRUG INTERACTIONS

Because patients with HIV infection and substance use disorders may require treatment with multiple medications at the same time, consideration of potential medication interactions is essential. Patient complaints about side effects or reduced efficacy of medications may be one indication of drug–drug interactions. Even in the absence of patient complaints, consideration of possible medication interactions is indicated whenever multiple medications are prescribed.

Potential interactions between seizure medications, rifampin, antiviral medications, and methadone are often of particular concern to patients. Some medications—most notably, carbamazepine and rifampin—induce more rapid metabolism of methadone and may precipitate withdrawal symptoms in methadone-maintained patients. Methadone-maintained patients are often quite anxious about the possibility of precipitated withdrawal when beginning any new medication, and anxiety symptoms may also be attributed to withdrawal. Patient complaints of AZT-precipitated withdrawal led to investigation of methadone–AZT interactions. Methadone leads to reduced renal clearance and increased blood levels of AZT, but AZT does not appear to affect methadone plasma levels (178,179). Increased AZT levels due to methadone, however, may be associated with troubling side effects and increased toxicity. Increased side effects may also contribute to patient noncompliance.

Hepatic cytochrome p450 3A4 is the major system involved in the N-demethylation of methadone. Methadone is also an inhibitor of cytochrome 2D6 isoforms. Protease inhibitors and many psychotropic medications are also metabolized by cytochrome p450 3A3/4 and 2D6 isoforms (176,180). Some medication interactions involving these systems are quite complex, since some medications (e.g., carbamazepine, rifampin) may induce these systems while others (e.g., naltrexone, disulfiram) may competitively inhibit them.

CONCLUSION

We have provided an overview of the epidemiology and prevention of HIV transmission in the substance abuse population. We have described the complexities of diagnosing and managing various psychiatric and substance use disorders in HIV-infected patients. This is a rapidly developing field with new advances taking place quickly; however, the human immunodeficiency virus remains a devastating threat to a young and vital segment of our society. It is important that clinicians specializing in the addictions continue in their attempt to understand and engage these patients, thereby reducing the psychosocial and economic consequences of this infection for both patient and society.

REFERENCES

1. Pneumocystis pneumonia—Los Angeles. MMWR 30:250–252, 1981.
2. Antibodies to a retrovirus etiologically associated with acquired immunodeficiency syndrome (AIDS) in populations with increased incidences of the syndrome. MMWR 33(27):377–379, 1984.
3. F Barre-Sinoussi, JC Chermann, F Rey, MT Nugeyre, S Chamaret, J Gruest, C Dauguet, C Axler-Blin, F Vezinet-Brun, C Rouzioux, W Rozenbaum, L Montagnier. Isolation of a T-lymphotropic retrovirus from a patient at risk for acquired immune deficiency syndrome (AIDS). Science 220(4599):868–871, 1983.
4. RC Gallo, SZ Salahuddin, M Popovic, GM Shearer, M Kaplan, BF Haynes, TJ Palker, R Redfield, J Oleske, B Safai, et al. Frequent detection and isolation of cytopathic retroviruses (HTLV-III) from patients with AIDS and at risk for AIDS. Science 224(4648):500–503, 1984.
5. Prevention of acquired immune deficiency syndrome (AIDS): report of interagency recommendations. MMWR 32(8):101–103, 1983.
6. Provisional Public Health Service inter-agency recommendations for screening donated blood and plasma for antibody to the virus causing acquired immunodeficiency syndrome. MMWR 34(1):1–5, 1985.
7. RM Selik, HW Haverkos, FW Curran. Acquired immune deficiency syndrome (AIDS) in the United States. Am J Med 38:229–236, 1984.
8. Revision of the case definition of acquired immunodeficiency syndrome for national reporting—United States. MMWR 34(25):373–375, 1985.
9. 1993 revised classification system for HIV infection and expanded surveillance case definition for AIDS among adolescents and adults. MMWR 41(RR-17):1–19, 1992.
10. SS Carpenter, MA Fischle, SM Hammer, et al. Antiretroviral therapy for HIV

infection in 1996: recommendations of an international panel. JAMA 276:146–154, 1996.
11. The status and trends of the Global HIV/AIDS Pandemic Symposium final report. In: International AFH, ed. UNAIDS. Vancouver, Canada: Harvard School of Public Health, 1996.
12. U.S. HIV and AIDS cases reported through December 1997. HIV AIDS Surveillance Report 9(2), 1997.
13. CDC. HIV/AIDS Surveillance Report: Year End Report 1996. Vol 8. Atlanta: Centers for Disease Control and Prevention, pp 1–39, 1997.
14. PS Rosenberg. Scope of the AIDS epidemic in the United States [comments]. Science 270(5240):1372–1375, 1995.
15. CDC. HIV/AIDS Surveillance Report: Results Through December 1995. Vol 7. Atlanta: Centers for Disease Control and Prevention, pp 1–39, 1996.
16. Holmberg SD. The estimated prevalence and incidence of HIV in 96 large metropolitan areas. Am J Public Health 1996; 86:643–654.
17. KE Nelson, D Vlahov, S Cohn, et al. Sexually transmitted diseases in a population of intravenous drug users: association with seropositivity to the human immunodeficiency virus (HIV). J Infect Dis 164:457–463, 1991.
18. T Diaz, SY Chu, RH Byers, et al. The types of drugs used by HIV-infected injection drug users in a multistate surveillance project: implications for intervention. Am J Public Health 84:1971–1975, 1994.
19. Human immunodeficiency virus infection in the United States. MMWR 36(suppl S-6):1–48, 1987.
20. Selected behaviors that increase risk for HIV infection, other sexually transmitted diseases, and unintended pregnancy among high school students—United States, 1991. MMWR 41(50):945–950, 1992.
21. CDC. National HIV Serosurveillance Summary: Results Through 1992. National HIV Surveillance Report. Vol 3. Atlanta: Centers for Disease Control and Prevention, 1992.
22. DC Des Jarlais, H Hagan, SR Friedman, P Friedmann, D Goldberg, M Frischer, S Green, K Tunving, B Ljungberg, A Wodak, et al. Maintaining low HIV seroprevalence in populations of injecting drug users. JAMA 274(15):1226–1231, 1995.
23. UNAIDS. WHO Report on the Global HIV/AIDS Epidemic: December 1997. Global HIV/AIDS and STD Surveillance, 1997.
24. AM Stimson GV, Rhodes T. The diffusion of drug injecting in developing countries. Int Drug Policy 7:245–255, 1996.
25. FF Hamers, V Batter, AM Downs, et al. The HIV epidemic associated with injecting drug use in Europe: geographic and time trends. AIDS 11:1365–1374, 1997.
26. SA Strathdee, EJC Van Ameijden, F Mesquita, S Rana, D Vlahov. Can HIV epidemic among injection drug users be prevented? AIDS 12(suppl A):S71–S79, 1998.

27. SR Friedman, DC Des Jarlais. HIV among drug injectors: the epidemic and the response. AIDS Care 3:239–250, 1991.
28. AIDS among racial/ethnic minorities—United States, 1993. MMWR 43(35):644–647, 1994.
29. T Diaz, JW Buehler, KG Castro, JW Ward. AIDS trends among Hispanics in the United States. Am J Public Health 83:504–509, 1993.
30. RM Selik, KG Castro, M Pappaioanou, JW Buehler. Birthplace and the risk of AIDS among Hispanics in the United States [comments]. Am J Public Health 79(7):836–839, 1989.
31. CDC. National HIV Serosurveillance Summary: Results through 1992. Vol 5. Atlanta: Centers for Disease Control and Prevention, 1994.
32. RJ Battjes, RW Pickens, HW Haverkos, Z Sloboda. HIV risk factors among injecting drug users in five US cities. AIDS 8:681–687, 1994.
33. RE Chaisson, P Bacchetti, D Osmond, B Brodie, MA Sande, AR Moss. Cocaine use and HIV infection in intravenous drug users in San Francisco. JAMA 261(4):561–565, 1989.
34. EE Schoenbaum, D Hartel, PA Selwyn, RS Klein, K Davenny, M Rogers, C Feiner, G Friedland. Risk factors for human immunodeficiency virus infection in intravenous drug users [comments]. N Engl J Med 321(13):874–879, 1989.
35. CDC. HIV AIDS Surveillance Report. U.S. HIV and AIDS Cases Reported Through December 1997. Vol 9. Atlanta: Centers for Disease Control and Prevention, pp 1–44, 1998.
36. BR Rosenberg PS, Goedert JJ. Declining age at HIV infection in the United States. N Engl J Med 330:789–790, 1994.
37. DR Prevots, DM Allen, JS Lehman, TA Green, LR Petersen, M Gwinn. Trends in human immunodeficiency virus seroprevalence among injection drug users entering drug treatment centers, United States, 1988–1993. Am J Epidemiol 143(7):733–742, 1996.
38. AIDS among children—United States, 1996. MMWR 45(46):1005–1010, 1996.
39. ME McCaul, M Lillie-Blanton, DS Svikis. Drug use, HIV status and reproduction. In: Societal Responses to Reproductive Choices of HIV Infected Women. R Faden, N Kass, eds. New York: Oxford University Press, 1996.
40. CA Chiriboga, M Vibbert, R Malouf, MS Suarez, EJ Abrams, MC Heagarty, JC Brust, WA Hauser. Neurological correlates of fetal cocaine exposure: transient hypertonia of infancy and early childhood. Pediatrics 96(6):1070–1077, 1995.
41. WD Lyman. Perinatal AIDS: drugs of abuse and transplacental infection. Adv Exp Med Biol 335:211–217, 1993.
42. EM Connor, RS Sperling, R Gelber, et. al. Reduction of maternal-infant transmission of human immunodeficiency virus type 1 with zidovudine treatment. N Engl J Med 331:1173–1180, 1994.
43. AA Wiznia, M Crane, G Lambert, J Sansary, A Harris, L Solomaon. Zidovudine use to reduce perinatal HIV type 1 transmission in an urban medical center. JAMA 275:1504–1506, 1996.
44. SH Landesman, LA Kalish, DN Burns, H Minkoff, HE Fox, C Zorilla, P Garcia,

MG Fowler, L Mofenson, R Toumala. Obstetrical factors and the transmission of Human Immunodeficiency Virus Type 1 from mother to child. N Engl J Med 334(25):1617–1623, 1996.
45. M Charwarski, J Pakes, R Schottenfeld. Effects of substance abuse treatments on AIDS risk behaviors. J Addict Dis 17(4):49–59, 1998.
46. S Darke, W Hall, N Heather, J Ward, A Wodak. The reliability and validity of a scale to measure HIV risk-taking behavior among intravenous drug users. AIDS 5(2):181–185, 1991.
47. DS Metzger, D Dephillippois, P Druley, CP O'Brien, AT McLellan, J Williams, H Navaline, S Dyanick, GE Woody. The impact of HIV testing on risk for AIDS behaviors. College on Problems of Drug Dependence, 58th Annual Scientific Meeting, 1991.
48. G Dowling Guyer, M Johnson, D Fisher, et al. Reliability of drug users' self-reported HIV risk behaviors and validity of self-reported recent drug use. Assessment 1:383–392, 1994.
49. R Needle, D Fischer, N Weatherby, et al. The reliability of self-reported HIV risk behaviors of drug users. Psychol Addict Behav 9:242–250, 1995.
50. MC Chawarski, J Pakes, RS Schottenfeld. Assessment of HIV risk. J Addict Dis 17(4):49–59, 1998.
51. JE Anderson, AM Hardy, K Cahill, S Aral. HIV antibody testing and posttest counseling in the United States: data from the 1989 National Health Interview Survey. Am J Public Health 82:1533–1535, 1992.
52. G Gerbert, BT Maguire, T Bleecker, TJ Coates, SJ McPhee. Primary care physicians and AIDS: attitudinal and structural barriers to care. JAMA 266:2837–2842, 1991.
53. PG O'Connor, S Molde, S Henry, WT Shockcor, RS Schottenfeld. Human immunodeficiency virus infection in intravenous drug users: a model for primary care. Am J Med 93:382–386, 1992.
54. JM Coffin. HIV population dynamics in vivo: implications for genetic variation, pathogenesis, and therapy. Science 267:483–489, 1995.
55. L Doyon, G Croteau, D Thibeault, et al. Second locus involved in human immunodefciency virus type 1 resistance to protease inhibitors. J Virol 70:3763–3769, 1996.
56. AJ Japour, S Welles, RT D'Aquila, et al. Prevalence and clinical significance of zidovudine resistance mutations in human immunodeficiency virus isolated from patients after long-term zidovudine treatment. J Infect Dis 171:1172–1179, 1995.
57. SM Schnittman, JJ Greenhouse, MC Psellidopoulos, et al. Increasing viral burden in $CD4^+$ T-cells from patients with human immunodeficiency virus (HIV) infection reflects rapidly progressive immunosuppression and clinical disease. Ann Intern Med 113:438–443, 1990.
58. RI Connor, H Mohri, Y Cao, et al. Increased viral burden and cytopathicity correlate temporally with $CD4^+$ T-lymphocyte decline and clinical progression in human immunodeficiency virus type 1-infected individuals. J Virol 67:1772–1777, 1993.

59. D Vlahov, N Graham, D Hoover, C Flynn, JG Barlett, JB Margolick, CM Lyles, KE Nelson, D Smith, S Holmberg, H Farzadegan. Prognostic indicators for AIDS and infectious disease death in HIV-infected injection drug users: plasma viral load and CD4+ cell count. JAMA 279(1):35–40, 1998.
60. JD Lipsitz, JB Williams, JG Rabkin, RH Remien, M Bradbury, W el Sadr, R Goetz, S Sorrell, JM Gorman. Psychopathology in male and female intravenous drug users with and without HIV infection. Am J Psychiatry 151(11):1662–1668, 1994.
61. SJ Ferrando, TL Wall, SL Batki, JL Sorenson. Psychiatric morbidity, illicit drug use, and adherence to zidovudine (AZT) among injection drug users with HIV disease. Am J Drug Alcohol Abuse 22:475–487 1996.
62. FM Regier DA, Rae DS, Locke BZ, Keith SJ, Judd LL, Goodwin FK. Comorbidity of mental disorders with alcohol and other drug abuse. JAMA 264(19):2511–2518, 1990.
63. MK Kessler RC, Zhao S, Nelson CB, Hughes M, Eshleman S, Wittchen HU, Kendler KS. Lifetime and 12-month prevalence of DSM-III-R psychiatric disorders in the United States: results from the National Comorbidity Survey. Arch Gen Psychiatry 51:8–19, 1994.
64. CR Kessler RC, Warner LA, Nelson CB, Schulenberg J, Anthony JC. Lifetime co-occurance of DSM-IIIR alcohol abuse and dependence with other psychiatric disorders in the national comorbidity survey. Arch Gen Psychiatry 54:313–321, 1997.
65. DJ Hu, R Byers, PL Fleming, WW Ward. Characteristics of persons with late AIDS diagnosis in the United States. Am J Prev Med 11(2):114–119, 1995.
66. S Ferrando, S Batki. HIV-infected intravenous drug users in methadone maintenance treatment: clinical problems and their management. J Psychoactive Drugs 23:217–224, 1991.
67. CA Wiley. Pathology of neurologic disease in AIDS. Psychiatr Clin North Am 17(1):1–15, 1994.
68. S Koeing, HE Gendelman, JM Orenstein, et al. Detection of AIDS virus in macrophages in brain tissue from AIDS with encephalopathy. Science 233:1089–1093, 1986.
69. A Nath, RA Padua, JD Geiger. HIV-1 coat protein gp120-induced increases in levels of intrasynaptosomal calcium. Brain Res 678:200–206, 1995.
70. B Brew, M Predices, P Darveniza, et al. The neurological features of early and "latent" human immunodeficiency virus infection. Aust N Z J Med 19:700–705, 1989.
71. J Berger, W Sherimata, L Resnick, et al. Multiple sclerosis–like leukoencephalopathy revealing human immunodeficiency virus infection. Neurology 39:324–329, 1989.
72. JC McArthur, DR Hoover, H Bacellar, EN Miller, BA Cohen, JT Becker, NM Graham, JH McArthur, OA Selnes, LP Jacobson, et al. Dementia in AIDS patients: incidence and risk factors. Multicenter AIDS Cohort Study. Neurology 43(11):2245–2252, 1993.

73. RS Janssen, OC Nwanyanwu, RM Selik, JK Stehr-Green. Epidemiology of human immunodeficiency virus encephalopathy in the U.S. Neurology 1990; 42:1472–1476.
74. P Portegies, RH Enting, J de Gans, PR Algra, MM Derix, JM Lange, et al. Presentation and course of AIDS dementia complex: 10 years of follow-up in Amsterdam, The Netherlands. AIDS 7:669–675, 1993.
75. J Meadows, J Catalan, AN Singh, AP Burgess. Prevalence of HIV associated dementia (HAD) in a central London Health District in 1991. 9th International Conference on AIDS. Berlin, 1993.
76. MJG Harrison, SP Newman, MA Hall-Craggs, CJ Fowler, R Miller, BE Kendall, M Paley, I Wilkinson, B Sweeney, S Lunn, S Carter, I Williams. Evidence of CNS impairment in HIV infection: clinical, neuropsychological, EEG, and MRI/MRS study. J Neurol Neurosurg Psychiatry 65(3):301–307, 1998.
77. JT Becker, R Caldararo, OL Lopez, MA Dew, SK Dorst, G Banks. Qualitative features of the memory deficit associated with HIV infection and AIDS: cross-validation of a discriminant function classification scheme. J Clin Exp Neuropsychol 17:134–142, 1995.
78. SW Perry. Organic mental disorders caused by HIV: update on early diagnosis and treatment. Am J Psychiatry 147:696–710 1990.
79. MC Wellman. Neuropsychological impairment among intravenous drug users in pre-AIDS stages of HIV infection. J Neuropsychiatry Clin Neurosci 64:183–194, 1992.
80. CH Silberstein, MA O'Dowd, P Chartock, et al. A prospective four-year follow-up of neuropsychological function in HIV seropositive and seronegative methadone-maintained patients. Gen Hosp Psychiatry 15:351–359, 1993.
81. M Concha, NMH Graham, A Munoz, et al. Effect of chronic substance abuse on the neuropsychological performance of intravenous drug users with a high prevalence of HIV-1 seropositivity. Am J Epidemiol 36:1338–1348, 1992.
82. OA Selnes, JC McArthur, W Royal, et al. HIV-1 infection and intravenous drug use: longitudinal neuropsychological evaluation of asymptomatic subjects. Neurology 42:1924–1930, 1992.
83. S Avants, A Margolin, T McMahon, T Kosten. Association between self-report of cognitive impairment, HIV status, and cocaine use in a sample of cocaine-dependent methadone-maintained patients. Addict Behav 22(5): 599–611, 1997.
84. MJG Harrison, SP Newman, MA Hall-Craggs, CJ Fowler, R Miller, BE Kendall, M Paley, I Wilkinson, B Sweeney, S Lunn, S Carter, I Williams. Evidence of CNS impairment in HIV infection: clinical neuropsychological, EEG, and MRI/MRS study. J Neurol Neurosurg Psychiatry 65(3):301–307, 1998.
85. R Ylikoski, A Ylikosle, T Erkinjuntii, et al. White matter changes in healthy elderly persons correlate with attention and speed of mental processing. Arch Neurol 50:818–824, 1993.
86. S Avants, A Margolin, D DePhilippis, T Kosten. A comprehensive pharmacologic-psychosocial treatment program for HIV-seropositive cocaine- and opioid-dependent patients. J Subst Abuse Treat 15(3):261–265, 1988.

87. JJ Sidtis, C Gatsonis, RW Price, EJ Singer, AC Collier, DD Richman, et al. Zidovudine treatment of the AIDS dementia complex: results of a placebo-controlled trial. Ann Neurol 33:343–349, 1993.
88. JD Hamilton, PM Hartigan, MS Simberkoff, PL Day, GR Diamond, GM Dickerson, et al. A controlled trial of early versus late treatment with zidovudine in symptomatic human immunodeficiency virus infection: results of the Veterans Affairs Cooperative Study. N Engl J Med 326:437–443, 1992.
89. T Baldeweg, J Catalan, BG Gazzard. Risk of dementia and opportunistic brain disease in AIDS and zidovudine therapy. J Neurol Neurosurg Psychiatry 65(1):34–41, 1998.
90. B Brew, N Dunbar, J Druett, et al. Pilot study of the efficacy of atevirdine in the treatment of AIDS dementia complex. AIDS 10:1357–1360, 1996.
91. J Pace, G Brown, J Rundell, S Paolucci, K Drexler, S McManis. Prevalence of psychiatric disorders in a mandatory screening program for HIV: a pilot study. Military Med 155:67–80, 1990.
92. DO Perkins, EJ Davidson, J Leserman, D Liao, DL Evans. Personality disorder in patients infected with HIV: a controlled study with implications for clinical care. Am J Psychiatry 150(2):309–315, 1993.
93. JG Johnson, JB Williams, JG Rabkin, RR Goetz, RH Remien. Axis I psychiatric symptoms associated with HIV infection and personality disorder. Am J Psychiatry 152(4):551–554 1995.
94. H Heard, M Linehan. Dialectic Behavioral Therapy: an integrated approach to the treatment of borderline personality disorder. J Psychother Integration 4(1):55–82, 1994.
95. M Maj, R Janssen, F Starace, M Zaudig, P Satz, B Sughondhabirom, MA Luabeya, R Riedel, D Ndetei, HM Calil, et al. WHO Neuropsychiatric AIDS study, cross-sectional phase I: study design and psychiatric findings. Arch Gen Psychiatry 51(1):39–49, 1994.
96. JH Atkinson, I Grant, CJ Kennedy, DD Richman, SA Spector, JA McCutchan. Prevalence of psychiatric disorders among men infected with human in-numodeficiency virus: a controlled study. Arch Gen Psychiatry 45:859–864, 1988.
97. FK Judd, AM Mijch. Depressive symptoms in patients with HIV infection. Aust N Z J Psychiatry 1996; 30(1):104–109, 1996.
98. N Singh, C Squier, C Sivek, MM Wagener, VL Yu. Psychological stress and depression in older patients with intravenous drug use and human immunodeficiency virus infection: implications for intervention. Int J STD AIDS 8(4):251–255, 1997.
99. MH Katz, JM Douglas, Jr, GA Bolan, R Marx, M Sweat, MS Park, SP Buchbinder. Depression and use of mental health services among HIV-infected men. AIDS Care 8(4):433–442, 1996.
100. I Fukunishi, T Hosaka, M Negishi, H Moriya, M Hayashi, T Matsumoto. Avoidance coping behaviors and low social support are related to depressive

symptoms in HIV-positive patients in Japan [comments]. Psychosomatics 38(2):113–118, 1997.
101. I Grant, JH Atkinson. The evolution of neurobehavioral complications of HIV infection. Psycholog Med 20:747–754, 1990.
102. JB McClure, SL Catz, J Prejean, PJ Brantley, GN Jones. Factors associated with depression in a heterogeneous HIV-infected sample. J Psychosom Res 40(4):407–415, 1996.
103. A Dannenburg, J McNeil, J Brundage, R Brookmeyer. Suicide and HIV infection: mortality and follow up of 4147 HIV seropositive military service applicants. JAMA 271:174–176, 1996.
104. JB Williams, JG Rabkin, RH Remien, JM Gorman, AA Ehrhardt. Multidisciplinary baseline assessment of homosexual men with and without human immunodeficiency virus infection. II. Standardized clinical assessment of current and lifetime psychopathology. Arch Gen Psychiatry 48(2):124–130, 1991.
105. M Maj. Depressive syndromes and symptoms in subjects with human immunodeficiency virus (HIV) infection. Br J Psychiatry 30(suppl):117–122, 1996.
106. J Catalan, A Burgess, I Klimes, B Gazzard. Psychological Medicine of HIV Infection. Oxford: Oxford University Press, 1995.
107. CG Lyketsos, DR Hoover, M Guccione, W Senterfitt, MA Dew, J Wesch, MJ VanRaden, GJ Treisman, H Morgenstern. Depressive symptoms as predictors of medical outcomes in HIV infection: Multicenter AIDS Cohort Study. JAMA 270(21):2563–2567, 1993.
108. JH Burack, DC Barrett, RD Stall, MA Chesney, ML Ekstrand, TJ Coates. Depressive symptoms and CD4 lymphocyte decline among HIV-infected men. JAMA 270(21):2568–2573, 1993.
109. M Perdices, N Dunbar, A Grunseit, W Hall, DA Cooper. Anxiety, depression and HIV related symptomatology across the spectrum of HIV disease. Aust N Z J Psychiatry 26(4):560–566, 1992.
110. D Mierlak, A Leon, S Perry. Does physical improvement reduce depressive symptoms in HIV-infected medical inpatients? Gen Hosp Psychiatry 17(5):380–384, 1995.
111. EP Zorrilla, JR McKay, L Luborsky, K Schmidt. Relation of stressors and depressive symptoms to clinical progression of viral illness. Am J Psychiatry 153(5):626–635, 1996.
112. I Fukunishi, T Matsumoto, M Negishi, M Hayashi, T Hosaka, H Moriya. Somatic complaints associated with depressive symptoms in HIV-positive patients. Psychother Psychosomatics 66(5):248–251, 1997.
113. DO Perkins, J Leserman, RA Stern, SF Baum, D Liao, RN Golden, DL Evans. Somatic symptoms and HIV infection: relationship to depressive symptoms and indicators of HIV disease. Am J Psychiatry 152(12):1776–1781, 1995.
114. JC Markowitz, JH Kocsis, B Fishman, LA Spielman, LB Jacobsberg, AJ Frances, GL Klerman, SW Perry. Treatment of depressive symptoms in human immunodeficiency virus–positive patients. Arch Gen Pychiatry 55(5):452–457, 1998.

115. B Grassi, O Gambini, G Garghentini, A Lazzarin, S Scarone. Efficacy of paroxetine for the treatment of depression in the context of HIV infection. Pharmacopsychiatry 30(2):70–71, 1997
116. VF Holmes, F Fernandez, JK Levy. Psychostimulant response in AIDS-related complex patients. J Clin Psychiatry 50:5–8, 1989
117. CG Lyketsos, J Schwartz, M Fishman, G Treisman. AIDS mania. J Neuropsychiatry Clin Neurosci 9(2):277–279, 1997
118. R Seth, K Granville-Grossman, D Goldmeier, S Lynch. Psychiatric illness in patients with HIV infection and AIDS referred to the liaison psychiatrist. Br J Psychiatry 159:347–355, 1991
119. HM Chochinov, KG Wilson, M Enn, S Lander. Prevalence of depression in terminally ill: effects of diagnostic criteria and symptom threshold judgements. Am J Psychiatry 151(4):537–540, 1994
120. SN Ghaemi, MD Katzow, SP Desai, MD Goodwin. Gabapentin treatment of mood disorders: a preliminary study. J Clin Psychiatry 59(8):426–429, 1998
121. MA Dew, JT Becker, J Sanchez, R Caldararo, OL Lopez, J Wess, SK Dorst, G Banks. Prevalence and predictors of depressive, anxiety and substance use disorders in HIV-infected and uninfected men. Psychol Med 27(2):395–409, 1997.
122. MA Dew. Psychiatric disorder in the context of physical illness. In: Adversity, Stress, and Psychopathology. BP Dohrenwend, ed. Washington, DC: American Psychiatric Press, 1997.
123. MA Dew, RG Simmmons, LH Roth, HC Schulberg, ME Thompson, JM Armitage, BP Griffith. Psychological predictors of vulnerability to distress in the year following heart transplantation. Psychol Med 24:929–945, 1994.
124. RD Canning, MA Dew, S Davidson. Psychological distress among caregivers to heart transplant recipients. Soc Sci Med 42:599–608, 1996.
125. PJ Abbott, BA Moore, SB Weller, HD Delaney. AIDS risk behavior in opioid dependent patients treated with community reinforcement approach and relationships with psychiatric disorders. J Addict Dis 17(4):33–48, 1998.
126. R Meibach, D Dunner, L Wilson, et al. Comparative efficacy of propranolol, chlordiazepoxide, and placebo in the treatment of anxiety: a double blind study. J Clin Psychiatry 9:22–27, 1989.
127. SM Brown, et al. Immunologic dysfunction in heroin addicts. Arch Intern Med 134:1001–1006, 1974.
128. J Heathcote, K Taylor. Immunity and nutrition in heroin addicts. Drug Alcohol Depend 8:245–255, 1981.
129. R Weber, A Pert. The periaqueductal gray matter mediates opiate-induced immunosuppression. Science 245:188–190, 1989.
130. A Falek, J Maden, D Shafer, R Donahoe. Individual differences in opiate-induced alterations at the cytogenetic, DNA repair, and immunologic levels: opportunity for genetic assessment. Natl Inst Drug Abuse Res Monogr Ser 66:11–24, 1986.
131. PS Dowd, RV Heatly. The influence of undernutrition on immunity. Clin Sci 66:241–248, 1984.

132. DM Novick, M Ochshirn, V Ghalli, TS Croxson, WD Mercer, N Chiorazzi, MJ Kreek. Natural killer cell activity and lymphocyte subsets in parenteral heroin abusers and long-term methadone maintenance patients. J Pharmacol Exp Ther 250:606–610, 1989.
133. C McLachlan, N Crofts, A Wodak, S Crowe. The effects of methadone on immune function among injecting drug users: a review. Addiction 88:257–263, 1993.
134. DS Metzger, GE Woody, AT McLellan, OB CP, P Druley, H Navaline, D DePhilippis, P Stolley, E Abrutyn. Human immunodeficiency virus seroconversion among intravenous drug users in- and out-of-treatment: an 18-month prospective follow-up. J AIDS 6(9):1049–1056, 1993.
135. E Drucker, P Lurie, A Wodak, P Alcabes. Measuring harm reduction: the effects of needle and syringe exchange programs and methadone maintenance on the ecology of HIV. AIDS 12(suppl A):S217–230, 1998.
136. PG O'Connor, PA Selwyn, RS Schottenfeld. Medical care for injection-drug users with human immunodeficiency virus infection. N Engl J Med 331:450–459, 1994.
137. A Kim, M Galanter, R Casteneda, et al. Crack cocaine use and sexual behavior among psychiatric inpatients. Am J Drug Alcohol Abuse 18:235–246, 1992.
138. RE Booth, JK Watters, DD Chitwood, RE Booth, JK Watters, DD Chitwood, RE Booth, JK Watters, DD Chitwood. HIV risk-related sex behaviors among injection drug users, crack smokers, and injection drug users who smoke crack. Am J Public Health 83(8):1144–1148, 1993.
139. BR Edlin, KL Irwin, S Faruque, CB McCoy, C Word, Y Serrano, JA Inciardi, BP Bowser, RF Schilling, SD Holmberg. Intersecting epidemics—crack cocaine use and HIV infection among inner-city young adults. Multicenter Crack Cocaine and HIV Infection Study Team. N Engl J Med 331(21):1422–1427, 1994.
140. SK Schwarcz, GA Bolan, M Fullilove, et al. Crack cocaine and the exchange of sex for money or drugs: risk factors for gonorrhea among black adolescents in San Francisco. Sex Transm Dis 19:7–13, 1992.
141. R Pillai, BS Nair, RR Watson. AIDS, drugs of abuse and the immune system: a complex immunotoxicological network. Arch Toxicol 65(8):609–617, 1991.
142. RM Donahoe, A Falek. Neuroimmunomodulation by opiates and other drugs of abuse: relationship to HIV infection and AIDS. Adv Biochem Psychopharmacol 1988; 44:145–158.
143. M Fiala, XH Gan, L Zhang, SD House, T Newton, MC Graves, P Shapshak, M Stins, KS Kim, M Witte, SL Chang. Cocaine enhances monocyte migration across the blood-brain barrier: cocaine's connection to AIDS dementia and vasculitis? Adv Exp Med Biol 1998; 437:199–205.
144. NS Siddiqui, LS Brown, Jr, RW Makuch. Short-term declines in CD4 levels associated with cocaine use in HIV-1 seropositive, minority injecting drug users. J Natl Med Assoc 85(4):293–296, 1993.
145. S Hintz, J Kuck, J Peterkin, D Volk, S Zisook. Depression in the context of

Human Immunodeficiency virus infection: implications for treatment. J Clin Psychiatry 51:497–501, 1990.
146. S Batki, L Manfredi, P Jacob, R Jones. Fluoxetine for cocaine dependence in methadone maintenance: quantitative plasma and urine cocaine/benzoylecgonine concentrations. J Clin Psychopharmacol 13(4):243–250, 1993.
147. BC Leigh, R Stall. Substance use and risky sexual behavior for exposure to HIV: issues in methodology, interpretation, and prevention. Am Psychologist 48(10):1035–1045, 1993.
148. AL Avins, WJ Woods, CP Lindan, ES Hudes, W Clark, SB Hulley. HIV infection and risk behaviors among heterosexuals in alcohol treatment programs. JAMA 271(7):515–518, 1994.
149. R Epstein. Cocaine and HIV prevalence in an alcohol treatment center. JAMA 272(6):10, 1994.
150. SJ Schleifer, SE Keller, JE Franklin, S LaFrarge, SI Miller. HIV seropositivity in inner-city alcoholics. Hosp Commun Med 41:248–254, 1990.
151. JM Jacobson, TM Worner, HS Sacks, CS Lieber. Human immunodeficiency virus and hepatitis B virus infections in a New York City alcoholic population. J Stud Alcohol 53(1):76–79, 1992.
152. J Mahler, D Yi, M Sacks, H Dermatis, A Stebinger, C Card, S Perry. Undetected HIV infection among patients admitted to an alcohol rehabilitation unit. Am J Psychiatry 151:439–440, 1994.
153. MT Fullilove, J Wiley, RE Fullilove, E Golden, J Catania, J Peterson, K Garrett, D Siegel, B Marin, S Kegeles, T Coates, S Hulley. Risk for AIDS in multiethnic neighborhoods in San Francisco, California. Western J Med 157:32–40, 1992.
154. B Critchlow. The powers of John Barleycorn: beliefs about the effects of alcohol on social behavior. Am Psychologist 41:751–764, 1986.
155. JA Boscarino, AL Avins, WJ Woods, CP Lindan, ES Hudes, W Clark. Alcohol-related risk factors associated with HIV infection among patients entering alcoholism treatment: implications for prevention. J Stud Alcohol 56:642–653, 1995.
156. BC Leigh. The relationship of sex-related alcohol expectancies to alcohol consumption and sexual behavior. Br J Addiction 85:919–928, 1990.
157. WJ Woods, AL Avins, CP Lindan, ES Hudes, JA Boscarino, WW Clark. Predictors of HIV-related risk behaviors among heterosexuals in alcoholism treatment. J Stud Alcohol 57(5):486–493, 1996.
158. SE Hyman. A man with alcoholism and HIV infection. JAMA 274(10):837–843, 1995.
159. JH Samet, KA Freedberg, MD Stein, R Lewis, J Savetsky, L Sullivan, SM Levenson, R Hingson. Trillion virion delay: time from testing positive for HIV to presentation for primary care. Arch Intern Med 158(7): 734–740, 1998.
160. J Tinsley, RE Finlayson, RM Morse. Developments in the treatment of alcoholism. Mayo Clin Proc 73(9):857–863, 1998.
161. J Mann, DJ Tarantola. AIDS in the World II. 2nd ed. New York: Oxford Press, 1996.

162. JK Watters. Historical perspective on the use of bleach in HIV/AIDS prevention. J AIDS 7:743–747, 1994.
163. HW Haverkos, ST Jones. HIV, drug-use paraphernalia, and bleach. J AIDS 7:741–742, 1994.
164. RS Schottenfeld, S O'Malley, K Abdul-Salaam, PG O'Connor. Decline in intravenous drug use among treatment-seeking opiate users. J Subst Abuse Treat 10:5–10, 1993.
165. P Griffiths, M Gossop, B Powis, J Strang. Transitions in patterns of heroin administration: a study of heroin chasers and heroin injectors. Addiction 89(3):301–309, 1994.
166. P Lurie, AL Reingold, B Bowser, et al. The Public Health Impact of Needle Exchange Programs in the United States and Abroad. San Francisco: University of California, 1993.
167. HW Haverkos, PF Pinsky, DPP Drotman, DJ Bergman. Disease manifestation among homosexual men with acquired immunodeficiency syndrome: a possible role of nitrates in Kaposi's sarcoma. Sex Transm Dis 14(1):29–40, 1988.
168. DA Calsyn, AJ Saxon, G Freeman, Jr, S Whittaker. Ineffectiveness of AIDS education and HIV antibody testing in reducing high-risk behaviors among injection drug users. Am J Public Health 82(4):573–575, 1992.
169. ML Kamb, M Fishbein, JM Douglas, Jr, F Rhodes, J Rogers, G Bolan, J Zenilman, T Hoxworth, CK Malotte, M Iatesta, C Kent, A Lentz, S Graziano, RH Byers, TA Peterman. Efficacy of risk-reduction counseling to prevent human immunodeficiency virus and sexually transmitted diseases: a randomized controlled trial. Project RESPECT Study Group. JAMA 280(13):1161–1167, 1998.
170. DD Celentano, D Vlahov, S Cohn, VM Shadle, O Obasanjo, RD Moore. Self-reported antiretroviral therapy in injection drug users. JAMA 280(6):544–546, 1998.
171. SA Strathdee, A Palepu, PGA Cornelisse, et al. Barriers to use of free antiretroviral therapy in injection drug users. JAMA 280:547–549, 1998.
172. RE Chaisson, JC Keruly, RD Moore. Race, sex, drug use, and progression of HIV disease. N Engl J Med 333:751–756, 1995.
173. R Baker. 3-Drug therapy reduces deaths and new AIDS-related illnesses by 50%. BETA 3–4, 1997.
174. JPA Ioannidis, HS Sacks, JC Cappellen, et al. Clinical efficacy of antiretroviral changes in treatment-experienced HIV-infected patients: a meta-analysis. 4th Annual Conference on Retroviruses and Opportunistic Infections. Washington, DC, 1997.
175. GF Vanhove, JM Schapiro, MA Winters, TC Merigan, TF Blaschke. Patient compliance and drug failure in protease inhibitor monotherapy [letter]. JAMA 276:1955–1956, 1996.
176. SG Deeks, M Smith, M Holodniy, JO Kahn. HIV-1 Protease inhibitors: a review for clinicians. JAMA 277(2):145–153, 1997.
177. GJ Treisman. A behavioral approach for the promotion of adherence in compli-

cated patient populations. 37th Interscience Congress on Antimicrobial Agents and Chemotherapy Symposium. Toronto, Ontario, 1997.
178. EL Schwartz, AB Brechbuhl, P Kahl, MA Miller, PA Selwyn, GH Friedland. Pharmacokinetic interactions of zidovudine and methadone in intravenous drug-using patients with HIV infection. J AIDS 5(6):619–626, 1992.
179. EF McCance-Katz, PM Rainey, P Jatlow, G Friedland. Methadone effects on zidovudine disposition (AIDS Clinical Trials Group 262). J AIDS Hum Retrovirol 18(5):435–443, 1998.
180. CB Nemeroff, CL Devane, BG Pollack. Newer antidepressants and the cytochrome P450 system. Am J Psychiatry 153:311–320, 1986.

11
Chronic Pain and Substance-Related Disorders

John R. Hubbard*
*Vanderbilt University Medical Center
and Nashville VA Medical Center
Nashville, Tennessee*

Edward A. Workman
*Pain Medicine & Neuropsychiatry Associates of Tennessee
and Lakeshore Mental Health Institute
Knoxville, Tennessee*

OVERVIEW

Chronic pain is a heterogeneous problem, which differs among patients in etiology, body location, duration, severity, and other important variables (1,2). Nearly 20% of the population will have chronic pain sometime in their life. The cost of chronic pain to the patient, their families, and society is enormous.

According to most current definitions, the syndrome of "chronic pain" (regardless of specific etiology) requires at least 6 months' duration of pain (1,3). Unlike acute pain, whose cause is usually known, the source of chronic pain is often less well defined and can be adjacent to or distal from the original site of the injury. Almost by definition, chronic pain is unrelenting and often unable to be "cured" in the usual sense of that term. The pain can, however, be minimized by proper treatment.

---

*Currently in private practice.

Chronic pain patients represent a subpopulation who are at increased risk for substance abuse and chemical dependence. In this chapter, the term "abuse" is generally used for convenience to refer to any substance-related problem(s) unless otherwise indicated. Other terms, such as "dependence" and "misuse," are used when appropriate. The term "abuse," as specifically defined by the fourth edition of the *Diagnostic and Statistical Manual of Mental Disorders* (DSM-IV), is more rigidly defined when studies compare "abuse" with another DSM-IV-defined problem such as "dependence."

When a patient has a substance abuse problem plus a chronic pain disorder, the treatment issues become even more difficult than the already complex problems associated with either of these disorders alone. Some patients will complain of pain who are actually drug seeking, and others with a history of substance abuse may appropriately request pain medications for their physical pain (not due to craving). Sorting out which patients may be drug seeking from those who need more pain control is a very difficult matter with no perfect answers. Knowing the pain patient well and having a thoughtful stepwise system for pain control will help optimize treatment.

The increased risk of substance abuse in the chronic pain population comes from many sources, including:

1. Exposure to pain medications with potential for abuse (particularly opiates and benzodiazepines), with inadequate screening and medical monitoring
2. Inappropriate self-medication of physical pain with substances of abuse
3. Inappropriate self-medication of pain-associated stress and emotional and relationship problems with substances of abuse
4. Inappropriate self-medication of comorbid psychiatric disorders (such as depression) with substances of abuse

The estimated prevalence of alcohol/drug problems in chronic pain patients ranges widely between different studies and subpopulations. In seven studies reviewed by Fishbain et al. (4) in 1992, the prevalence of substance-related disorders in chronic pain patients varied from 3% to 19%. These data suggest that while most pain patients will not develop an alcohol or drug problem, substance abuse occurs in a significant number of these patients.

The presence of other comorbid psychiatric problems together with a substance abuse problem should be carefully considered in the evaluation of chronic pain patients (5–10). Chronic pain patients often have resulting depression and anxiety problems. Treatment of comorbid psychiatric disorders is essential to the overall health of these patients and impacts on the outcome of both chronic pain and substance abuse treatment. Interestingly, many of the medications commonly used for psychiatric purposes, such as antidepressants and mood-stabilizing medications, also appear to reduce baseline chronic pain levels independent of their effects on the psychiatric illnesses.

In this chapter, we discuss basic concepts in chronic pain, the association between chronic pain and substance-related disorders, and treatment strategies for comorbidity. In addition, we address the difficulties of doing research on this topic, as well as discuss important areas for future investigations.

CLASSIFICATION OF CHRONIC PAIN

Chronic pain has a variety of etiologies, such as trauma, malformation, and disease. The pain sites most often involve the lower back, neck, and head (1). The major neuronal pain conduction pathways include the lateral spinothalamic tract, dorsal lateral tract, and dorsal column (3,11,12). Pain pathways travel to the posterior thalamus in the brain. The posterior thalamus is also influenced by the limbic system (which contributes an emotional integration of the pain) and cortical system (which provides contextual integration of the pain) (2,3,11,12). In this regard, Malzack and Casey (13) subdivided the pain experiences into three divisions: 1) sensory-discriminative, 2) motivational-affective, and 3) cognitive-evaluative. "Sensory-discriminative" refers to the basic neuronal information rapidly conducting afferent nerves sensing that damage has occurred. The motivational-affective component comprises more of the emotional reaction to the pain. The cognitive-evaluation division places this pain information into context of a person's life via interconnection with the cerebral cortex (2,13).

Chronic pain can be categorized in other ways, as shown in Table 1. For example, it can be conceptualized by the etiologies of the pain, such as nerve damage versus muscle damage (neurophysiological classification). Terminal (often cancer) versus nonterminal pain distinctions are very important. Another classification is based on the influence of psychological factors on pain (the DSM-IV approach). Naturally, any particular source of pain may be classified by several different systems (discussed above and elsewhere).

Terminal Versus Nonterminal Etiology

One important way chronic pain can be classified is by terminal versus nonterminal etiology of the pain. In most cases the terminal etiology is malignant cancer, whereas nonterminal causes of chronic pain are numerous (such as disc disease, trauma, and arthritis). As discussed below, such a differentiation often impacts on treatment choices (such as the use of chronic

Table 1. Chronic Pain Classifications

1. Terminal versus nonterminal etiology—usually malignant or nonmalignant
2. Muscle versus nerve etiology

    Myofacial (muscle) pain

    Rotator cuff injury
    Tendinitis
    Tension headache
    Temporomandibular joint disorder
    Muscle strain
    Fibromyalgia

    Neuropathy (nerve) pain

    Diabetic neuropathy
    Carpal tunnel syndrome
    Reflex sympathetic dystrophy
    Postherpetic neurolgia
    Phantom pain
    Thoracic outlet syndrome
    Causalgia

3. DSM-IV-Based Classification
    1. Chronic pain associated with psychological factors
    2. Chronic pain associated with both psychological factors and a general medical condition

Source: Refs. 1, 14, 63.

opiate narcotics). Generally, there is little concern about chronic opiate use in terminal patients, however, much more consideration of the long-term risk/benefits is needed for nonterminal chronic pain patients since sedation, cognitive slowing, tolerance, future withdrawal symptoms, and possible chemical dependency on opiates could have a significant impact on the patient's life.

Neurophysiological Classification

Chronic pain can also be categorized neurophysiologically. According to neurophysiological criteria, chronic pain can be divided into "neuropathic" or "myofascial" pain as described below (1):

1. *Neuropathic pain* involves damage, irritation, or impingement of nerves. Classic neuropathic pain syndromes (Table 1) include diabetic neuropathy, carpal tunnel syndrome, thoracic outlet syndrome, causalgia in a specific nerve or nerve root, phantom pain, reflex sympathetic dystrophy, and postherpetic neuralgia

2. *Myofascial pain* is believed to be due to disruption of muscle or adjacent soft-tissue structures, such as tendons and ligaments (1). This type of pain is often caused by tissue strain or muscle-fiber rupture, leading to the destruction of microvascular structures in muscle tissue. This, in turn, leads to fibrosis within the muscle. Myofascial pain syndromes (Table 1) include rotator cuff injury, tendinitis, tension headache, temporomandibular joint dysfunction syndrome (TMJ), fibromyalgia, and muscle-strain syndromes.

DSM-IV Classification of Pain Syndromes

The DSM-IV (14) divides chronic pain disorders into two categories:

1. *Pain disorder associated with psychological factors*—when emotional issues are believed to be the dominant source of the chronic pain, while general medical problems (i.e., the physical basis of the pain) are of less significance
2. *Pain disorder associated with both psychological factors and a general medical condition*—when physical illness and emotional issues both have major roles in the pain syndrome

Pain itself is a major stressor that results in typical emotional sequelae, and, sometimes, full-blown mood and/or anxiety disorders (15). Depressive and anxiety symptoms develop in a majority of chronic pain patients as feelings of loss and hopelessness grow, and a significant proportion (about 40–60%) develop a full blown depressive spectrum disorder (such as major depressive disorder or dysthymia) (5–10). In most cases, these depressive conditions stem from pain, rather than vice versa. That is, the chronic pain acts as a severe stressor, and chronic stress can lead to development of depression. Thus, pain is more likely to cause psychiatric sequelae than to be caused by psychiatric processes. This is contrary to common folklore suggesting that "psychosomatic" or "psychogenic" pain (i.e., with psychological rather than physiological causes) is the rule rather than the exception.

CHRONIC PAIN TREATMENT STRATEGIES

Overview

Treatment of chronic pain patients should involve a well-coordinated, multidisciplinary team, consisting of a primary care physician, pain specialist, psychiatrist, anesthesiologist, physiatrist (physical and rehabilitation medicine doctor), physical therapist, social worker, psychologist, and possibly others (1,2). In some cases such a large team may not be required, or may not be possible to arrange. However, attempts should be made to utilize the healthcare professionals who are needed and available, and to communicate with those involved in the care of the patient. Coordinated care not only maximizes pain control but also decreases the risk of related problems such as multiple doctors prescribing the same or related medications.

Common problems associated with providing medical care to chronic pain patients include:

1. Limited access to medical care
2. Secondary-gain issues (such as possible litigation and disability claims)
3. Lack of coordination of professional staff
4. Frustration with unfulfilled and possibly unrealistic expectations of patients
5. Untreated comorbid substance abuse and/or other psychiatric disorders
6. Insufficient accessibility of healthcare providers in busy practices
7. Misunderstanding by staff of patient "needs" versus "wants," and/or lack of knowledge about the nature and optimal treatment of chronic pain

Although there are both important medication and nonmedication treatment modalities for chronic pain, we focus in this chapter on the pharmacological options, as drug choices can influence the risk of substance abuse in chronic pain patients (1). Other important treatment modalities should not be minimized and in fact can help reduce and/or help prevent the need for medications. Some nonpharmacological approaches to pain management are shown in Table 2.

Nonopiate Medications in Treatment of Chronic Pain

Optimizing the use of nonopiate pain medication can be an important means of preventing substance abuse problems arising from prescription nar-

Table 2. Nonpharmacological Treatment Options for Chronic Pain

Trigger point injection	Radiation therapy
Surgery	TENS Unit
Psychotherapy	Whirlpool
Nerve blocks	Massage therapy
Physical therapy	Acupuncture
Occupational therapy	Hypnosis
Relaxation training	Heat/cold
Biofeedback	

Source: Refs. 1, 2, 16, 17, 27, 31, 64–68.

cotics in chronic pain patients. In some cases nonopiate pain medications can be used alone, and in other circumstances they may be used in combination with opiate pain medications. Pharmacological treatment options for neuropathic pain and myofascial pain overlap, but differ to a certain extent as described below (1).

Nonopiate pharmacological treatment of *neuropathic chronic pain* primarily includes tricyclic antidepressants (TCAs), anticonvulsant medications, and nonsteroidal anti-inflammatory drugs (NSAIDs) (1,2,16). Although the mechanism of TCAs and anticonvulsants in treatment of chronic pain is uncertain, some studies indicate that their effect occurs even in the absence of depression or other mood disorders. Presumably, antidepressants act via their impact on serotonin and/or norepinephrine neuronal systems. The anticonvulsants (such as valproic acid, gabapentin, and carbamazepine) appear to modulate sodium channels in nerve fibers, preventing hyperalgesia (1). NSAIDs decrease the inflammatory processes (as described below) that are often associated with pain (1,2,16).

Treatment of *myofascial chronic pain* syndromes primarily includes NSAIDs, TCAs, muscle relaxants, and antispasmodic agents (1,2). NSAIDs are of particular importance because inflammation is often a major contributor to this type of pain. NSAIDs, such as aspirin and ibuprofen, act by inhibiting cylo-oxygenase, an enzyme used in the biosynthesis of prostaglandins, which sensitize nociceptors in peripheral nerve cells (2,17). A CNS mechanism of action is also suspected for NSAIDs (2,17,18).

Meclofenamate is an NSAID that appears to have particular efficacy in myofascial pain syndromes. Some adverse effects of NSAIDs include blood-clotting changes (especially aspirin), renal problems, and gastrointestinal (such as bleeding of ulcers) (1,2). Misoprostol is often used with meclofenamate (and other NSAIDs) to prevent gastrointestinal side effects (17). Acetaminophen can be used for pain control and has few side effects, except for hepatotoxicity at high doses.

Clonazepam, and other benzodiazepines, enhance the GABA neurotransmitter system and may be prescribed to reduce muscle spasms and promote sleep in appropriate patients. Interestingly, the benefits of benzodiazepines are not always demonstrated in pain patients. For example, Gracely et al. (19) reported that diazepam lowered the affective response to an electrical pain stimulus but did not diminish pain sensory stimulation. In a 1990 study, 38% of 114 chronic pain patients were using benzodiazepines (20). Of these, 93% started benzodiazepine use after pain onset. Most (86%) were using these medications for sleep (20). Despite benzodiazepine use, the majority of chronic pain patients continued to experience sleep difficulties similar to those of the non–benzodiazepine group (20). In addition, results of Hendler et al. (21) indicated that benzodiazepines caused greater cognitive impairment and associated EEG changes than opiates in chronic pain patients. Some reports suggest that benzodiazepines may actually worsen the chronic pain syndrome, possibly by inhibiting serotonin release (20).

The primary advantage of nonopiate medications is their lack of tolerance and chemical dependence (except for benzodiazepines) (17). Unfortunately, nonopiate pain medications have a "ceiling effect" whereby pain control is limited and may not be totally eliminated (2,17). It is therefore important to optimize the nonpharmacological treatment options, and, if necessary, opiate pain medications may be administered. Although a ceiling effect may limit effectiveness of a drug, it is important to remember that the ceiling dose differs between individuals and may be more than the usual dose (2). Although not commonly suspected, it is interesting to note that nonnarcotic analgestics can be abused, especially by females in lower socioeconomic situations (22–24).

Opiate Treatment of Chronic Pain

The term "opiate" originates from the "opium poppy," *Papaver Somniferum*. Numerous natural and synthetic opiates (opioids) are currently available for clinical use. Opiates can be properly and effectively used for most sufferers of chronic pain (2,25). However, it is also important to recognize that these medications can lead to serious problems such as substance abuse in some patients. It is because of their potential for abuse that opiate medications are highly regulated. Some animal studies suggest that chronic morphine use can stimulate factors that increase pain sensitization (26).

Chronic Pain

In general, opiates are the most potent and rapid-acting medications for pain. Traditionally, opiate medications have been prescribed for acute trauma, postsurgical pain, and chronic pain associated with malignancy. Opiates may also be used in cases of nonmalignant chronic pain if other treatment options are not successful. Unlike alcohol, marijuana, cocaine, and other substances of abuse, opiates are generally obtained directly from physicians (although they can be purchased illegally on the street) and so manipulation of medical professionals often occurs. In many, if not most, cases the prescribing clinican never realizes that he or she has been used as a source of drugs for recreational purposes. Some patients sell their medications on the street to obtain the revenue needed to purchase other substances of abuse such as cocaine. In accordance with the philosophy "first do no harm," most doctors are very cautious about prescribing opiates for nonterminal chronic pain conditions. On the other hand, some doctors argue that chronic pain is often undertreated and tend to more readily prescribe narcotics for nonmalignant chronic pain patients. Thus, the use of opiates in nonmalignant chronic pain management continues to be a source of considerable and often heated debate (27). Ultimately every case must be examined on an individual basis to determine the risk/benefits of opiates for the patient.

Abuse of opiates is reported to be low in prevalence for the general population, but may occur in higher numbers in certain subpopulations. People in urban settings, healthcare professionals, and males appear to be higher-risk groups (28). Chronic narcotic use in nonmalignant chronic pain patients requires caution, appropriate patient education, close monitoring, and clear warnings to the patient of potential risks to diminish the chance of abuse, dependence, and other side effects. In instances when chronic narcotics are used, some general guidelines include (1,29):

1. *Alternative* pharmacological approaches (such as NSAIDs, TCAs, and mood stabilizers) and nonpharmacological means (such as physical therapy, heat/cold, and transcutaneous electrical nerve stimulation) of pain management should be attempted (and failed) prior to chronic use of narcotics.
2. *Rule out* a history of past or current problems with alcohol and/or other drugs. If a history of a substance use disorder(s) exists, avoid narcotics if possible. Use of a substance of possible abuse, such as opiates, can (but does not always) escalate and trigger a relapse of substance abuse problems.
3. Use the *lowest dose* of the opiate with the *lowest potential for abuse* that effectively treats the pain. If possible, use slow-onset, long-

acting opiates, as they tend to have less abuse potential, and avoid p.r.n. scheduling. Opiates should be used on a specific and fixed schedule to avoid "pill popping" in response to stress and increased pain. Careful monitoring will dictate if the medication dose is too high or too low.
4. *Re-evaluate* the need for narcotic analgesics at frequent office visits (initially at least every 2–4 weeks). If opiates are not needed, taper them off as appropriate.
5. *Titrate* analgesic medications carefully and slowly in either direction. Abrupt changes can cause withdrawal or other consequences.
6. *Monitor for side effects* of opiates, including chemical dependence (such as tolerance and/or withdrawal symptoms), abuse, sedation, respiration problems, visual motor deficits, cognitive slowing, and others.
7. Obtain *informed consent*, and consider a written contract when prescribing chronic opiates, indicating that the medications will be used only as prescribed and are to be prescribed by only *one doctor*.
8. Consider *confirmation* of no drug abuse/dependence by other sources as appropriate (such as occasional discussions with patient's family members with the patient's consent). Although we would like to trust all our patients to properly use medications, this is not always the case. It is important for doctors to remember that when abuse occurs, it is generally hidden from them (they are the source of the drug), but abuse may be suspected by a spouse or other family member.
9. Use a *coordinated approach* if other clinicians are involved with care to prevent several doctors from prescribing the same or similar medications and to optimize pain control. A patient who has no intention of abusing medications may simply not be aware that two medications from different physicians may both be opiates that taken together can lead to chemical dependence and/or abuse.
10. Set up an agreement to allow for random urine *drug screening*. If this is presented within the context of a larger program rather than as an individual issue, patients will generally be understanding and cooperative.

In addition to the general guidelines above, screening tools for substance abuse can be helpful. For example, a 42-question monitor was published by Compton et al. (30) in 1998 that focuses on evaluating possible prescription drug abuse in chronic pain patients.

Specific Opiate Medications

Opiate pain medications (Table 3) are effective analgesics and do not cause major organ damage when properly used. Toxic doses and certain side effects (such as constipation, oversedation, and cognitive slowing) are the primary concerns along with possible dependence and abuse (27). Withdrawal, tolerance, and physical dependence to opiates can develop very quickly and should be monitored (31,32). In some cases the effective treatment of pain outweighs the potential development of physical dependence (31). Schofferman (33) suggested that chronic pain patients can be divided into three groups, with Type 1 being "typical" chronic pain patients who have disability and pain sensation out of proportion to the etiology of pain, Type 2 having moderate refractory pain proportional to the stimulus, and Type 3 with severe pain proportional with severity of etiology. While long-term opiate use was not suggested for Type 1 patients, Type 2 and 3 patients are considered for chronic opiate use in this report (33).

When a physician has come to the decision of using a narcotic, an "analgesic ladder," similar to that of the Cancer Pain Relief Program of the World Health Organization, can be helpful (17,34). Doctors should initially try mixed agonist–antagonist opiates and weak opiates because they have less abuse potential than the strong opiate agonists (19,35). Mixed opiate agonist–antagonists include medications such as pentazocine (Talwin), nalbuphine (Nubain), and butorphanol (Stadol). " Weak" narcotics include drugs such as hydrocodone, codeine, dihyrocodeine, and propoxyphene (Darvon)

Table 3. Opiate Pain Medications

Pure opiate agonists	Mixed agonists/antagonists
Morphine	Nalbuphine
MS Contin (long-acting morphine sulfate)	Pentazocine
Hydromorphine	Butorphanol
Oxycodone	
Oxycontin (long-acting oxycodone)	Partial Opiate Agonists
Codeine (weak)	Buprenorphine
Dihydocodeine (weak)	
Merperidine	
Fentanyl	
Methadone	
Hydrocodone (weak)	
Propoxyphene (weak)	

Source: Refs. 17, 64.

(1,17,34,35). A "ceiling effect" may occur with weak opiates and agonists–antagonist opiates.

If pain severity necessitates, the physician may move up the analgesic ladder to prescribe stronger opiate pain medications until the desired effect is achieved (34,35). The more powerful opiate agonists such as oxycodone (Roxicodone), levorphenol (Levo-Dromoran), fentanyl (Sublimimaze), hydromorphone (Dilaudid), morphine, and methadone (Dolophine) may be needed, but are more prone to potential abuse/dependence and should be used with caution (17). In most cases morphine and other strong analgesics can be used safely (25). Fentanyl is an effective long-acting semisynthetic agonist analgesic that is available in transdermal form and is often useful for providing a more constant level of analgesia (1,17,35). In one report, nearly 75% of nonmalignant chronic pain patients were able to achieve moderate to very good pain control with transdermal fentanyl (27,36). Using a stepwise medication approach, 70–90% of patients can have effective pain control (17,35). If, after careful consideration, chronic opiates are required, scheduled dosing is generally better than a p.r.n. approach, except for occassional "rescue dosing" (17).

CHRONIC PAIN AND SUBSTANCE-RELATED DISORDERS

Opiate Abuse and Chronic Pain

Although the vast majority of patients who use opiate medications do not develop substance-related problems, those who do abuse or become dependent on opiates often have great difficulties staying off these medications. Opiate-dependent patients may experience significant morbidity during withdrawal (cramping, nausea, vomiting, anxiety, and craving). If opiate abuse occurs, problems can develop in patients' physical health, self-esteem, marital relationships, work capacity, friendships, and almost every other area of their lives. Some patients express surprise, and even outrage, when they find themselves dependent on opiate pain medications if proper education was not provided by their doctor(s).

Opiate abuse is low in the general population, but prolonged use of opiate medications in chronic pain patients is an area of concern. When using opiates in chronic pain patients, the treating physician must evaluate the patient's clinical need for use, diagnosis, history, comorbid disorders, psychological stability, and reliability, as well as the relative risk of dependence and/or abuse and alternative treatment options (37). Generally, only one physician should prescribe medications of possible abuse, and predetermined goals should be agreed upon by the patient and prescribing physician (37).

Chronic pain patients who have opiate, alcohol, and/or other drug-related problems may be particularly prone to worsening of their substance-related disorder(s) by prolonged exposure to opiate pain medications. Opiate abuse is a serious problem for some patients, and a major factor in prolonging illness behavior in chronic pain patients (38). Chemical dependence to opiates often occurs, but does not have to lead to problems if properly handled with patient education and cautious tapering of opiates. Withdrawal symptoms—common side effects of opiate use—should be minimized, and patients warned that they may occur. In 1994, Ralphs et al. (39) showed that most (about 55%), but not all, severely disabled chronic pain patients with long-term medication use were able to remain off narcotics 6 months after tapering by two different methods, and many more significantly reduced opiate use. The average narcotic dose level was the best predictor of follow-up abstinence (39).

It is important to remember that the treating physicians(s) may not be aware of opiate abuse by their patients. These problems are generally concealed from doctors to enable drug-abusing patients to obtain more narcotics from the same doctor in the future, because of shame and guilt, and/or because the topic of possible abuse has not been discussed between the patient and doctor. "Doctor-shopping" patients may use several doctors, perhaps even in different states, who all believe they are prescribing the appropriate amount and dose of opiate medications for a real medical condition with little or no knowledge of prescriptions by other doctors. The patient may thus be abusing large amounts of opiates even though it appears to each doctor that appropriate amounts are being used without evidence of abuse. Sometimes the opiates are not abused themselves, but rather sold on the street for money to buy other drugs such as cocaine. Another possibility, which can be quite surprising to doctors to find out—if they do find out—is that even the nice elderly patient to whom they provide opiates for vague back problems may be selling the drug to younger abusers in exchange for needed cash.

A history of drug-related problems, early prescription refills, somatization, and evidence of doctor shopping are red flags of possible drug misuse and should stimulate greater caution in prescribing opiates to such a patient. Current drug-related problems or knowledge that a patient is already in a methadone maintenance program should also prohibit chronic opiate use in most cases (35). If opiate abuse is discovered, re-evaluation of opiate prescribing and prompt referral to a substance abuse treatment program are suggested.

The craving for opiates can be very strong in opiate-dependent people, and relapse can occur months or even years after discontinuation if a powerful trigger presents itself. A 12-year follow-up study of opiate-abusing/-dependent subjects in a government treatment program found a relapse rate of 98% within the first year after discharge from treatment (28). The methadone maintenance programs are helpful in decreasing criminal and other harmful behavior of opiate addicts, but are also a testimony to the great difficulty of keeping opiate abusers off these drugs.

In the case of opiate-related disorders, it is important to try to distinguish abuse from chemical dependence. In some cases, the benefit of pain reduction will outweigh the development of physical dependence (tolerance and/or withdrawal symptoms). This is particularly true of pain associated with terminal illnesses. Although physiological dependence to opiates may occur in some cases without causing significant distress or harm, in other cases it can become a serious and destructive problem.

Prevalence

The prevalence of opiate abuse/dependence is difficult to determine in any population, but is particularly problematic for chronic pain patients, who may have secondary-gain issues and many other inherent complications to accurate reporting. An overview of reported prevalence rates is shown in Table 4. In a 1979 study of 144 chronic pain patients with nonmalignant etiologies, 41% had abused drugs and 24% were currently drug-dependent; only about 35% did not have a drug problem (40). Codeine was the drug cited most frequently, with abuse and dependence prevalence being approximately 39% and 43%, respectively (40). Oxycodone had a dependence rate of 31% and an abuse rate

Table 4. Opiate-Related Disorders in Chronic Pain Patients

N[a]	Opiate abuse (%)	Opiate dependence (%)	Year published	Ref.
144	41	24	1979	40
37	5	19	1985	6
283	—	11	1985	42
414	2	13	1995	43
61	5	—	1996	44
403	28	—	1997	45

[a]Total number of patients in this group, with or without the disorder.

of 20% (40), and patients abusing oxycodone reportedly had a particular difficulty discontinuing their medications (40). Abuse rates of propoxphene, pentozocine, and meperidine were 14%, 10%, and 8%, respectively, and dependence rates 17%, 6%, and 29%. Although there was no control group, the nonabuse group (35% of the subjects) did not significantly differ from the abuse and dependence groups with regard to age, education, marriage, IQ, and family history of alcoholism (40). These authors concluded that prescription drug problems were a significant problem in chronic pain patients (40).

Halpern (41) estimated in 1982 that as many as 30–50% of chronic pain patients had a chemical dependence on narcotics and/or sedative medications. In a 1985 study of 37 inpatient chronic pain patients, about 19% were found to be opiate-dependent according to the NIMH Diagnostic Interview Schedule (6). The authors also found that slightly over 5% of the patients met criteria for opiate abuse (6). Similarly, in a 1986 study of 283 chronic pain patients, Fishbain et al. (42) reported that criteria for current opiate "dependence" were met by about 11% of the patients.

In a 1995 Swedish study of 414 chronic pain patients, about 13% met DSM-III-R criteria (using a Swedish form of the Substance Use Disorder Diagnostic Schedule) for current opiate dependence, and about 2% for current misuse (43). Past "misuse" and dependence are reported to be 2.9% and 1.7%, respectively (43).

In more recent studies, including a 1996 survey of 61 chronic back pain patients and 181 controls in a primary care setting, no differences were found in the lifetime prevalence of heroin use (3.3% for each group) or analgesic abuse (which was reportedly negligible) (44). In a 1997 study by Chabal et al. (45), 76 (19%) of 403 nonmalignant chronic pain VA patients were on chronic opiates (longer than 6 months). About 34% (26 of 76) of the patients using opiates met one criterion of abuse, and nearly 28% (21 of 76) met three or more criteria of abuse on a five-point checklist derived from the DSM-III-R (45). Unexpectedly, past alcohol or opiate abuse did not predict those who developed opiate abuse in their study. In addition, abusers and nonabusers of opiates had similar pain levels and symptoms of depression.

In a preliminary study of 40 chronic pain patients by Workman et al. (5), about 10% met the Diagnostic Interview Schedule criteria for opiate abuse. Importantly, the presence of substance abuse appeared to negatively impact on treatment outcome for their chronic pain (5). Thus, while about 52% met the research criteria for improvement in the no-substance-abuse group, only 27% improved significantly in the opiate or alcohol abuse group (5). Among primary care chronic back pain patients, Brown et al. (44) reported in 1996 that current analgesic abuse or dependence was about 5% in the pain group ($n = 61$), but only 1% in the control group using the Composite International Diagnostic Interview–Substance Abuse Module (CIDI-SAM). Lifetime analgesic abuse or dependence was about 11% for the pain patients and 6% for nonpain patients (44).

Interestingly, it has been suggested that in some patients opiates should be discontinued not so much because of worries about drug abuse as because chronic opiate use is not always the most effective treatment (4,38,46). For example, in some headache patients, an opiate-withdrawal rebound of headache pain has been reported (4).

Benzodiazepines (and Other Hypnosedatives) and Chronic Pain

Benzodiazepines and other hypnosedatives are among the most commonly prescribed medications in the United States. These medications are frequently used in chronic pain patients to relieve muscle spasm, induce sleep, and reduce anxiety (43,47). For example, in 1979, Ziesat et al. (48) reported that 53% of chronic pain patients in several medical settings were using minor tranquilizers. A report from 1990 indicated that of 114 patients at a university pain clinic, 38% were taking benzodiazepines at initial evaluation (20). As with opiates, chronic pain patients are more frequently exposed to these medications with potential for abuse, and, again as with opiates, persons who abuse benzodiazepines often obtain their supply from unsuspecting physicians.

Although abuse and chemical dependence can occur with benzodiazepines, knowledge about misuse of this class of drugs in chronic pain patients is limited. In 1979 Maruta et al. (40) reported that of 144 nonmalignant chronic pain patients, 14% abused diazepam and 11% were dependent on that benzodiazepine. In a 1995 Swedish study, 3.4% reported sedative dependence in remission, and current misuse of sedative was reported to be 1.2 % (43). Some of the same safety guidelines listed above for opiate use should be applied to benzodiazepines to minimize the risk of chemical dependency and abuse.

Alcohol and Chronic Pain

Alcohol-related problems and chronic pain are often found to coexist. Some patients report using alcohol to suppress their physical and emotional pain. However, in most cases, the alcohol-related problems start before the chronic pain syndrome (6). In 1985, Katon et al. (6) reported alcohol problems in about 41% of the 37 chronic pain patients studied. About 5% had current alcohol abuse problems and 22% were alcohol-dependent according to the NIMH Diagnostic Interview Schedule (6). Approximately 35% reported a history of past alcohol abuse. Another 16% of these patients reported a history of alcohol dependence (6).

In 1991, Atkinson et al. (49) showed that the lifetime rate of alcohol use disorder was about 65% in chronic low back pain (CLBP) patients, but only approximately 39% in controls (age- and demographically matched) (49). The 6-month prevalence of alcohol abuse/dependence was about 12% in CLBP patients, and only about 2% in controls (49). However, 81% of the cases had alcohol problems prior to CLBP, suggesting that alcohol use increased the risk of later CLBP rather than vice versa (49).

More recently, in 1995, a study of over 400 Swedish chronic pain patients (using a structured diagnostic interview for DSM-III-R criteria) reported a prevalence of about 10% for current alcohol dependence, 6% for alcohol dependence in remission, approximately 1.0% for alcohol misuse, and nearly another 1% for alcohol misuse in remission (43).

In a study by Workman et al. (5), 15% of 40 patients in a chronic pain program had an alcohol-related problem. The presence of alcohol abuse reduced the success rate of the program from 52% in those without substance abuse problems to 33% in those with an alcohol (only) problem (5).

Development of alcohol-related pancreatitis generally requires many years of heavy alcohol intake (generally at least 7g/day for at least 7 years) (50). Continued alcohol use is associated with increased frequency of pain episodes in patients with chronic pancreatitis (51). Although this illness is progressive, if alcohol consumption is stopped, the rate of pancreatic function decline appears to be reduced (50).

Illicit Drugs

Marijuana

Because marijuana has analgesic, antispasticity, and anxiolytic properties, its frequent use by chronic pain patients would not be surprising. The analgesic effects of marijuana appear to be associated with brain stem circuitry similar to that of opiates and act via new central mechanism (52). However, little work has been done in this area and mixed data have been reported with this population. In addition, interpretation of results may be difficult because control groups selected may vary widely in their marijuana use, and secondary issues associated with use of a popular but illegal substance that reduces pain may make data gathering less reliable. In a 1990 study of over 260 chronic pain patients, Steele-Rosomoff et al. (53) found that of the nine subjects who lied about their substance use, eight lied about marijuana.

In a 1991 study, nonalcohol substance abuse (mainly of cannabis) was 6% in nonpain controls compared to 11% in CLBP patients (49). In a 1996 report of primary care patients, the lifetime use of marijuana was slightly higher in chronic pain patients than in controls (about 69% for CBP patients and 59% for controls) (44). The percentage who used marijuana in the prior month and the number of lifetime-use episodes were reported to actually be higher in the control group (44).

A 1997 article indicated that 30–97% of multiple sclerosis patients reported decreased chronic pain and spasticity with cannabis use (29). Although this difference was statistically significant, the percentage who used cannabis in the past month and the number of episodes of lifetime use were both reported to be significantly higher in the control group (44). It is obvious that a great deal more work is needed to understand the prevalence of marijuana abuse in chronic pain patients, and how marijuana affects their overall status.

Cocaine and Other Psychostimulants

Because chronic pain patients have high rates of depression, use of cocaine and other stimulants may be expected as inappropriate attempts to acutely improve their mood and energy. For example, a 1996 review suggested that a patient with chronic cancer pain used amphetamines to diminish sedation by opiates or other medications (54).

In a 1985 study of 37 chronic pain patients, 5.4% were found to abuse amphetamines and 2.7% met criteria for amphetamine dependence (6). More recently, in a 1996 study of about 61 primary care CBP patients, the lifetime cocaine use was not different from that by controls, and the number of episodes of use in a lifetime was actually greater in the control group (57 ± 74) than in the CBP group (22 ± 31) (44). The possible comorbidity rates and issues of chronic pain and psychostimulants clearly need further investigation.

RESEARCH PROBLEMS AND FUTURE DIRECTIONS

Although numerous studies have investigated the relationship between chronic pain and substance abuse, considerably more research is needed in this area. The issue of chronic opiate use in patients with a history of substance abuse is an area of heated debate, and large prospective studies are needed comparing the outcomes of nonmalignant chronic pain patients treated with opiates with those of patients treated without opiates. For now, decisions must be made on a case-by-case basis, preferably with a well-coordinated treatment team that is knowledgeable in the various treatment options and complicated chronic pain issues.

Numerous methodological problems exist in obtaining reliable data in the area of substance-related disorders and in the chronic pain field. Thus, obtaining accurate information when these two problems occur together in a patient population is a particularly difficult challenge. In the context of substance-related disorders, terms such as "misuse," "abuse," "dependence," and "addiction" have been defined in numerous ways, changed over time, and frequently used interchangeably (55,56). In fact, although numerous definitions have been put forth, there is still no absolute consensus as to what is actually meant by these terms. In the psychiatric/medical community, definitions of abuse and dependence usually adhere to those provided by DSM-IV (14). This source does not, however, define "addiction" or "misuse." Patient reports of drug use can vary greatly in accuracy because of poor recall, denial, guilt, secondary-gain issues, and other reasons.

Chronic pain is also difficult to study. It is as much a subjective feeling (which is difficult to accurately measure) as it is an objective physical phenomenon. Chronic pain is not a homogeneous disorder, but it has many sites, causes, levels of severity, prognoses, and other aspects. These multiple factors make these patients difficult to compare between groups and between studies. In addition, many studies provide data on chronic pain patients, but do not use appropriate controls and report important demographic information. Although much attention has been given to the relationship between chronic pain and opiate or alcohol abuse, much less is known about chronic pain and abuse of other substances such as marijuana and cocaine.

In many cases, opiate abuse is totally unknown to a prescribing physician. In other patients, apparent abuse of pain medications may lead to undertreatment of the chronic pain (i.e., "pseudoaddiction"). Such dilemmas make clinical work in this area as difficult as the research.

The psychological characteristics of patients with comorbid substance abuse and chronic pain patients are also in need of further investigation. In 1976 altered MMPI profiles were seen in chronic pain patients (57). Turner et al. (58) reported in 1982 that chronic pain patients who tended to misuse narcotics also scored higher on the hypochondriasis and hysteria scales on the MMPI than other subjects. Finlayson et al. (59) showed that the MMPI profiles of 41 Mayo Clinic patients with substance abuse and chronic pain also significantly differed from those of a large general medical control group. Statistically significant differences were observed on all scales except social introversion and masculinity–femininity for males, and all scales except social introversion for females (59). A 1988 study of 25 women with chronic pelvic pain indicated that this group not only had more substance abuse problems than their controls, but had more somatization, adult sexual problems, reported history of sexual abuse, and depression (60,61). Others have reported similar associations between substance abuse and sexual/physical abuse histories in chronic pelvic pain patients (62). Understanding how psychological perspectives develop, change over time (with and without effective treatment), and affect treatment success could provide valuable information for development of effective treatment programs.

One of the most important goals in this area is the development of more effective pain control medications that have little or no abuse/dependence potential. Clearly the comorbidity of chronic pain and alcohol/drug abuse represents a very difficult medical, social, and scientific challenge that warrants considerable future effort.

REFERENCES

1. EA Workman, JR Hubbard. Chronic pain. In: Primary Care Medicine for Psychiatrists: A Practitioner's Guide. JR Hubbard, D Short, ed. New York: Quantum, 1997, pp 231–242, 1997.
2. RK Portenoy. Chronic pain management. In: Psychiatric Care of the Medical Patient. New York: Oxford University Press, pp 341–363, 1993.
3. JJ Bergman, MN Werblun. Chronic pain: a review for the family physician. J Fam Practice 7:685–693, 1978.
4. DA Fishbain, HL Rosomoff, RS Rosomoff. Drug abuse, dependence, and addiction in chronic pain patients. Clinic J Pain 8:77–85, 1992.
5. EA Workman, JR Hubbard, DD Short. Incidence of psychiatric disorders and predictions of pain management success. Submitted.
6. W Katon, I Egan, D Miller. Chronic pain: lifetime psychiatric diagnosis and family history. Am J Psychiatry 142:1156–1160, 1985.
7. J Reich, J Tupin, S Abramowitz, et al. Psychiatric diagnosis of chronic pain patients. Am J Psychiatry 140:1495–1498, 1983.
8. J Atkinson, M Slater, T Patterson, I Grant, S Garfin. Prevalence, onset, and risk of psychiatric disorders in men with chronic low back pain: a controlled study. Pain 45:111–121, 1991.
9. K Fassbender, W Samborsky, M Kellner, W Muller, S Lautenbacher. Tender points, depressive and functional symptoms: comparison between fibromyalgia and major depression. Clin Rheumatol 16:76–79, 1997.
10. W Katon, RK Ries, A Klienman. The prevalence of somatization in primary care. Compr Psychiatry 25:208–215, 1984.

11. JJ Bonica. Considerations in Management of Pain. New York: Hospital Practice, pp 4–13, 1977.
12. KL Casey. The neurophysiologic basis of pain. Postgrad Med 6:58, 1973.
13. R Melzack, KL Casey. Neurophysiology of pain. In: The Psychology of Pain. New York: Raven Press, pp 1–24, 1968.
14. American Psychiatric Association. Diagnostic and Statistical Manual of Mental Disorders. 4th ed. Washington, DC: American Psychiatric Press, 1994.
15. WB Hodges, EA Workman. Pain and stress. In: Handbook of Stress Medicine: An Organ System Approach. Boca Raton, FL: CRC Press, pp 251–269, 1998.
16. D Jones, S Sherg. Opiates in chronic pain of non-malignant origin: an interim consensus [letter]. N Z Med J 108: 492, 1995.
17. NI Cherny, KM Foley. Nonopioid and opioid analgesic pharmacotherapy of cancer pain. Hematol Oncol North Am 10:70–103, 1996.
18. AB Malmbert, TL Yaksh. Hyperalgesia medicated by spinal glutamate and substance P receptors, blocked by spinal cyclooxygenase inhibition. Science 92:1276–1279, 1992.
19. RH Gracely, P McGrath, R Dubner. Validity and sensitivity of ratio scales of sensory and affective verbal pain descriptors: manipulation of affect by diazepam. Pain 5:19–29, 1978.
20. SA King, JJ Strain. Benzodiazepine use by chronic pain patients. Clin J Pain 6:143–147, 1990.
21. N Hendler, C Cimini, A Terence, D Long. A comparison of cognitive impairment due to benzodiazepines and to narcotics. Am J Psychiatry 137:828–830, 1980.
22. RM Gallagher III, FI Stewart, T Weissbein, A Weissbein. Nonnarcotic analgesic abuse: a common biopsychsocial problem. Gen Hosp Psychiatry 9:102–107, 1988.
23. RS Nanra. Analgesic nephropathy. Med J Aust 1:745–748, 1976.
24. JM Duggan. The analgesic syndrome. Aust N Z J Med 4:365–372, 1974.
25. M Zenz. Morphine myths: sedation, tolerance, addiction. Postgrad Med J 67: S100–S102, 1991.
26. L Stinus, M Allard, L Gold, G Simmonnet. Changes in CNS neuropeptide FF-like material, pain sensitivity, and opiate dependence following morphine treatment. Peptides 16:1235–1241, 1995.
27. A. Kaplan. Opiates for non-malignant pain: from taboo to treatment. Psych Times, March 28–31, 1999.
28. N Adreasen, DW Black. Introductory Textbook of Psychiatry. 2nd ed. Washington, DC: American Psychiatric Press, 1995.
29. P Conscoe, R Masty, J Rein, W Tillery, R Pertwee. The perceived effects of smoked cannabis on patients with multiple sclerosis. Eur Neurol 38:44–48, 1997.
30. P Compton, J Darakjian, K Miotto. Screening for addiction in patients with chronic pain and "problematic" substance use: evaluation of a pilot assessment tool. J Pain Symptom Manage 16:355–363, 1998.
31. KL Sees, HW Clark. Opioid use in the treatment of chronic pain: assessment of addiction. J Pain Symptom Manage 8:257–264, 1993.

32. RE Enck. Understanding tolerance, physical dependence and addiction in the use of opioid Analgesics. Am J Hospice Palliative Care Jan–Feb:9–11, 1991.
33. J Schofferman. Long-term use of opioid analgesics for the treatment of chronic pain of nonmalignant origin. J Pain Symptom Manage 8:279–288, 1993.
34. World Health Organization. Cancer Pain Relief. Geneva: World Health Organization, 1986.
35. RK Portenoy, R Payne. Acute and chronic pain. In: Substance Abuse: A Comprehensive Textbook. 2nd ed. JH Lowinson, P Ruiz, RB Millman, JG Langrod, eds. Philadelphia: Williams and Wilkins, pp 691–721, 1992.
36. E Kalso, H Hays, H Allen, et al. Subject preferences for transdermal fentanyl or sustained release morphine: a crossover efficacy, tolerability and quality-of-life trial in chronic pain patients. 17th Annual Scientific Meeting of the American Pain Society, San Diego, Nov 1998.
37. PJ Graziotti, CR Goucke. The use of oral opioids in patients with chronic non-cancer pain: management strategies. Med J Aust 167:30–34, 1997.
38. RG Black. The chronic pain syndrome. Surg Clin N Amer 55:999–1011, 1975.
39. JA Ralphs, AC de C Williams, PH Richardson, CE Pither, MK Nicholas. Opiate reduction in chronic pain patients: a comparison of patient-controlled reduction and staff controlled cocktail methods. Pain 56:279–288, 1994.
40. T Maruta, DW Swanson, RE Finlayson. Drug abuse and dependency in patients with chronic pain. Mayo Clin Proc 54:241–244, 1979.
41. L Halpern. Substitution-detoxification and its role in the management of chronic benign pain. J Clin Psychiatry 43:10–14, 1985.
42. DA Fishbain, M Goldberg, BR Meaghen, R Steele-Rosomoff. Male and female chronic pain patients categorized by DSM-III and psychiatric diagnostic criteria. Pain 16:181–197, 1986.
43. NG Hoffmann, O. Olofssom, B Salen, L Wickrstrom. Problems of abuse and dependency in chronic pain patients. Int J Addict 30(8):919–927, 1995.
44. RL Brown, JJ Patterson, LA Rounds, O Papasovliotis. Substance abuse among patients with chronic back pain. J Fam Practice 43:152–160, 1996.
45. C Chabal, MK Erjavec, L Jacobson, A Marionio, E Chaney. Prescription, opiate abuse in chronic pain patients: clinical criteria, incidence and predictors. Clin J Pain 13:150–155, 1997.
46. AC de C Williams. Inpatient management of chronic pain, In: Psychological Treatment in Disease and Illness. M Hodes, S Moorey, eds. London: Gaskell Press, 1993.
47. LE Hollister, FK Conley, RH Britt, L Sher. Long-term use of diazepam. JAMA 246:1568–1570, 1980.
48. HA Ziesat, HV Angle, WD Gentry, EH Ellinwood. Drug use and misuse in operant pain patients. Addict Behav 4:263–266, 1979.
49. JH Atkinson, MA Slater, TL Patterson, I Grant, SR Garfin. Prevalence, onset and risk of psychiatric disorders in men with chronic low back pain: a controlled study. Pain 45:111–121, 191.

50. WB Strum. Abstinence in alcoholic chronic pancreatitis. J Clin Gastroentrol 20(1):37–41, 1995.
51. G de las Heras, J de la Pena. Drinking patterns and hepatitis. J Clin Drug Abuse 20:33–36, 1995.
52. ID Meng, BH Manning, WJ Martin, HL Fields. An analgesia circuit activated by cannabinoids. Nature 395:381–383, 1998.
53. R Steele-Rosomoff, DA Fishbain, M Goldberg, H Rosomoff. Chronic pain patients who lie in their psychiatric examination about current drug/abuse. Pain (suppl):S 299, 1990.
54. MG Reich, D Razavi. Role of amphetamines in cancerology: a review of the literature. Bull Cancer 83:891–900, 1996.
55. RC Rinaldi, EM Steindler, BB Wilford, D Goodwin. Clarification and standardization of substance abuse terminology. JAMA 259:557–562, 1988.
56. RG Newman. The need to redefine "addiction." N Engl J Med 18:1096–1098, 1983.
57. DW Swanson, WM Swenson, T Maruta, MC McPhee. Program for managing chronic pain. I. Program description and characteristics of patients. Mayo Clin Proc 51:401–408, 1976.
58. JA Turner, DA Calsyn, WE Fordyce, LB Ready. Drug utilization patterns in chronic pain patients. Pain 12:257–263, 1982.
59. RE Finlayson, T Maruta, RM Morse, WM Swenson, MA Martin. Substance abuse and chronic pain: profile of 50 patients in alcohol and drug dependence unit. Pain 26:167–174, 1986.
60. J Harrop-Griffiths, W Katon, E Walker, L Hom, J Russo, LR Hickok. The association between chronic pelvic pain, psychiatry diagnosis, and childhood sexual abuse. Obstet-Gynecol 71:589–594, 1988.
61. E Walker, W Katon, J Harrop-Griffiths, L Holm, J Russo, LR Hickok. Relationship of chronic pelvic pain to psychiatric diagnoses and childhood sexual abuse. Am J Psychiatry 145:75–80, 1988.
62. AS Badura, RC Reiter, EM Altmaier, A Rhomberg, D Elas. Dissociation, somatization, substance abuse and coping in women with chronic pelvic pain. Obstet Gynecol 90:405–410, 1997.
63. AM Ludwig. Principles of Clinical Psychiatry. New York: Free Press, 1980.
64. EA Workman, FF Tellian. Practical Handbook of Psychopharmacology: A Clinician's Guide. Ann Arbor, MI: CRC Press, 1994.
65. JM Portnow, JD Strassman. Medically induced drug addiction. Int J Addictions 20:605–611, 1985.
66. RD Hicks. Pain management in the chemically dependent patient. Hawaii Med J 48:491–495, 1989.
67. GE Ruoff, GB Berry. Chronic pain, characteristics, assessment and treatment plans. Postgrad Med 78:91–97, 1985.
68. KM Foley, CE Inturrisi. Analgesic drug therapy in cancer pain: principles and practice. Med Clin North Am 71:207–232, 1987.

12
Substance Dependence in the Elderly

Richard R. Irons
Professional Renewal Center
Lawrence, Kansas

Donald E. Rosen
Oregon Health Sciences University
Portland, Oregon

EPIDEMIOLOGY

Aging is a time of diminished physical capacity, recurrent loss, and increased psychological dependence on others. The desire to find refuge from the angst, loneliness, and despair associated with the challenge of aging will often lead one to seek comfort and solace through the use of a pill, potion, drink, or substance. For many this is a temporary escape. However, some members of our society habitually pursue this course of action, despite formidable consequences. They will come to meet the diagnostic criteria for substance abuse or dependency in the fourth edition of the *Diagnostic and Statistical Manual of Mental Disorders* (DSM-IV).

The incidence and prevalence of substance-related disorders in those 65 or older have always been difficult to measure. Prevalence studies have used divergent definitions of alcohol dependency or abuse, populations (community-, clinic-, or hospital-based) and age range; over the past three decades they have presented contrasting conclusions and recommendations. In community studies, rates in the elderly are not substantially different from estimates for entire adult populations; of the 50% or so of the adult population who do drink, between one in six and one in seven meet the diagnostic criteria for alcohol dependency. In other words, the prevalence of "heavy" drinking in the elderly was generally found to be 6%. Fewer older women consume alcohol or have problem drinking, but they may be more prone to abuse psychoactive drugs than older men (1–3).

In contrast, surveys conducted in clinics or hospitals have consistently found increasing prevalence of alcoholism in the elderly population. Alcohol-related hospitalization of elderly people is common in the United States. Using hospital claims data from the Health Care Financing Administration, one study found that alcohol-related discharge diagnoses occurred as frequently as myocardial infarction (4). Substance abuse in the elderly is positively correlated with being male, tobacco smoking, and life in a suburban/urban setting. It is most negatively correlated with health orientation. It is also negatively correlated with increasing age, especially into the octogenarian years and beyond, being female, and socioeconomic status (5,6). Actual prevalence is difficult to assess because of variance in the definition of substance abuse and dependence. Instruments for definition of this needed information have not been validated for an older age group (7,8).

Two types of patients with substance-related disorders would be found in this population. The first encompasses those who have been treated for alcoholism or addiction earlier in life, and those who accumulated significant life consequences from substance use but never were given the diagnosis of substance dependency. The second includes those who before the age of 60 never experienced significant development of tolerance, physiological or psychological withdrawal, or mental preoccupation with any substance. They present with a relatively short, intense period of substance use that meets the criteria for substance dependence. Distinctions between these two types have not been studied extensively, but between one-half and two-thirds of elderly alcoholic patients are estimated to be in the first group (9,10). Further research and investigation will likely show significant differences in prognosis and the benefit from different approaches to treatment in these groups.

RISK FACTORS

Superimposed on a biopsychosocial substrate that predisposes one to stumble into the pathology of an addiction are a number of factors unique to the individual that should define and tailor the necessary rehabilitation process. Some of these are listed in Table 1.

As older adults undergo life transitions or undertake stressful roles, vulnerability to alcohol and prescription drugs may increase. Transitions that may increase risk include menopause; failure to maintain limits socially or

Substance Dependence in the Elderly

Table 1. Problems Commonly Associated with Substance Abuse in the Elderly

Axis I mental disorders
Axis II personality disorders
Cognitive deficits or disorders
Social stressors and changes
Unresolved loss
Family obligations, conflicts, and separations
Chronic medical problems
Acute medical problems
Physical limitations
Sensory deterioration (sight, hearing, etc.)
Financial constraints

vocationally; recognition of the "empty nest" after children leave; accepting the "traumatic nest" associated with taking into the home adult children who have major life problems or illnesses; unplanned and/or unwanted retirement from a profession, business, or vocation; significant and, especially, sudden changes in physical, emotional or intellectual functioning; and major moves to new houses or new communities. Assuming care for relatives or grandchildren, confronting the deaths of siblings or close friends, or adjusting to a new environment may trigger increased desire to medicate associated feelings, conflicts, forced choices, and fears with a mood-altering substance. In addition, many older adults have diminished cognitive skills and difficulties with recent memory. They may slip into drug dependence from uncertainty regarding the indications, dosing, and frequency of prescribed psychoactive substances, as well as being unsure when they took their last dose. Many seniors are slow to ask for help because it reinforces their fear of loss of independence and they feel ashamed. The adult says to his parent, "There's no need to feel embarrassed; we're family." The parent responds, "Who can I be more embarrassed in front of?"

INTERVENTION CHALLENGES

The despair of substance dependency in the elderly is clearly felt if one will only mindfully pause to contemplate one's own fate while looking at a patient ravaged by an addictive disorder in this season of life. The aging addict hopes that all we will do is ignore him or her. This conscious wish to be ignored and to disappear hides a latent plea for relief from their despair—a wish to be held in a containing, loving, safe, and supportive environment. The price we pay for standing by witnessing or colluding with this dance of self-destruction grows over time, and the situation becomes a nightmare filled with guilt and frustration. A case example is provided below:

> Jed Stone is a 73-year-old retired pharmacist. He has been a pillar of his community for more than 50 years, and never had any major afflictions or mental disorders to contend with until after his retirement six years ago. He reluctantly seeks treatment for substance dependency to appease his family and placate his wife of 54 years. He does not view alcoholism as a disease but rather a lack of willpower and strength. He recalls the Old Testament descriptions of alcohol dependency as sinful gluttony. He grudgingly acknowledges signs and symptoms of alcohol dependency. During treatment he discloses his surreptitious use of pharmaceutical samples and purloined tablets from the drugstore he used to own. He has maintained a large supply of pharmaceuticals and has a pill for almost anything that has afflicted, or might afflict, him.
>
> He was intervened upon by his wife and children after he had spent the better part of a week on his own, "fishing up north." A state trooper found him bewildered and afraid, sitting next to the site where his Jeep Cherokee had left the highway and struck a guardrail. The trooper conducted a field sobriety test, which showed that Jed was impaired in his ability to operate a motor vehicle. Because the breathalyzer test showed a blood alcohol level below the legal limit, the trooper gave him a ticket for reckless operation. His Jeep had to be towed, and Jed blustered as he tried to explain the accident to his wife and asked for someone to come and take him home. She knew he sounded "different" that day, with the changes in speech pattern and behavior that she and others had recognized on occasion over the past five or six years. When she and one of her children picked up Jed at the police station, it was apparent that he had not maintained his usual level of personal grooming, and had been eating erratically. This "binge" was associated with minimal use of alcohol and the family was concerned about his health. He returned home and had a comprehensive physical and laboratory examination. He even saw a neurologist to rule out a blackout or transient stroke, and completed a CT scan, which was normal. Over the next few days he began to tell his wife about all the pills he had been taking for various aches and pains. More than a decade and a half ago, he began to hide the extent of his use from his wife, as he did not want to worry her. When his wife related this story of sequestered medications to her children, they became very concerned and an intervention followed rather quickly thereafter.

Physicians often unknowingly create and support barriers to intervening effectively upon patients such as Jed. They fail to remember that even minor

Substance Dependence in the Elderly

or truncated interventions in the office or hospital bear considerable weight with an elderly patient, especially if made in the presence of family or friends.

Denial is an extremely effective defense against addiction. It runs the gamut from the obvious primitive denial to the selective and sophisticated manifestations that can deceive experienced clinicians and loved ones alike. It courses through the patient, the family, social network, and even professional contacts. Treaters are often slow to detect addiction in the elderly, and questions are often phrased in a way that promotes the patient's denial. One could easily imagine the trepidation Jed's family doctor over many years might have had when inquiring about his drug use. "You don't take any illicit substances, do you, Jed?" It is all too easy to collude with patients' denial out of respect for their position as senior members of our community. In addition, the higher a patient's socioeconomic level and professional background, the easier it is for the clinician to miss the diagnosis. Images of the elderly alcoholic are not well ingrained in our society, and the conventional stereotypes such as the skid-row bum, the loud obnoxious boozer, or the careless lush who is clearly intoxicated in public do not apply to this population. In fact, attempts to apply such stereotypes may lead to rather pathetic humor. The elderly alcoholic is seldom drunk and disorderly, rarely arrested for driving under the influence, and rarely becomes physically or emotionally aggressive or menacing. They are not often the perpetrators of family violence or sexual abuse, yet they frequently become victims. These are not the squeaky wheels, and because of this are all too often ignored (as they long to be).

Inquiries should be made in a confidential setting. Questions should be posed in a nonjudgmental manner, for many patients will be extremely sensitive to being identified as abusive or imprudent in their use of these substances. Older adults are far more willing to address a medical problem than a substance-related disorder or other mental health problem. Approaching the issue as a reasonable behavior that got out of control is often an effective technique. The sleeping pill or tranquilizer that a patient has developed tolerance to is a way of identifying the problem in nonmoralizing terms.

ASSESSMENT

The CAGE Questionnaire (11) and the Michigan Alcoholism Screening Test–Geriatric Version (MAST-G) (12) are the two most widely used alcohol screening self-evaluation tests that have been validated for use and apply directly to older adults. The four-question CAGE (has tried to **C**ut back, is **A**nnoyed by criticism, feels **G**uilty about drinking, desires **E**ye-opener drinks) questionnaire is easily adapted for use with other drugs or problem behavior, and is readily administered informally in an interview without the need to bring out a reference paper or disrupt the general flow of the information-gathering process. Remember that for CAGE questions the questions should be posed "Have you ever . . . ", referring to any time in life, not just currently. Although two or more positive responses are considered an indicator for potential addiction, elucidation of a positive response should trigger further inquiry into this area. In a large study of 5065 consecutive patients, 15% of men and 12% of women aged 60 and older self-reported regularly drinking in excess of 14 ounces of alcohol and 7 ounces of alcohol weekly, respectively. In this study the CAGE questionnaire detected less than half of the heavy or binge drinkers, but rarely misclassified a non–problem drinker as a problem drinker. Screening questions can be added to a self-administered medical history questionnaire that many primary care clinicians regularly use. It appears that a combination of screening tools, including questions on quantity and frequency of drinking as well as the CAGE, should be used to maximize the number of problem drinkers detected (13). In one study, the MAST was able to define 5% of the respondents as alcohol-dependent, but when the CAGE was given to the same group, only 1.4% had two or more positive responses. The Geriatric Depression Scale proved a more effective screening tool for detecting depression than either the CAGE or MAST for alcohol dependency (14).

Many older adults do not believe that alcohol consumption is creating problems in their daily living and adversely affecting their health. The consumption level that brings an individual to the threshold of dependency is considerably lower for older drinkers (15). Chronic medical conditions associated with significant decreases in functional capacity and quality of life may obscure the role of alcohol in their pattern of deterioration. Many prescribed medications and over-the-counter remedies interact with alcohol and each other, producing unexpected and confusing mental and physical iatrogenic effects, toxicity, and intoxication. Elderly patients come to rely on certain medications to ameliorate troublesome symptoms or pain and are reluctant or frankly opposed to changes, especially if such medication has been prescribed for months or years by their family doctor.

Comorbid medical diseases and mental disorders will significantly influence the strength of the recommendation for abstinence and treatment, and will also have a direct negative effect on treatment outcome. A number of medical problems commonly found in older adults can be adversely influenced by alcohol use, such as hypertension, gastroesophogeal reflux, ulcers, pancreatitis, and diabetes mellitus. In these disorders medication may not be as effective until all alcohol consumption ceases. In addition, the combination of medications and alcohol can have a synergistic detrimental effect on consciousness

Table 2. Signs and Symptoms Associated with Substance Dependency in Older Adults

---
Abiding grief
Inability to cope with loss of occupation
Loss of physical mobility or ability
Progressive family and social isolation
Deterioration in personal hygiene
Changes in clothes and grooming
Insomnia or hypersomnia
Unexplained accidents or signs of trauma
Mood swings
Change in capacity to be socially engaged or approached
Changes in behavior

---

and judgment. It is also true that many older adults use alcohol to medicate insomnia, restless-leg syndrome, depression, and chronic pain problems. When effective alternative treatment can be initiated, then alcohol use can be dramatically tapered and discontinued.

MANAGEMENT ISSUES

Alcohol and drug dependence ravages the body and mind with recurrent use. Over time, the cost–benefit ratio for using substances that place a genetically susceptible individual at risk for dependency shifts dramatically. Early in the relationship, many find there is little, if any, price to pay for altering one's neurobiochemistry. However, the complications often accumulate over time, especially with substances used on a daily basis. Sadly, and sometimes tragically, the physical consequences of use can be grave in proportion to the amount of a substance ingested in the late stages of this disease. Trauma research has expanded in the past few decades, and we know that certain types of trauma are frequently associated with a given substance. For example, the risk of sustaining a subdural hematoma increases dramatically as alcohol dependency progresses. The risk of having an accident, either in an automobile or at home, increases significantly in active substance dependency. Textbooks in multiple subspecialties of medicine have audited and explained the protean medical consequences of alcohol use. A discussion of this material is beyond the scope of this chapter. Far less is known about the medical consequences of the abuse of and dependency on prescription medications.

Once it becomes apparent that an older adult may benefit from substantial reduction of alcohol consumption—or complete abstention—then it is also important to review and critically determine whether the prescription and nonprescription medications the patient is taking, or even just has in his home, are medically necessary, and whether the dosage of any mood-altering substances could be reduced. Gradual increases in the number and dosage of medications, often from a variety of practitioners, often go unchallenged and can lead to major problems if the trend continues. The clinician and other concerned parties must help the patient to understand the need for these changes and assess the patient's level of comprehension and need. Acute alcohol-withdrawal syndrome is more protracted and severe in the elderly than in younger patients with equivalent disease severity (16). Careful evaluation of physical and mental health is needed to determine whether inpatient detoxification is medically necessary, because a higher percentage of elderly patients will require such service. Hemodynamic and neurological instability often necessitate inpatient detoxification. Outpatient detoxification may not be appropriate for older adults who live alone, are fragile, have limited family support, or have multiple medical problems and medications (17).

TREATMENT

Patients with high degrees of medical or mental health impairment or who need close monitoring should receive primary medical/addiction medicine/psychiatric care at an inpatient facility. Ensuring adequate hydration, monitoring ambulation, and closely monitoring chronic medical conditions (often in poor control) require the vigilance and facilities available at an inpatient setting. With recent changes in the healthcare system (even with Medicare), availability of this level of care is rapidly diminishing. In addition, "gatekeepers" for managed-care organizations may not understand or be easily convinced that certain combinations of multiple medical needs of the aged with addiction/mental health demand necessitate a level of care greater than the sum of the care requirements for each illness. Inpatient rehabilitation programs for alcohol and substance dependency are no longer readily available in the community and are too often no longer covered by health insurance. The distance that one may be required to travel for rehabilitation, and the expenses, become major problems for many older adults. Inpatient care, when available, is now often on medical wards or geriatric psychiatric units.

Treatment is effective, however, only if it is individualized to address the unique combination of triggers and factors associated with the addiction together with addressing life-stage issues. Most elderly addicts drink or medicate to cope (and manage anxiety), not to become intoxicated. They are upset about specific losses or realities that have to be faced every day. The older adult addict usually comes to treatment worn out from worry and struggles concerning events they do not have the power to control or significantly influence. The anxiety associated with loss awakens longstanding conflicts regarding independence, autonomy, and dependence. For those who relied on demonstrating power and influence over events as a means of reassuring themselves that they are safe and in control, such anxiety can be unnerving. Many "drink at" or "act out" over these situations.

Many are spiritually bankrupt. The Eriksonian stage of ego integrity versus despair leaves them with a profound sense of fragmentation and hopelessness. Treatment must address the importance of abstinence and recovery in this life stage. The spiritual and existential underpinnings of the question "What do I have to live for?" must be addressed. Seniors frequently wish to avoid facing issues related to their legacy to family and community, or coming to terms with their spirituality. This repair in one's core sense of ego integrity is a key component to recovery. When these issues are overlooked, abstinence often becomes superficial compliance with the demands and expectations of others. Coming to grips with the dual aspects of the first step is crucial. It is one thing to acknowledge that one is powerless over the substance, but it is frequently much harder to admit that life has become unmanageable, for this represents not only another loss but the fear that the ability to live independently may be coming to a close.

For many patients, a critical point in the treatment is reached when the individual must determine if there is something to live for that is dear enough and significant enough to make the commitment to live their lives free of mood-altering substances worth the time, effort, and expense. A significant and often fairly subtle shift in perception is required. Life must have renewed meaning and purpose if genuine recovery is to emerge. The key to this shift, often experienced in Alcoholics Anonymous members as a genuine realization of the eleventh and twelfth steps, is elusive but well worth pursuing. At least two studies demonstrate that older adults are more compliant with treatment and have as good, if not better, treatment outcomes than matched patients who were much younger (18,19). It appears that their success rate in recovery is at least as great as that for the general population.

CONTINUING REHABILITATION

The multiple challenges many older adults face upon discharge from an intensive rehabilitation program or therapeutic community require multiple linkages to community services, agencies, and resources as well as healthcare providers. No treatment program can continue to meet the needs of an individual after discharge, and when compensatory services are not provided for an extended period of time, the recidivism rate is very high.

Effective case management involves implementation of discharge plans. Many patients are discharged into a life of meager social networks, tenuous family connections, and real physical and mental limitations. Family members and friends are lost through death or drift away. Basic resources may be difficult to access because of inability to effectively use the telephone, fill out necessary paperwork, or use a computer. Limitations in sight and hearing impede the ability to even know that one cannot perform complex tasks or executive functions. Standard features of continuing-care plans for older adults in early recovery from substance dependency include:

Age-appropriate, accessible Alcoholics Anonymous, or other 12-step groups. Transportation to meetings, use of a temporary sponsor until a defined sponsor is found, and locating someone to accompany the patient to the first few meetings are extremely helpful.

Removal from the home of unneeded medications, including over-the-counter drugs, prior to or at the time of return. A reliable means of monitoring medication compliance is often important.

Establishment of a network of friends and family that will support and assist during the early weeks and months of recovery. If the patient is living alone, regular visits should be established.

Setting up a daily, weekly, and monthly calendar with scheduled visits, activities, and meetings. For a patient who has limited mobility or is shut in, the use of tapes, large-type books, videos, and even computer on-line meetings can become vital links with the recovering community and help to maintain growth in recovery.

Ongoing monitoring of recovery by the primary care/addiction medicine clinician. This must include an evolving management plan to ensure the prescription of and compliance with needed medication.

Sharing the patient's relapse prevention plan (which includes an essential "what happens if I drink/drug/act out again" provision) with members of his or her support network and family.

Socialization and maintenance of a healthy peer group should be encouraged and promoted. The availability and use of social supports help diminish the isolation, anxiety, and despair associated with late-life addictive disease. Early recovery in late life is especially difficult given the physical and psychological stresses of aging. Leading seniors to recognize their needs—and to allow them to be met—requires treatment with skill, sensitivity, and respect.

FUTURE RESEARCH

So little has been adequately researched in this area. Studies on the incidence and prevalence of substance dependency in the elderly need to be completed. Prescription-medication dependency patterns are not well understood. If a person uses a "drug" (such as acetaminophen and butalbital, but also orally administered narcotics or benzodiazepines) on an intermittent basis for 30 or 40 years to assuage symptoms with safety, is there still risk of dependency in the future?

REFERENCES

1. Gomberg ES. Older women and alcohol: use and abuse. Recent Dev Alcohol 12:61–79, 1995.
2. Hill SY. Mental and physical consequences of alcohol use in women. Recent Dev Alcohol 12:181–197, 1995.
3. Brennan PL, Moos RH, Kim JY. Gender differences in the individual characteristics and life contexts of late middle-aged and older problem drinkers. Addiction 88:781–790, 1993.
4. Adams WL, Yuan Z, Barboriak JJ, Rimm AA. Alcohol-related hospitalizations of elderly people. JAMA 270:1222–1225, 1993.
5. Bercsi SJ, Brickner PW, Saha DC. Alcohol use and abuse in the frail, homebound elderly: a clinical analysis of 103 persons. Drug Alcohol Depend 33(2):139–149, 1993.
6. Mirmand AL, Welte JW. Alcohol consumption among the elderly in a general population in Eric Co., New York. Am J Public Health 86(7):978–984, 1996.
7. Fulop G, Reinhardt J, Strain JJ, Paris B, Miller M, Fillit H. Identification of alcohol and depression in a geriatric medicine outpatient clinic. J Am Geriatr Soc 41:737–41, 1993.
8. Lakhani N. Alcohol use amongst community dwelling elderly people: a review of the literature. J Adv Nursing 25(6):1227–32, 1997.

9. Gulino C, Kadin M. Aging and reactive alcoholism. Geriatr Nursing 7:148–151, 1986.
10. Atkinson RM, Tolson RL, Turner JA. Late versus early onset problem drinking in older men. Alcohol Clin Exp Res 14(4):574–579, 1990.
11. Ewing JA. Detecting alcoholism: the CAGE Questionnaire. JAMA 252:1905–1907, 1984.
12. Blow FC, Cook CA, Booth BM, Falcon SP, Friedman MJ. Age related psychiatric co-morbidities and level of functioning in alcoholic veterans seeking treatment. Hosp Commun Psychiatry 43:990–995, 1992.
13. Abrams WL, Barry KL, Fleming MF. Screening for problem drinking in older primary care patients. JAMA 276:1964–1967, 1996.
14. Fulop G, Reinhardt J, Strain JJ, Paris B, Miller M., Fillit H. Identification of alcohol and depression in a geriatric medicine outpatient clinic. J Am Geriatr Soc 41:737–741, 1993.
15. Cermak ST, Blow FC, Hill EM, Mudd SA. The relationship between alcohol symptoms and consumption among older drinkers. Alcoholism Clin Exp Res 20(7):1153–1158, 1996.
16. Brower KJ, Mudd S, Blow FC, Young JP, Hill EM. Severity and treatment of alcohol withdrawal in elderly versus younger patients. Alcoholism Clin Exp Res 18(1):196–201, 1994.
17. Liskow BI, Rinck C, Campbell J, DeSousa C. Alcohol withdrawal in the elderly. J Stud Alcohol 50:414–421, 1989.
18. Oslin DW, Pettonati H, Volpicelli JR, Katz IR. Enhancing treatment compliance in elderly alcoholics: a new psychosocial treatment model. Presented at the annual meeting of the Gerontologic Society of America, 1997.
19. Atkinson RM. Treatment programs for aging alcoholics. In: Alcohol and Aging. Beresford T, Gomberg E, eds. New York: Oxford University Press, pp 186–210, 1995.

13
Neurological Disorders and Head Injuries

David D. Weinstein and Peter R. Martin
Vanderbilt University Medical Center
Nashville, Tennessee

INTRODUCTION

> For once in his life he got a scare. The only thing he ever feared was losing his mind or destroying the responses or functions of his brain, and it looked as if he might be doing just that.
>
> *The Lost Weekend* (1)

The observations on alcohol written about decades ago in *The Lost Weekend* have with the passage of time and events become applicable to a much broader range of substances and their effects on individuals, some of which can result in short-lived or permanent central nervous system injury. In present-day psychiatry, use of the term "substance" not only refers to the 11 classes of drugs listed in the fourth edition of the *Diagnostic and Statistical Manual of Mental Disorders* (DSM-IV) (alcohol, amphetamines, cocaine, etc.) but may also include medications (prescription and over-the-counter) and toxin exposure (2). In this chapter we review some of the more common neurological consequences that may arise as a result of substance use. In addition, we consider the effects that substance abuse may have on individuals with concurrent neurological disorders. Given the complexity and interwoven nature of the substance abuse and neurological disorder interface, we hope this

TRAUMATIC BRAIN INJURY

Association with Alcohol and Drug Abuse

Traumatic brain injuries (TBIs) resulted in 34% of the injury deaths that occured in the United States in 1992 (3). A recent report that summarized TBI statistics in four states noted that transportation-related events (i.e., involving motor vehicles, bicycles, recreational vehicles, and pedestrians) were the "external cause of injury" in 48%, and falls were involved in 23% of injuries (4), findings consistent with earlier data (5).

A key factor in the association between accidents and TBI is alcohol abuse, since it places individuals at greater risk for head injury than any other factor examined, including age and occupation (5). Other studies have provided additional support for the connection between alcohol intoxication and head trauma (6–13). A host of factors contribute to this association, including the physiological effect of an increased blood alcohol concentration on trauma-avoidance behaviors, psychopathology, and acute stressful life events (14,15). Drugs other than alcohol can also result in significant perceptual disturbances in association with intoxication or withdrawal states (16), thereby contributing to TBI. In DSM-IV the nosology of substance-induced perceptual problems is divided into substance intoxication with perceptual disturbances, substance withdrawal with perceptual disturbances, and substance-induced psychotic disorder with hallucinations (2). Compared to alcohol, there are fewer studies examining non-alcohol substance-abuse-related trauma, but the available data appear to be consistent with such a link (17).

Mechanisms of Brain Injury in Substance Abuse

Clinical/Mechanical Factors

The majority of TBIs seen in civilian settings are closed head injuries (CHIs), as opposed to missile (penetrating) wounds (18). CHI can be described in terms of primary and secondary brain injury. Primary brain injury in CHI refers to damage to the brain that occurs at the moment of trauma; secondary brain injury in CHI describes injury to the brain due to events following the initial trauma. A detailed review of these issues is beyond the scope of this chapter

Neurological Disorders and Head Injuries

but can be located in the references (18–22). In the context of this subject we start with a brief review of primary brain injury in CHI, as this process is a common pathway for brain injury involving trauma—substance-abuse-related or otherwise.

Contact injuries are a category of primary brain injury that occur when the head (in a static position) is hit by a blunt object. These forces may result in skull deformation, fracture, and brain contusions directly under the area of impact. Contusions represent regions of perivascular hemorrhage of small blood vessels and brain necrosis, often located on the gyral crests, sometimes extending down to the white matter. If the damage includes disruption of the pia and arachnoid membranes, the injury is described as a cerebral laceration. Under some circumstances, contact injuries can distort the entire skull during the time of impact and lead to vault fractures in the cranium and brain contusions distant from the original site of contact. These events may be magnified further in the presence of chronic alcohol consumption, which may result in a decrease in osteoblast function with significant decrease in bone mass, resulting in a higher incidence of skeletal fractures (23–26) and exacerbation of contact trauma.

The other major etiology of primary brain injury in CHI is acceleration/deceleration forces. Since the brain is enclosed in a fluid-filled environment and attached to the cranium via the meninges, acute changes in cranial velocity and direction can lead to brain location and movement lagging behind those of the dura and skull, resulting in collision of the brain on the bony projections on the floor of the cranium (27). The anterior and inferior surfaces of the frontal and temporal lobes are the most vulnerable to acceleration/deceleration contusions from impact on the lesser wing of the sphenoid (20). These findings were reflected in an autopsy series published by Adams and coworkers, (28,29), who studied individuals with fatal CHI and found that brain contusions were most common in the frontal lobes, followed by the temporal lobes, regardless of the area of external impact. A recent study looking at neuropsychological and PET evaluations of a group of individuals with lesions of the prefrontal cortex suggested that performance of executive tasks appears to be associated with the dorsolateral prefrontal cortex (30), while orbitofrontal cortex lesions were manifested by irritability and disinhibited behaviors. Concerning temporal-lobe lesions (bilateral), apathy, affective disorders, and problems with short-term memory have been described (31); additional information on this topic is provided later in the chapter. Primary brain injury may also result in diffuse damage when rotational movement(s) are added to acceleration/deceleration forces, causing stretching and subsequent shearing of axonal tissue (diffuse axonal injury), and is associated with loss of consciousness (32–34).

Secondary brain injury occurs as a result of aftereffects of mechanical trauma causing both focal and diffuse ischemic lesions in the brain. Compromise of cerebral circulation leading to ischemia may occur from intracranial hematomas (epidural and subdural), brain swelling, increased intracranial pressure, and herniation. Hyperpyrexia, with infection or seizure activity, can increase metabolic demand and produce a relative form of ischemia (18–20). Systemic hypoxia and hypotension are frequently associated with TBI and may contribute further to this problem (18,20,21,35).

Chronic alcohol consumption can add to damage through "brain shrinkage," making bridging veins in the subdural space more vulnerable to tearing and subsequent subdural hematoma (36). Bleeding can also be exacerbated in chronic alcohol consumption by affecting platelet function, causing thrombocytopenia, and lowering liver-derived clotting factors (37,38).

Neurochemical Factors

Excitatory amino acids such as glutamate may be involved in TBI on a cellular level. Glutamate is an amino acid that is widely distributed in the brain and plays an important role in excitatory neurotransmission and memory acquisition and developmental plasticity (39–41). Different receptors for glutamate have been identified according to their varying affinities for specific glutamate agonists. One of these is the NMDA receptor, defined by the glutamate agonist N-methyl-D-aspartate (42). When glutamate binds to NMDA receptors, one of its functions is to allow intracellular influx of calcium ions through its receptor-gated channels (43). Under normal physiological circumstances, glutamatergic excitatory neurotransmission is balanced by activation of $GABA_A$, receptor-associated chloride-ion channels that augment inhibitory postsynaptic potentials (44,45). As discussed below, if this system is disrupted (with chronic ethanol use or TBI), a shift toward excitatory neurotransmission can occur, resulting in cellular damage or destruction through influx of excess calcium ions and subsequent generation of free radicals.

Free radicals of oxygen are generated as a byproduct of normal tissue metabolism (46–48). These molecules, which contain an unpaired electron, may damage membrane lipids, cellular proteins, nucleic acids, etc., through oxidation (oxidative stress). Endogenous enzymes (e.g., superoxide dismutase and glutathione peroxidase) work together with exogenous antioxidants (i.e., vitamin C and vitamin E) to inactivate free radicals and limit oxidative stress in the cellular environment (48,49).

CHI can precipitate oxidative injury via primary (mechanical) or secondary (ischemic) means since both promote calcium ion influx into neurons. Mechanical defects in neuronal membranes lead to the influx of calcium ions across a concentration gradient from the extracellular space (32,50, 51). A concurrent hypoxic/ischemic environment can elevate the extracellular level of glutamate in the brain several-fold above baseline levels (52,53), causing a supraphysiological influx of calcium ions into neurons through NMDA receptors and resulting in metabolic cell injury and death (excitotoxicity) (54–57). Voltage-dependent calcium-ion channels may join with NMDA-receptor channels to compound the calcium-ion influx into neurons (58).

This convergence of excess calcium ions inside neurons leads to activation of phospholipase A_2 with subsequent production of superoxide anions (46) and nitric oxide. Superoxide anions can then interact with nitric oxide to form highly reactive hydroxyl radicals. Arachidonic acid (59), free radicals of oxygen (60), and nitric oxide (61–63) may diffuse from their postsynaptic location, across the synaptic gap to the presynaptic area and augment further release of glutamate from the presynaptic terminal in a vicious circle (47).

Chronic alcohol consumption contributes to excitotoxicity by causing inhibition of $GABA_A$ chloride channels and thus shifting the balance toward the neuroexcitatory threshold in neurons (64,65). Other important membrane receptor changes that occur under the influence of chronic ethanol ingestion are an increase in the number of NMDA-receptor-mediated calcium-ion channels (66,67) and functional increase of calcium-ion flux through these NMDA-mediated channels (68,69). In addition, there may be an increase in the number and functional activity of a subtype of voltage-mediated neuronal-membrane calcium channels (70).

Other factors to consider as possible contributors to excitotoxicity include thiamine deficiency resulting from malnutrition (71,72) and elevated circulating glucocorticoids related to alcohol withdrawal (73). Chronic alcohol use may also interfere with defenses against oxidative injury by reducing levels of vitamin E (74,75) and decreasing activity of superoxide dismutase (76).

Neuropsychological Effects

Studies evaluating the neuropsychological effects of chronic alcohol abuse and concurrent TBI are relatively few, but are consistent in suggesting that individuals with a history of heavy ethanol use and a history of TBI reveal problem-solving and memory deficits on testing consistent with frontal-lobe and/or temporal-lobe injury (77–79), and the injury patterns caused by heavy ethanol consumption and TBI appear to be cumulative (78,80,81).

Areas of damage in the prefrontal and temporal lobes can be manifested in behavioral changes, including reduced attention, memory, and executive functioning (i.e., judgment and impulse control) (79). From a neurobehavioral viewpoint, the prefrontal lobe can be separated into four sections: superior mesial, inferior mesial, dorsolateral, and orbital (Table 1) (82). Superior mesial lesions bilaterally lead to mutism and akinesia without spontaneity. Destruction of the inferior mesial region causes memory loss, in particular, "temporal-spatial" facets of recent memory, confabulation, disinhibition, decreased motivation, and inattention.

Injury to the dorsolateral region results in cognitive deficits with decreased ability to process information, perseveration, rigidity, and poor planning. Focal damage of the orbital frontal region may cause significant changes in personality characterized by problems with adaptation to social situations and poor social judgment. The temporal lobes tend to be most affected by TBI with contusions to the anterior-inferior areas and involve control of emotions. If damage to the temporal lobes is more extensive (i.e., affecting the medial temporal and posterior inferior temporal regions), memory deficits may occur. The clinical findings described for prefrontal- and temporal-lobe lesions can also occur or be exacerbated in the presence of diffuse axonal injury due to disruption of axonal projections going to and coming from these areas of the brain (82).

Traumatic Brain Injury and Rehabilitation

The National Head Injury Foundation (NHIF) Task Force published the results of a survey on substance abuse it had conducted at head-injury rehabilitation centers across the United States (81). Seventy percent of the centers responded, constituting a patient population of more than 1500. Of note was that 55% of the respondents mentioned problems with substance abuse up to the time of

Table 1. Neurobehavioral Manifestations Seen with Frontal-Lobe Injury Sites

Site of injury	Deficits
Superior mesial	Akinesia, mutism, lack of spontaneity
Inferior mesial	Amnesia, confabulation, disinhibition, decreased motivation, inattention
Dorsolateral	Decreased ability to process information, perseveration, rigidity, poor planning
Orbital	Personality changes, poor social judgment, problems adapting to social situations

Source: Modified from Ref. 82.

their head injury (40% had moderate to severe problems with substance abuse and 15% had mild to moderate substance abuse). The NHIF study also noted that the substance of choice was alcohol in over 95% of survey responses. In a review of alcohol and drug abuse studies in physically disabled patients in rehabilitation, alcohol-associated traumatic injuries made up 79% of one rehabilitation patient population (83). Regarding studies of drugs of abuse other than alcohol, differences in data collection and outcome and small numbers of patients limit the clinical conclusions that can be drawn (83,84).

Kreutzer and coworkers surveyed patients with a history of TBI for alchol consumption before and after injury and discovered that 8–14% of participants appeared to be problem drinkers and 20% were moderate to heavy drinkers after injury (85).

Individuals with TBI and associated neuropsychological disorders may have difficulties processing information and learning new behaviors in traditional alcohol treatment programs (81,86,87). Efforts to treat substance abuse in the TBI population have been described (88–90), but their long-term results have yet to be established. A recent paper on this issue, however, suggests that structured cognitive-behavioral group psychotherapy (especially for individuals with frontal-lobe and limbic functioning affected by brain injury) may be the most effective way to treat substance abuse and anger dyscontrol, especially if combined with effective community case management (91).

SEIZURES

Determining the prevalence of specific complications in individuals who abuse substances is problematic in terms of both identifying and following them. Therefore, it is very difficult to determine the rate at which drugs of abuse precipitate seizures (92) or cause other neurological complications. In general, for clinical and etiological reasons described later, seizures associated with substance abuse can be divided into two major groups: the CNS-depressant class (i.e., alcohol/sedatives), which causes seizures as a result of withdrawal, and substances that directly cause seizure activity (e.g., cocaine and amphetamines) (92,93).

Sedative/Hypnotic Withdrawal

In 1953, Victor and Adams published a study that evaluated the clinical course of patients admitted to a hospital with alcohol-related neurological complications (94). Their report initially included 88 patients who experienced seizures characterized as being "grand mal" in type ("major generalized motor seizures with loss of consciousness"). The majority of seizures occurred within 48 hours of cessation of alcohol use. In a continuation of this study, they reported on 241 "alcoholic" patients whose course was complicated by seizure(s). Over 90% of the seizures occurred within 7 to 48 hours after cessation of drinking (95). Within the patient population described, three clinically distinct groups emerged (see Table 2). The first group of 213 patients (88.4%) was characterized as having grand mal seizures that occurred as a single seizure or in short bursts and were related to withdrawal from alcohol after chronic intoxication. Their EEG was described as normal, except in relation to their seizure(s). The two smaller groups consisted of seven patients (2.9%) with idiopathic epilepsy who developed alcoholism after occurrence of seizures and 21 patients (8.7%) with posttraumatic epilepsy and alcoholism whose seizures preceded their alcoholism. The posttraumatic group was also distinguished by a significant incidence of focal seizures and EEG abnormalities. In each of these smaller groups, seizures occurred "with or without drinking," but were more frequent and severe in withdrawal.

Isbell and coworkers (96), in the 1950s, administered alcohol to six patients on a closed ward for a minimum of 48 days and followed them after discontinuation of alcohol. "All had tremor, weakness, perspiration, nausea, vomiting, diarrhea, hyperreflexia, slight fever, elevated blood pressure and insomnia. Convulsions occurred in two." The study thus revealed under controlled conditions that the length of intoxication and the amount of alcohol consumed were directly related to the severity of the abovementioned withdrawal symptoms. Subsequent to this clinical study, a series of experiments in mice (97), dogs (98), and rhesus monkeys (99,100) confirmed the concept of the alcohol withdrawal syndrome (AWS) (101,102) and its association with seizures. Of note is that acute alcohol ingestion with high blood-alcohol concentrations can also cause seizures (103).

With the availability of newer neuroimaging techniques, (e.g., CT and MRI) it is easier to determine whether there are structural brain causes of

Table 2. Patients Whose Hospital Course Was Complicated by Alcohol-Withdrawal Seizure(s) ($n = 241$)

Alcoholic patients with seizures only following withdrawal	213 (88.4%)
Alcoholic patients with idiopathic epilepsy	7 (2.9%)
Alcoholic patients with posttraumatic epilepsy	21 (8.7%)

Source: Modified from Ref. 95.

seizures. Accordingly, the above percentage of seizures attributed to alcohol withdrawal has decreased, with approximately 70% of alcohol-related seizures secondary to withdrawal, 20% with history of head trauma as a significant potential contributing element, and the residual 10% attributed to other causes (in only 2–4% of the total did alcohol abuse precede the epilepsy) (93).

Barbiturate withdrawal syndrome is similar to AWS. It starts with tremulousness and diaphoresis, sometimes followed by seizures and delirium, and can be fatal (104,105). With benzodiazepines, withdrawal symptoms also include autonomic hyperactivity but are generally less severe (104,106,107).

As mentioned earlier, excessive, long-term ethanol consumption, with increase in number and function of NMDA and voltage-mediated calcium channels and reduction in $GABA_A$ chloride channel function, may play an important role in precipitating seizures in AWS (108,109). Use of a standardized and validated withdrawal-assessment instrument—e.g., the Clinical Institute Withdrawal Assessment for Alcohol Scale (revised) (CIWA-Ar)—can assist the clinician in determining the need to treat alcohol withdrawal and whether pharmacotherapy (i.e., benzodiazepines) is indicated (110,111). Repeated episodes of alcohol withdrawal may result in an increase in severity of the signs and symptoms of subsequent episodes of alcohol withdrawal and increase the possibility of withdrawal seizures as predicted by the kindling model (112,113). Similar effects in benzodiazepine and barbiturate withdrawal syndromes are thought to occur (114), but affect the $GABA_A$ channel in a somewhat different manner than alcohol, and require different treatment approaches (115,116).

CNS Stimulants

A second group of drugs thought to cause seizures—either as a direct effect of their actions on the CNS or secondary to their systemic effects—is further characterized below.

The largest study available on recreational drug abuse and associated seizures was conducted at San Francisco General Hospital from 1975 to 1987. This study sought to investigate the types of recreational drugs associated with acute intoxication and seizures, characterize the types of seizures, and identify possible neurological sequelae secondary to drug-induced seizures (117). During that 12-year period, 49 cases of seizures were noted in 47 patients in the series. All the seizures were described as generalized tonic-clonic, and two of the patients presented in status epilepticus (refer to Table 3 for the recreational drugs identified). Of note was that seizures occurred regardless of route of administration and in first-time as well as chronic users (all with close temporal relationship with drug use), and 46 of the 47 patients showed no

Table 3. Seizure(s) Related to Recreational Drug Use

Recreational drugs identified	Number of cases
Cocaine	32
Amphetamine	11
Heroin	7
Phencyclidine	4

Source: Modified from Ref. 117.

short-term neurological deficit following seizure(s) (117). Other surveys have also looked at cocaine-related seizures (118–121), and, based on the available literature, cocaine appears to be the most common cause of seizures related to drug intoxication (93,122). Cocaine-related seizures may be secondary to other cocaine-related complications (i.e., cerebral infarction and intracranial hemorrhage) (119) discussed later.

At the level of the synapse, cocaine acts to block reuptake of dopamine, norepinephrine, and serotonin by attaching to cocaine-specific binding sites on bioamine-uptake transporters. Cocaine also promotes the release of dopamine from granular storage vesicles (123). Despite cocaine's role of elevating intrasynaptic levels of neurotransmitters, the etiology of cocaine-related seizures appears to be the result of other etiologies (124). The sodium-channel-blocking effects of cocaine and electrophysiological data suggest that changes in sodium-channel function of CA1 hippocampal neurons occur as a consequence of chronic exposure to cocaine, resulting in an increase in voltage-dependent sodium-channel function that may precipitate/increase the potential of seizures with exposure to cocaine (125). Cocaine-induced pharmacological kindling may be involved as well. Post and coworkers reported that repetition of a previously subconvulsant dose of cocaine might cause seizures in a rat model (126). In 1992, Itzhak and Stein introduced data indicating that the NMDA receptor may be involved in cocaine kindling (127). In cortical membranes from mice treated for 7 days with cocaine, in vitro receptor binding demonstrated an increase in the number of NMDA receptors (139% over the control group). More recently, Itzhak (128) showed that cocaine-kindled mice were significantly more sensitive to the convulsive actions of an NMDA receptor agonist than saline controls.

Amphetamines appear to be a less common source of seizures based on a limited literature (117,129). Of note is that in a survey of 127 cases of amphetamine toxicity seen in an emergency department, only 3% were listed as having had seizures (130).

Amphetamines have their main effect by causing the release of catecholamines, especially norepinephrine and dopamine, from presynaptic nerve terminals in the CNS. The so-called designer amphetamines, e.g., 3,4 methylenedioxymethamphetamine (MDMA), have much the same effect in addition to release of serotonin (131). The possible mechanism resulting in amphetamine-associated seizures may also involve NMDA receptors and kindling (132). Other cortical stimulants that may cause seizures include methylphenidate and ephedrine (133).

Other Drugs

Other drugs of abuse have been associated with seizures—for example, heroin, although there is some speculation on the actual causative agents, including contaminants or other concurrent conditions (134). Meperidine (Demerol) is thought to cause seizures secondary to a potentially toxic metabolite (normeperidine). Of note is that naloxone does not treat normeperidine toxicity, and may actually worsen the situation by countering its depressant actions (135).

Intravenous mixtures of pentazocine (Talwin) and tripelennamine (pyribenzamine), also known as "Ts and Blues," have been associated with seizures. The suspension (made by crushing tablets of both drugs), even after filtering, contains particles of cellulose (used as a binder in pentazocine) and magnesium silicate/talc (used as a binder in tripelennamine). These foreign materials can cause a granulomatous reaction in the lungs and result in the formation of pulmonary arteriovenous fistulas, leading to foreign body emboli in the CNS (136).

Some patients may be receiving isoniazid for either prophylaxis or treatment of tuberculosis. Isoniazid can contribute to seizures by depleting GABA in the CNS (103).

Including the abovementioned issues, other etiologies have also been associated with alcohol-drug-induced seizures (Table 4).

Management

Presentation of a patient for management of an alcohol- or drug-related seizure involves an interdisciplinary approach, with emergency medicine, neurology, and psychiatry staff often collaborating on the diagnosis and treatment issues involved. The most important step in diagnosing such a seizure is obtaining a

Table 4. Etiologies of Alcohol-/Drug-Induced Seizures

Direct CNS toxicity
Withdrawal hyperactivity
Ischemia effects (infarct/hemorrhage)
CNS infections (systemic/embolic)
Systemic metabolic disorders
Epilepsy (idiopathic/traumatic)

Source: Modified from Ref. 93.

comprehensive history (93). Adolescents or adults who present with a first seizure should be asked about any use of over-the-counter, prescription, alcohol, or street drugs. Questioning family or friends on this (if possible) might provide valuable information, even if the patient gives a negative history. Signs of intravenous drug use or excess somnolence/confusion in the postictal state may provide important information for a diagnosis (93). Appropriate toxicology studies (i.e., blood-alcohol level and urine drug screen) are also very important in establishing an etiology. If a seizure is thought to be drug-related, psychiatric evaluation would be helpful to clarify the issue and screen for other concurrent psychiatric illnesses (e.g., mood disorder or psychosis). Acute care for drug-/alcohol-related seizure is beyond the scope of this chapter, but references are listed for further information (137–139). Treatment should be planned prior to discharge from the emergency room to provide medical and psychiatric follow-up, that is, alcohol and/or drug treatment if indicated.

STROKE

Thrombotic/Hemorrhagic Stroke

Cigarette smoking and alcohol consumption are the primary drugs of abuse associated with stroke (140,141). Also of note is the role of elevated blood pressure in the etiology of stroke. A review of several prospective studies revealed that increased systolic and diastolic blood pressure were independent risk factors for stroke and that the greater the blood pressure the greater the risk for stroke, and relative risk nearly doubles for every 10-mm elevation of diastolic blood pressure (141). Meta-analysis of 32 studies revealed a dose response between the number of cigarettes smoked and relative risk, with an overall relative risk of 50% for stroke (142). Increased stroke risk may be partly attributable to carbon monoxide in cigarette smoke, which decreases the oxygen-carrying capacity of the blood (143). Smoking increases platelet reactivity (144); chronic smoking reduces cerebral blood flow in neurologically normal individuals (145) and elevates the circulating endothelial cell count (revealing endothelial injury) (146). A potential mechanism contributing to this injury pattern may be smoking-mediated oxidative injury (147). The factors of increased platelet reactivity, decreased blood flow, and injury to the endothelium of the arterial wall all promote platelet obstruction of the vessel. This, in turn, causes platelet release of serotonin and thromboxane, leading to vasoconstriction (148). Vessels may also be affected by smoking-released enzymes that may damage elastin and collagen in their walls and possibly contribute to hemorrhage (149).

As mentioned earlier, stroke has been linked with heavy alcohol intake (150,151), possibly moderate drinking (150,152), and even occasional intoxication (153). Alcohol and withdrawal can cause cardiac-rhythm disturbances and cardiomyopathy, which both may lead to CNS emboli (154). Chronic alcohol consumption is associated with hypertension, the "dominant risk factor for stroke" (154), and may act through increasing the levels of cortisol, renin, aldosterone, and argenine vasopressin in the circulation along with increasing adrenergic activity (154). Chronic ethanol intake is also linked with decreased regional cerebral blood flow (154). When ethanol use is discontinued, post-AWS hypertension may resolve (155). With a setting of increased blood pressure and decreased platelet function, as mentioned earlier, risk of spontaneous intracranial hemorrhage is elevated (156). If a subarachnoid bleed occurs, oxyhemoglobin can release superoxide anion as it is autoxidized to methhemoglobin (148). This can result in lipid peroxidation in the arterial wall and cause endothelial damage and subsequent vasospasm, as discussed above (148).

A 9-year study of patients aged 15–44 years admitted to San Franciso General Hospital with a diagnosis of stroke (ischemic or hemorrhagic) was conducted by Kaku and Lowenstein (157). They collected data on 214 patients and found that 34% were drug abusers compared with 8% of their control group. In patients under 35, drug abuse was the most common predisposing condition (47% of patients). The risk for stroke was highest within hours of drug use. The drugs most often associated with drug-related stroke were cocaine and amphetamines, with cocaine being the most common drug used (157).

A multicenter study compared the cerebrovascular effects of cocaine hydrochloride with the alkaloidal form of cocaine, "crack" (158). The authors of that study noted that cerebral infarction was significantly higher among the crack users in their study than the cocaine hydrochloride group (even the parenteral users of the drug). A possible reason for this difference may be that, in "bypassing" hepatic metabolism, crack cocaine users can reach high brain levels of cocaine quickly (159) and potentiate some of the possible mechanisms for stroke listed below.

Strokes resulting from cocaine use are considered to be multifactorial in their etiology (160) and common factors described include vasospasm with thrombosis, intracerebral hemorrhage, and embolic strokes, each to be briefly described. Konzen and coworkers, (161) noted that cocaine potentiates the interactions of catecholamines with postsynaptic receptors and can result in vasospasm, causing ischemia. Cocaine also increases serotonin levels, which can contribute to vasoconstriction of large and medium-sized arteries of the cerebral circulation. Studies of cocaine administration in animals and cerebral angiography in patients with cocaine-associated ischemic strokes are consistent with this data, and the authors conclude that some brain infarcts among crack cocaine users result from this mechanism, in addition to secondary thrombosis (161).

Intracerebral arterioles can, under normal conditions, change their diameter with alterations in perfusion pressure to maintain cerebral blood flow at acceptable levels over a range of arterial pressures (autoregulation). If the upper limit of autoregulation is exceeded, cerebral vessels widen, blood flow increases, and risk of rupture of arterial vessels increases. Cocaine can decrease the upper limit of autoregulation and thus increase the possibility of vessel rupture at lower blood pressures (162). In addition to its effect on cerebral vascular autoregulation, cocaine can also cause an acute elevation of blood pressure and precipitate intracerebral hemorrhage (163,164). In addition to the abovementioned potential stroke factors, embolic stroke from cocaine-related cardiomyopathy with associated left ventricular thrombus (165) and septic embolic stroke from endocarditis are other possibilities to be listed in the differential diagnosis of cocaine-related stroke. Other sympathomimetics have also been linked to both ischemic and hemorrhagic cerebral infarction, including amphetamine (166), methamphetamine (167), and ephedrine (168), a nonprescription, over-the-counter drug.

Systemic Effects

Other drugs that have been associated with stroke because of their vasoconstrictive properties are lysergic acid diethylamide (LSD) (169), phencyclidine (PCP) (169), and sniffing glue containing trichlorethylene, which is known to sensitize end-organ receptors in the walls of blood vessels to the action of circulating catecholamines (170). Heroin has been associated with strokes with different etiological possibilities described, including emboli from bacterial or fungal endocarditis, ischemia due to overdose with associated hypoventilation, and drug allergy or "vessel toxicity" (171). As mentioned earlier, "T's and Blues" used intravenously (chronically) can cause pulmonary arteriovenous fistulas and subsequent embolic stroke(s) (136).

Treatment of stroke may change in the future whether secondary to substance abuse or another etiology. Increasing knowledge of the mechanisms of cell injury suggests the possibility of new and more effective treatment options for patients. Kosten (172) recently reviewed this issue and mentioned the possibility of using excitatory amino acid antagonists as well as other pharmacotherapy options in future clinical trials.

MOVEMENT DISORDERS

Alcohol

The extrapyramidal system modifies movements and maintains muscle tone and posture. In terms of clinical discussion, the most important element is the nigrostriatal system (173). As its name implies, it extends from the substantia nigra to the striatum to provide dopamine at its synapses and subsequently effects inhibition of neostriatal neurons (174). Alcohol use has been associated with both parkinsonism and dyskinesias (175,176). One group of authors commented that they had often seen "older alcoholic patients in early withdrawal with subtle signs of parkinsonism along with the more usual postural tremor, confusion, and ataxia" (175). Although the mechanism for these observations has not been resolved, some evidence points to a connection between alcohol and dopamine in the basal ganglia (175,176). Darden and Hunt (177) demonstrated a reduction in dopamine secretion from the striatum in laboratory animals administered ethanol. In addition to alcohol's apparent inhibition of striatal dopamine release, other studies have revealed striatal dopamine receptor hypersensitivity in conjunction with chronic alcohol consumption (178–180). The hypersensitivity noted was consistent with increased numbers of striatal dopamine receptors, and no change in binding affinity of these receptors was found (179).

GABA, as mentioned previously, is the main inhibitory neurotransmitter in the CNS, and one of its locations is in neurons in the striatum that project to the substantia nigra through a nigrostriatal tract. GABA may play an important role in the above-noted parkinsonian effects linked to chronic alcohol consumption by decreasing dopamine secretion in the striatum, leading to up-regulation of dopamine receptors in the striatum. Smolders and coworkers (181), presented data supporting a "tonic" inhibition by GABA of dopamine release in rat striatum. They described the dopaminergic terminals in the striatum as appearing to be controlled by GABA: "The effects via the $GABA_A$ receptor seem to be postsynaptic and dependent on an unimpaired striatonigral $GABA_A$-ergic feedback loop or striatal interneurons" (181). With these relationships in mind, one could speculate that ethanol exerts its inhibitory action on dopamine secretion in the striatum through its agonist actions on $GABA_A$.

Stimulants

Cocaine has been linked to a number of movement disorders with features that appear to be associated with excess dopamine activity (173,182). Case reports have been published that presented patients with a history of Tourette's syndrome who experienced significant exacerbation of their symptoms following cocaine use (183–185). Two of the patients in one report had no previous history of tics, but both had a history of chronic cocaine use prior to onset of tics (185). Cocaine may also precipitate choreoathetosis and akathisia, described by cocaine users as "crack dancing" (186).

Acute dystonic reactions have also been reported following chronic cocaine use. Some of these reports mention onset of dystonia shortly after discontinuation of cocaine (187,191). Others describe a significantly increased risk of dystonia in cocaine users treated with neuroleptics (192,193). The pathophysiology for these episodes is still not clear, but a recent paper summarizes the literature in addition to presenting data from an autopsy study on the brains of 12 chronic cocaine users (194). The results from the autopsy study suggested that chronic cocaine use was associated with "modestly reduced levels of striatal dopamine and the dopamine transporter in some subjects and that these changes might contribute to the neurological and psychiatric effects of the drug" (194).

Amphetamine use has also been associated with movement disorders. The presence of continuous buccal-oral movements was noted to be a characteristic sign of amphetamine abusers and thought to be helpful in diagnosis (195). In a study of the influence of amphetamine on chorea (196), patients with Huntington's chorea, patients with Sydenham's chorea, and one patient with lupus erythematosus (with right hemichorea), in addition to normal volunteers, were each given one 10-mg dose of D-amphetamine intravenously. The amphetamine worsened the chorea of the Huntington's and Sydenham's patients, but caused no movement disorders in the control group or in the unaffected side of the patient with hemichorea. Some of the patients with chorea were subsequently treated with Haldol for 1 month and then rechallenged with a dose of D-amphetamine, leading to a significant reduction in the amphetamine-induced worsening of their chorea. Given the effects of an indirect dopamine agonist (D-amphetamine) and a dopamine antagonist (Haldol), this study is consistent with a dopamine-mediated role in amphetamine-exacerbated chorea. It was also important in demonstrating that amphetamine did not produce chorea in subjects with a normal striatum, and raises the question of why amphetamine produces chorea in chronic amphetamine abusers (196).

In another paper (197), four case studies of chronic amphetamine users demonstrated choreiform/athetoid movements and ataxia. These movements began during amphetamine use and resolved in some of the patients after they stopped but in others persisted after years of abstinence (197). Choreoathetosis also appears to have been precipitated by methamphetamine use (198). In summary, the above data suggest that amphetamine-related compounds can produce movement disorders only in individuals with a striatal abnormality and that chronic amphetamine abuse may cause significant loss of function or damage to this brain region. In terms of possible mechanisms, Bartzokis and coworkers have noted that "bursts of increased dopamine metabolism increase free radical production and can cause neurotoxicity" (159). Despite suggestive clinical data and possible mechanism(s) for amphetamine-related neurotoxicity, investigations of the effects of chronic use of such compounds on dopamine receptors have been unclear, possibly because of differences in methodology (199).

Toxin Exposure

The importance of opiates in movement disorders is due mainly to the role of methyl-phenyl-tetrahydropyridine (MPTP), a synthetic opiate that can cause a parkinsonian syndrome and has been used in animals as a model for Parkinson's disease. Recent summaries of MPTP-related parkinsonism can be found in the reference section (176,200). Briefly, in terms of its clinical features, the severity of MPTP-induced parkinsonism appears to be directly related to the amount of the drug consumed. Compared to patients with Parkinson's disease, patients with MPTP-induced parkinsonism have less rest tremor but more features of depression, loss of motivation, decreased mentation, and "aberrant" sensation (176). Pathological evaluation of these patients has been limited, but appears to demonstrate loss of the neurons in the pars compacta of the substantia nigra (176,200). Biochemical studies of its neurotoxicity on dopaminergic neurons showed that MPTP is oxidized in the CNS by monoamine oxidase type B (MAOb) to 1-methyl-4-phenylpyridinium (MPP+), which is taken up by and accumulates in nigral neurons (in their striatal terminal). MPP+ then accumulates in the mitochondria of these neurons, where it inhibits cellular respiration and causes neuronal injury/destruction, resulting in its clinical manifestations of parkinsonism (176,200). The evaluation/diagnosis and treatment of this and other drug-induced movement disorders would, again, suggest a multidisciplinary approach.

REFERENCES

1. C Jackson. The Lost Weekend. New York: Farrar & Reinhart, p 233, 1944.
2. American Psychiatric Association. Diagnostic and Statistical Manual of Mental Disorders. 4th ed. Washington, DC: American Psychiatric Press, 1994.
3. DM Sosin, JE Sniezek, RJ Waxweiler. Trends in death associated with traumatic brain injury, 1979 through 1992: success and failure. JAMA 273:1778–1780, 1995.
4. Traumatic Brain Injury—Colorado, Missouri, Oklahoma, and Utah, 1990–1993. MMWR 46(1), 1997.
5. SB Sorenson, JF Kraus. Occurrence, severity, and outcomes of brain injury. Head Trauma Rehab 6:1–10, 1991.
6. Alcohol Alert—Drinking and Driving. NIAAA, no. 31, 1996.
7. G Li, GS Smith, SP Baker. Drinking behavior in relation to cause of death among US adults. Am J Public Health 84:1402–1406, 1994.
8. WH Ruthford. Diagnosis of alcohol ingestion in mild head injuries. Lancet i:1021–1023, 1977.
9. S Galbraith, AR Murray, R Knill-Jones. The relationship between alcohol and head injury and its effects on the conscious level. Br J Surg 63:128–130, 1976.
10. R Honaken, G Smith. Impact of acute alcohol intoxication on patterns of non-fatal trauma: cause specific analysis of head injury effect. Injury 22:225–229, 1991.
11. W Wechsler, EH Kasey, D Thum, HW Demone Jr. Alcohol level and home accidents. Public Health Rep 84:1043–1050, 1969.
12. HW Demone Jr, EH Kasey. Alcohol and non-motor vehicle injuries. Public Health Rep 81:585–590, 1966.
13. J Shepherd, M Irish, C Scully, L Leslie. Alcohol intoxication and severity of injury in victims of assault (brief report). Br Med J 296:1299, 1988.
14. Eighth Special Report to the U.S. Congress on Alcohol and Health from the Secretary of Health and Human Services, Sept 1993.
15. DD Weinstein, PR Martin. Psychiatric implications of alcoholism and traumatic brain injury. Am J Addictions 4:285–296, 1995.
16. RM Weinrieb, CP O'Brien. Persistent cognitive deficits attributed to substance

abuse. In: Neurologic Complications of Drug and Alcohol Abuse. Neurol Clin 11:663–691, 1993.
17. AJ Twerski. Substance abuse in head injury rehabilitation. Legal Med 93–108, 1992.
18. DI Graham, JH Adams, TA Gennarelli. Pathology of brain damage in head injury. In: Head Injury. 3rd ed. PR Cooper, ed. Baltimore: Williams and Wilkins, 1993.
19. TA Gennarelli. Mechanisms of cerebral concussion, contusion, and other effects of head injury. In: Neurological Surgery. 3rd ed. J Youmans, ed. Philadelphia: WB Saunders, 1990.
20. GF Gade, DP Becker, JD Miller, PS Dwan. Pathology and pathophysiology of head injury. In: Neurological Surgery. 3rd ed. Youmans JR, ed. Philadelphia: WB Saunders, 1990.
21. G Teasdale, D Mendelow. Pathophysiology of head injuries. In: Closed Head Injury: Psychological, Social, and Family Consequences. DN Brooks, ed. Oxford: Oxford University Press, 1984.
22. TA Gennarelli. Head injury in man and experimental animals: clinical aspects. Acta Neurochir 32(suppl):1–13, 1983.
23. DD Bickle, HK Genant, C Cann, RR Recker, BP Halloran, GJ Strewler. Bone disease in alcohol abuse. Ann Intern Med 103:42–48, 1985.
24. T Diamond, D Stiel, M Lunzer, M Wilkinson, S Posen. Ethanol reduces bone formation and may cause osteoporosis. Am J Med 86:282–288, 1989.
25. JL Gonzalez-Calvin, A Garcia-Sanchez, V Bellot, M Munoz-Torres, E Raya-Alvarez, D Salvatierra-Rios. Mineral metabolism, osteoblastic function, and bone mass in chronic alcoholism. Alcohol Alcohol 28:571–579, 1993.
26. A Garcia-Sanchez, JL Gonzalez-Calvin, A Diez-Ruiz, JL Casals, F Gallego-Ro-Jo, D Salvatierra. Effect of acute alcohol ingestion on mineral metabolism and osteoblastic function. Alcohol Alcohol 30:449–453, 1995.
27. AHS Holbourn. Mechanics of head injuries. Lancet ii:438–441, 1943.
28. JH Adams, G Scott, LS Parker, DI Graham, D Doyle. The Contusion Index: a quantitative approach to cerebral contusions in head injury. Neuropathol Appl Neurobiol 6:319–324, 1980.
29. JH Adams, D Doyle, DI Graham, AE Lawrence, DR Mc Lellan, TA Gennerelli, M Pastuszko, T Sakamoto. The Contusion Index: a reappraisal in human and experimental non-missle head injury. Neuropathol Appl Neurobiol 11:299–308, 1985.
30. M Sarazin, B Pillon, P Giannakopoulos, G Rancurel, Y Samson, B Dubois. Clinicometabolic dissociation of cognitive functions and social behavior in frontal lobe lesions. Neurology 51:142–148, 1998.
31. R Formisano, B Schmidhuber-Eiler, L Saltuari, E Cigany, G Birbauer, F Gerstenbrand. Neuropsychological outcome after traumatic temporal lobe damage. Acta Neuroclin 109:1–4, 1991.
32. TA Gennarelli. Cerebral concussion and diffuse brain injuries. In: Head Injury. 3rd ed. Cooper PR, ed. Baltimore: Williams and Wilkins, 1993.
33. TA Gennarelli, LE Thibault, JH Adams, DL Graham, CJ Thompson, RP Marcin-

cin. Diffuse axonal injury and traumatic coma in the primate. Ann Neurol 12:564–574, 1982.
34. JH Adams, DI Graham, LS Murry, G Scott. Diffuse axonal injury due to non-missle head injury in humans: an analysis of 45 cases. Ann Neurol 12:557–563, 1982.
35. J Rose, S Valtonen, B Jennett. Avoidable factors contributing to death after head injury. Br Med J 2:615–618, 1977.
36. RM Ruff, LF Marshall, MR Klauber, et al. Alcohol abuse and neurological outcome of the severely head-injured. J Head Trauma Rehab 5:21–31, 1990.
37. O Elmér, G Göransson, E Zoucas. Impairment of primary hemostasis and platelet function after alcohol ingestion in man. Haemostsis 14:223–228, 1984.
38. DH Cowan. The platelet defeat in alcoholism. Ann NY Acad Sci 252:328–341, 1975.
39. DR Curtis, GAR Johnston. Amino acid transmitters in the mammalian central nervous system. Ergebnisse der Physiologie Biologischen Chemie und Experimentellen Pharmakologie 69:98–188, 1974.
40. F Fonnum. Glutamate: a neurotransmitter in mammalian brain. J Neurochem 42:1–11, 1984.
41. JR Cooper, FE Bloom, HR Roth. The Biochemical Basis of Neuropharmacology. 6th ed. New York: Oxford University Press, 1991.
42. JC Watkins, P Krogsgaard-Larsen, T Honore. Structure-activity relationships in the development of excitatory amino acid receptor agonists and competitive antagonists [review]. Trends Pharmacol Sci 1:25–33, 1990.
43. AB MacDermott, ML Mayer, GL Westbrook, SJ Smith, JL Barker. NMDA-receptor activation increases cytoplasmic calcium concentration in cultural spinal cord neurones. Nature 321:519–522, 1986.
44. DM Lovinger. Excitotoxicity and alcohol-related brain damage. Alcohol Clin Exp Res 17:19–27, 1993.
45. RW Olsen, AJ Tobin. Molecular biology of GABA$_A$ receptors. FASEB J 4:1469–1480, 1990.
46. RA Floyd. Role of oxygen free radicals in carcinogenesis and brain ischemia. FASEB J 4:2587–2597, 1990.
47. JT Coyle, P Puttfarken. Oxidative stress, glutamate, and neurodegenerative disorders. Science 262:689–695, 1993.
48. A Bjørneboe, GEA Bjørneboe. Antioxidant status and alcohol-related diseases. Alcohol Alcohol 28:111–116, 1993.
49. WA Hunt. Role of free-radical reactions in ethanol-induced brain damage: an introduction. In: Alcohol-Induced Brain Damage. Hunt WA, Nixon SJ, eds. Washington, DC: NIAAA Research Monograph 22, 1993.
50. BK Siesjö. Cell damage in the brain: a speculative syntheses. J Cereb Blood Flow Metab 1:155–185, 1981.
51. W Young, V Yen, A Blight. Extracellular calcium ionic activity in experimental spinal cord contusion. Brain Res 253:105–113, 1982.
52. B Meldrum, MH Millan, TP Obrenovitch. Excitatory amino acid release in-

duced by injury. In: The Role of Neurotransmitters in Brain Injury. M Globus, WD Dietrich, eds. New York: Plenum, 1992.
53. R Bullock, S Butcher, D Graham, G Teasdale. Excitatory amino acid release after focal cerebral ischemia: infarct volume determines E.A.A. release. In: The Role of Neurotransmitters in Brain Injury. M Globus, WD Dietrich, eds. New York: Plenum, 1992.
54. DW Choi. Glutamate neurotoxicity in cortical cell culture is calcium-dependent, Neurosci Lett 58:293–297, 1985.
55. DW Choi. Calcium: still center-stage in hypoxic-ischemic neuronal death. Trends Neurosci 18:58–60, 1995.
56. SM Rothman, JW Olney. Excitotoxicity and the NMDA receptor-still lethal after eight years. Trends Neurosci 18:57–58, 1995.
57. WJ Goldberg, RM Kandingo, JN Barrett. Effects of ischemia-like condition on cultured neurons: protection by low Na^+, low Ca^{+2} solutions. J Neurosci 6:3144–3151, 1986.
58. A Frandsen, AJ Shousboe. Excitatory amino acid-mediated cytotoxicity and calcium homeostasis in cultured neurons. J Neurochem 60:1202–1211, 1993.
59. JH Williams, ML Errington, MA Lynch, TV Bliss. Arachidonic acid induces a long-term activity-dependent enhancement of synaptic transmission in the hippocampus. Nature 341:739–742, 1989.
60. DE Pellegrini-Giampietro, G Cherici, M Alesiani, V Carla, F Moroni. Excitatory amino acid release form rat hippocampal slices as a consequence of free-radical formation. J Neurochem 51:1960–1963, 1988.
61. FE Lancaster. Nitric oxide and ethanol-induced brain damage: a hypothesis. In: Alcohol-Induced Brain Damage. WA Hunt, SJ Nixon, eds. Washington, DC: NIAAA Research Monograph 22, 1993.
62. TJ O'Dell, RD Hawkins, ER Kandel, O Arancio. Tests of the roles of two diffusable substances in long-term potentiation: evidence for nitric oxide as a possible early retrograde messenger. Proc Natl Acad Sci USA 88:11285–11289, 1991.
63. VL Dawson, TM Dawson, ED London, DS Bredt, SH Snyder. Nitric oxide mediates glutamate neurotoxicity in primary cortical cultures. Proc Natl Acad Sci USA 88:6368–6371, 1991.
64. FT Crews, LJ Chandler. Excitotoxicity and the neuropathology of ethanol. In: Alcohol-Induced Brain Damage. WA Hunt, SJ Nixon, eds. Washington, DC: NIAAA Research Monograph 22, 1993.
65. RA Harris, AM Allan. Alcohol intoxication: ion channels and genetics. FASEB J 3:1689–1695, 1989.
66. KA Grant, P Valverins, M Hudspith, B Tabakoff. Ethanol withdrawal seizures and the NMDA receptor complex. Eur J Pharmacol 176:289–296, 1990.
67. EK Michaelis, WJ Freed, N Galton, J Foye, ML Michaelis, I Phillips, JE Kleinman. Glutamate receptor changes in brain synaptic membranes from human alcoholics. Neurochem Res 15:1055–1063, 1990.
68. KR Iorio, L Reinlib, B Tabakoff, PL Hoffman. Chronic exposure of cerebellar

granule cells to ethanol results in increased N-methyl-D-aspartate receptor function. Mol Pharmacol 41:1142–1148, 1992.
69. CT Smothers, JJ Mrotek, DM Lovinger. Chronic ethanol exposure leads to a selective enbardment of N-methyl-D-aspartate receptor function in cultured hippocampal neurons. J Pharmacol Exp Ther 283:1214–1222, 1997.
70. S Dolin, H Little, M Hudspith, C Pagonis, J Littleton. Increased dihydropyridine-sensitive calcium channels in rat brain may underlie ethanol physical dependence. Neuropharmacology 26:275–279, 1987.
71. PR Martin, BA McCool, CK Singleton. Genetic sensitivity to thiamine deficiency and development of alcoholic organic brain disease. Alcohol Clin Exp Res 17:31–37, 1993.
72. PJ Langlais, SX Zhang. Extracellular glutamate is increased in the thalamus during thiamine deficiency-induced lesions and is blocked by MK-801. J Neurochem 61:2175–2182, 1993.
73. MP Armanini, C Hutchins, BA Stein, RM Sapolsky. Glucocorticoid endangerment of hippocampal neurons is NMDA-receptor-dependent. Brain Res 532:7–12, 1990.
74. SK Majumdar, GK Shaw, AD Thomson. Plasma vitamin E status in chronic alcoholic patients. Drug Alcohol Depend 12:269–272, 1983.
75. GAE Bjørneboe, J Johnsen, A Bjørneboe, JE Bache-Wiig, J Morland, CA Drevon. Diminished serum concentration of vitamin E in alcoholics. Ann Nutr Metab 32:56–61, 1988.
76. M Ledig, J-R M'Paria, P Mandel. Superoxide dismutase activity in rat brain during acute and chronic alcohol intoxication. Neurochem Res 6:385–390, 1981.
77. BC Chandler, A Vega, OA Parsons. Dichotic listening in alcoholics with and without a history of possible brain injury. Q J Stud Alcohol 34:1099–1109, 1973.
78. DA Solomon, PF Malloy. Alcohol, head injury, and neuropsychological function. Neuropsycholog Rev 3:249–280, 1992.
79. M Oscar-Berman. The experimental analysis of cognitive deficit after head injury: perspectives from other neurological disorders and nonhuman animal research. In: Neurobehavioral Recovery from Head Injury. HS Levin, J Grafman, HM Eisberg, eds. New York: Oxford University Press, pp 178–188, 1987.
80. MP Kelly, CT Johnson, N Knoller, DA Drubach, MM Winslow. Substance abuse, traumatic brain injury and neuropsychological outcome. Brain Injury 11:391–402, 1997.
81. National Head Injury Foundation. Substance abuse task force report: white paper. Southborough, MA: NHIF, 1988.
82. ML Dombouy 1997. Tramatic brain injury. In: Principles of Neurologic Rehabilitation. RB Lazar, ed. New York: McGraw-Hill, 1997.
83. JR Hubbard, AS Everett, MA Khan. Alcohol and drug abuse in patients with physical disabilities. Am J Drug Alcohol Abuse 22(2):215–231, 1996.
84. JD Corrigan. Substance abuse as a mediating factor in outcome from traumatic brain injury. Arch Phys Med Rehabil 76:302–309, 1995.

85. JS Kreutzer, KR Doherty, JA Harris, et al. Alcohol use among persons with traumatic brain injury. J Head Trauma Rehab 5:9–20, 1990.
86. T Kupke, W O'Brien. Neuropsychological impairment and behavioral limitations exhibited within an alcohol treatment program. J Clin Exp Neuropsychol 7:292–304, 1985.
87. FR Sparadeo, D Strauss, JT Barth. The incidence, impact, and treatment of substance abuse in head trauma rehabilitation. J Head Trauma Rehab 5:1–8, 1990.
88. WF Blackerby, A Baumgarten. A model treatment program for the head injured substance abuser: preliminary findings. J Head Trauma Rehab 5:47–59, 1990.
89. M Langley, W Lindsay, C Lam, DA Priddy. A comprehensive alcohol abuse treatment program for persons with traumatic brain injury. Brain Injury 4:77–86, 1990.
90. JD Corrigan, GL Lamb-Hart, E Rust. A program of intervention for substance abuse following traumatic brain injury. Brain Injury 9:221–236, 1995.
91. RL Delmonico, P Hanley-Peterson, J Englander. Group psychotherapy for persons with traumatic brain injury: management of frustration and substance abuse. J Head Trauma Rehab 13:10–22, 1998.
92. PA Garcia, BK Alldredge. Drug-induced seizures. In: Epilepsy II: Special Issues. Neurol Clin 12:85–89, 1994.
93. MP Earnest. Seizures. In: Neurologic Complications of Drug and Alcohol Abuse. Neurol Clin 11:563–575, 1993.
94. M Victor, RD Adams. The effect of alcohol on the nervous system. Res Publ Assoc Nerv Ment Dis 32:526–573, 1953.
95. M Victor, C Brausch. The role of abstinence in the genesis of alcoholic epilepsy. Epilepsia 8:1–20, 1967.
96. H Isbell, HF Fraser, A Wikler, et al. An experimental study of the etiology of "rum fits" and delirium tremens. Q J Stud Alcohol 16:1–33, 1955.
97. DG McQuarrie, E Fingl. Effects of single doses and chronic administration of ethanol on experimental seizures in mice. J Pharmacol Exp Ther 124:264–271, 1958.
98. CF Essig, RC Lam. Convulsions and hallucinatory behavior following alcohol withdrawal in the dog. Arch Neurol 18:626–632, 1968.
99. FW Ellis, JR Pick. Ethanol-induced withdrawal reactions in rhesus monkeys. Pharmacologist 11:256, 1969.
100. FW Ellis, JR Pick. Experimentally induced ethanol dependence in rhesus monkeys. J Pharmac Exp Ther 175:88–93, 1970.
101. M Victor. Alcohol withdrawal seizures: an overview. In: Alcohol and Seizures: Basic Mechanisms and Clinical Concepts. RJ Porter, RH Mattson, JA Cramer, I Diamond, eds. Philadelphia: FA Davis, 1990.
102. M Victor. Summary: questions answered and unanswered. In: Alcohol and Seizures: Basic Mechanisms and Clinical Concepts. RJ Porter, RH Mattson, JA Cramer, I Diamond, eds. Philadelphia: FA Davis, 1990.

103. N Delanty, CJ Vaughan, JA French. Medical causes of seizures. Lancet 352:383–390, 1998.
104. FG Hofman, JH Woods, G Winger. Depressants of the central nervous system: alcohol, barbiturates, and benzodiazepines. In: A Handbook of Drug and Alcohol Abuse: Biomedical Aspects. 3rd ed. New York: Oxford University Press, 1992.
105. H Isbell, S Altschul, CH Kormetsky, AJ Eisenman, HG Flanary, HF Fraser. Chronic barbiturate intoxication. Arch Neurol Psychiatry 64:1–28, 1950.
106. RT Owen, P Tyrer. Benzodiazepine dependence: a review of the evidence. Drugs 25:385–398, 1983.
107. PR Martin, BM Kapur, EA Whiteside, EM Sellers. Intravenous phenobarbital therapy in barbiturate and other hypnosedative withdrawal reactions: a kinetic approach. Clin Pharmacol Ther 26:256–264, 1979.
108. PL Hoffman, KA Grant, LD Snell, L Reinlib, K Iorio, B Tabakoff. NMDA receptors: role in ethanol withdrawal seizures. Ann NY Acad Sci 654:52–60, 1992.
109. MA Whittington, JDC Lambert, HJ Little. Increased NMDA receptor and calcium channel activity underlying ethanol withdrawal hyperexcitability. Alcohol Alcohol 30:105–114, 1995.
110. MF Mayo-Smith. Pharmacological management of alcohol withdrawal: a meta-analysis and evidence-based practice guideline. JAMA 278:144–151, 1997.
111. RH Lohr. Treatment of alcohol withdrawal in hospitalized patients. Mayo Clin Proc 70:777–782, 1995.
112. J Ballenger, R Post. Carbanazepine in alcohol withdrawal syndromes and schizophrenic psychoses. Psychopharmacol Bull 20:572–584, 1984.
113. M Brown, R Anton, R Malcom, JC Ballenger. Alcohol detoxification and withdrawal seizures: clinical support for a kindling hypothesis. Biol Psychiatry 23:507–514, 1988.
114. DA Greenberg. Ethanol and sedatives. In: Neurologic Complications of Drug and Alcohol Abuse. Neurol Clin 11:523–534, 1993.
115. PR Martin, DM Lovinger, GR Breese. Alcohol and other abused substances. In: P Munson, RA Mueller, GR Breese, eds. Principles of Pharmacology: Basic concepts and clinical applications. New York: Chapman & Hall, pp 417–452, 1995.
116. MA Schuckit. Drug and Alcohol Abuse. 4th ed. New York: Plenum Medical, 1995.
117. BK Alldredge, DH Lowenstein, RP Simon. Seizures associated with recreational drug abuse. Neurology 39:1037–1039, 1989.
118. DH Lowenstein, SM Massa, MC Rowbotham, SD Collins, HE McKinney, RP Simon. Acute neurologic and psychiatric complications associated with cocaine abuse. Am J Med 83:841–846, 1987.
119. E Brown, J Prager, HY Lee, RG Ramsey. CNS complications of cocaine abuse: prevalence, pathophysiology, and neuroradiology. Am J Roentgenol 159:137–147, 1992.

120. M Choy-Kwong, RB Lipton. Seizures in hospitalized cocaine users. Neurology 39:425–427, 1989.
121. A Pascual-Leone, A Dhuna, I Altafullah, DC Anderson. Cocaine-induced seizures. Neurology 40:404–407, 1990.
122. RL Rodnitzky, DL Keyser. Neurologic complications of drugs: tardive dyskinesias, neuroleptic malignant syndrome, and cocaine-related syndromes. Psychiatr Clin North Am 15:491–510, 1992.
123. JCM Brust. Cocaine. In: Neurological Aspects of Substance Abuse. Woburn, MA: Butterworth-Heinemann, 1993.
124. HC Jacobson, DM Ball, DJ Nutt. Noradrenergic mechanisms appear not to be involved in cocaine-induced seizures and lethality. Life Sci 47:353–359, 1990.
125. J Zhai, SJ Wieland, FM Sessler. Chronic cocaine intoxication alters hippocampal sodium channel function. Neurosci Lett 229:121–124, 1997.
126. RM Post, SRB Weiss, A Pert. Cocaine-induced behavioral sensitization and kindling: implications for the emergence of psychopathology and seizures. In: The Mesocorticolimbic Dopamine System. PW Kalivas, CB Nemeroff, eds. Ann NY Acad Sci 537:292–308, 1988.
127. Y Itzhak, I Stein. Sensitization to the toxic effects of cocaine in mice is associated with the regulation of N-methyl-D-aspartate receptors in the cortex. J Pharmacol Exp Ther 262:464–470, 1992.
128. Y Itzhak. Cocaine kindling in mice. Mol Neurobiology 11:217–222, 1995.
129. KA Olson, TE Kearney, JE Dyer, NL Benowitz, PD Blanc. Seizures associated with poisoning and drug overdose. Am J Emerg Med 11:565–568, 1993.
130. RW Derlet, P Rice, BZ Horowitz, RV Lord. Amphetamine toxicity: experience with 127 cases. J Emerg Med 7:157–161, 1989.
131. HI Kaplan, BJ Sadock, JA Grebb. Kaplan and Sadock's Synopsis of Psychiatry: Behavioral Sciences, Clinical Psychiatry. 7th ed. Baltimore: Williams and Wilkins, 1994.
132. TB Borowski, RD Kirby, L Kokkinidis. Amphetamine and antidepressant drug effects on GABAA- and NMDA-related seizures. Brain Res Bull 30:607–610, 1993.
133. KK Jain. Drug-Induced Neurological Disorders. Seattle, WA: Hogrefe and Huber, 1996.
134. SKC Ng, JC Brust, WA Hauser, M Susser. Illicit drug use and the risk of new-onset seizures. Am J Epidemiol 132:47–57, 1990.
135. PJ Armstrong, A Bersten. Normeperidine toxicity. Anesth Analg 65:536–538, 1986.
136. LR Caplan, C Thomas, G Banks. Central nervous system complications of addiction to "T's and Blues." Neurology 32:623–628, 1982.
137. ES Freedland, DB McMicken. Alcohol-related seizures. I. Pathophysiology, differential diagnosis, and evaluation. J Emerg Med 11:463–473, 1993.
138. ES Freedland, DB McMicken. Alcohol-related seizures. II. Clinical presentation and management. J Emerg Med 11:605–618, 1993.

139. A Jagoda, L Richardson. The evaluation and treatment of seizures in the emergency department. Mt Sinai J Med 64:249–257, 1997.
140. DE Grobbee, PJ Koudstaal, ML Bots, LA Amaducci, PC Elwood, J Ferro, A Freire de Concalves, O Kruger, D Inzitari, Y Nikitin, JT Salonen, J Sivenius, W Scheuermann, DS Thelle, A Trichopoulou, JT Tuomilehto. Incidence and risk factors of ischemic and haemorrhagic stroke in Europe. Neuroepidemiology 15:291–300, 1996.
141. K-T Khaw. Epidemiology of stroke. J Neurol Neurosurg Psychiatry 61:333–338, 1996.
142. R Shinton, G Beevers. Meta-analysis of relation between cigarette smoking and stroke. Br Med J 298:789–794, 1989.
143. NL Benowitz. Pharmacologic aspects of cigarette smoking and nicotine addiction. N Engl J Med 319:1318–1330, 1988.
144. S Renaud, D Blanche, E Dumont, C Thevenon, T Wissendanger. Platelet function after cigarette smoking in relation to nicotine and carbon monoxide. Clin Pharmacol Ther 36:389–395, 1984.
145. K Kubota, T Yamaguchi, Y Abe, T Fujiwara, J Hatazawa, T Matsuzawa. Effects of smoking on regional cerebral blood flow in neurologically normal subjects. Stroke 14:720–724, 1983.
146. JW Davis, L Shelton, DA Eigenberg, CE Hignite, IS Watanabe. Effects of tobacco and non-tobacco cigarette smoking on endothelium and platelets. Clin Pharmacol Ther 37:529–533, 1985.
147. JD Morrow, B Frei, AW Longmire, JM Goziaro, SM Lynch, Y Shyr, WE Strauss, JA Oates, LJ Roberts II. Increase in circulating products of lipid peroxidation (F2-isoprostanes) in smokers. N Engl J Med 332:1198–1203, 1995.
148. T Shishido, R Suzuki, L Qian, K Hirakawa. The role of superoxide anions in the pathogenesis of cerebral vasospasm. Stroke 25:864–868, 1994.
149. R Fogelholm, K Murros. Cigarette smoking and subarachnoid hemorrhage: a population-based case-control study. J Neurol Neurosurg Psychiatry 50:78–80, 1987.
150. S Junela, M Hillbom, H Palomaki. Risk factors for spontaneous intracerebral hemorrhage. Stroke 26:1558–1564, 1995.
151. SG Wannamethee, AG Shaper. Patterns of alcohol intake and risk of stroke in middle-aged British men. Stroke 27:1033–1039, 1996.
152. CA Camargo. Moderate alcohol consumption and stroke: the epidemiologic evidence. Stroke 20:1611–1626, 1989.
153. M Hillbom, M Kaste. Ethanol intoxification: a risk factor for ischemic brain infarction. Stroke 14:694–699, 1983.
154. PB Gorelick. Alcohol and stroke. Stroke 18:268–271, 1987.
155. WT Longstraeth Jr, TD Koepsell, MS Yerby, G Van Belle. Risk factors for subarachnoid hemorrhage. Stroke 16:377–385, 1985.
156. JM MacKenzie. Intracerebral hemorrhage. J Clin Pathol 49:360–364, 1996.
157. DA Kaku, DH Lowenstein. Emergence of recreational drug abuse as a major risk factor for stroke in young adults. Ann Intern Med 113:821–827, 1990.

158. SR Levine, JCM Brust, N Futrell, LM Brass, D Blake, P Fayad, LR Shultz, CH Millikan, KL Ho, KM Welch. A comparative study of the cerebrovascular complications of cocaine: alkaloidal versus hydrochloride—a review. Neurology 41:1173–1177, 1991.
159. G Bartzokis, M Beckson, W Ling. Clinical and MRI evaluation of psychostimulant neurotoxicity. In: Neurotoxicity and Neuropathology Associated with Cocaine Abuse. MD Majewska, ed. Rockville, MD: NIDA Research Monograph 163, 1996.
160. N Martinez, E Diez-Tejedor, A Frank. Vasospasm/thrombus in cerebral ischemia related to cocaine abuse [letter]. Stroke 27:147–148, 1996.
161. JP Konzen, SR Levine, JH Garcia. Vasospasm and thrombus formation as possible mechanisms of stroke related to alkaloidal cocaine. Stroke 26:1114–1118, 1995.
162. K Kibayashi, A Mastri, C Hirsch. Cocaine induced intracerebral hemorrhage: analysis of predisposing factors and mechanisms causing hemorrnagic strokes. Hum Pathol 26:659–663, 1995.
163. L Caplan. Intracerebral hemorrhage revisited. Neurology 38:624–627, 1988.
164. JR Mangiardi, M Daras, ME Geller, I Weitzner, AJ Tuckman. Cocaine related intracranial hemorrage: report of nine cases and review. Acta Neurol Scand 77:177–180, 1988.
165. CM Sauer. Recurrent embolic stroke and cocaine-related cardiomyopathy. Stroke 22:1203–1205, 1991.
166. MM El-Omar, K Ray, R Geary. Intracerebral haemorrhage in a young adult: consider amphetamine abuse. Br J Clin Pract 50:115–116, 1996.
167. DJ Yen, SJ Wang, TH Ju, CC Chen, KK Liao, JL Fuh, HH Hu. Stroke associated with methamphetamine inhalation. Eur Neurol 34:16–22, 1994.
168. A Bruno, KB Nolte, J Chapin. Stroke associated with ephedrine use. Neurology 43:1313–1316, 1993.
169. BT Altura, BM Altura. Phencyclidine, lysergic acid diethylamide, and mescaline: cerebral artery spasms and hallucinogenic activity. Science 212:1051–1052, 1981.
170. MJ Parker, MJ Tarlow, JM Anderson. Glue sniffing and cerebral infarction. Arch Dis Child 59:675–677, 1984.
171. JCM Brust, RW Richter. Stroke associated with addiction to heroin. J Neurol Neurosurg Psychiatry 39:194–199, 1976.
172. TR Kosten. Pharmacotherapy of cerebral ischemia in cocaine dependence. Drug Alcohol Depend 49:133–144, 1998.
173. DM Kaufman. Involuntary movement disorders. In: Clinical Neurology for Psychiatrists. 4th ed. Philadelphia: WB Saunders, 1995.
174. RD Adams, M Victor. Abnormalities of movement and posture due to disease of the extrapyramidal motor systems. In: Principles of Neurology. 5th ed. New York: McGraw-Hill, 1993.
175. J Neiman, AE Lang, L Fornazzari, PL Carlen. Movement disorders in alcoholism: a review. Neurology 40:741–746, 1990.

176. F Cardoso, J Jankovic. Movement disorders: neurologic complications of drug and alcohol abuse. Neurologic Clin 11:625–638, 1993.
177. JH Darden, WA Hunt. Reduction of striatal dopamine release during an ethanol withdrawal syndrome. J Neurochem 29:1143–1145, 1977.
178. S Liljequist. Changes in the sensitivity of dopamine receptors in the nucleus accumbens and in the striatum induced by chronic ethanol administration. Acta Pharmacol Toxicol 43:19–28, 1978.
179. H Lai, MA Carino, A Horita. Effects of ethanol on central dopamine functions. Life Sci 27:299–304, 1980.
180. J Balldin, C Alling, CG Gottfries, G Lindstedt, G Langstrom. Changes in dopamine receptor sensitivity in humans after heavy alcohol intake. Psychopharmacology 86:142–146, 1985.
181. I Smolders, N DeKlippel, S Sarre, G Ebinger, Y Michotte. Tonic GABAA-ergic modulation of striatal dopamine release studied by in vivo microdialysis in the freely moving rat. Eur J Pharmacol 284:83–91, 1995.
182. FEC Cardoso, J Jankovic. Cocaine-related movement disorders. Mov Disord 8:175–178, 1993.
183. MM Mesulam. Cocaine and Tourette's syndrome [letter]. N Engl J Med 315:398, 1986.
184. SA Factor, JR Sanchez-Ramos, WJ Weiner. Cocaine and Tourette's syndrome [letter]. Ann Neurol 23:423–424, 1988.
185. A Pascual-Leone, A Dhuna. Cocaine-associated multifocal tics. Neurology 40:999–1000, 1990.
186. M Daras, BS Koppel, E Atos-Radzion. Cocaine-induced choreoathetoid movements ("crack dancing"). Neurology 44:751–752, 1994.
187. J Merab. Acute dystonic reaction to cocaine [letter]. Am J Med 84:564, 1988.
188. D Rebischung, M Daras, AJ Tuchman. Dystonic movements associated with cocaine use [abstr]. Ann Neurol 28:266, 1990.
189. M Choy-Kwong, RB Lipton. Dystonia related to cocaine withdrawal: a case report and pathogenic hypothesis. Neurology 39:996–997, 1989.
190. K Kumor. Cocaine withdrawal dystonia [letter]. Neurology 40:863, 1990.
191. SL Satel, AL Swann. Extrapyramidal symptoms and cocaine abuse [letter]. Am J Psychiatry 150:347, 1993.
192. K Kumor, M Sherer, J Jaffe. Haloperidol-induced dystonia in cocaine addicts [letter]. Lancet ii:1341–1342, 1986.
193. AM Hegarty, RB Lipton, AE Merriam, K Freeman. Cocaine as a risk factor for acute dystonic reactions. Neurology 41:1670–1672, 1991.
194. JM Wilson, AI Levey, C Bergeron, K Kalasinsky, L Ang, F Peretti, VI Adams, J Smialek, WR Anderson, K Shannak, J Deck, HB Niznik, SJ Kish. Striatal dopamine, dopamine transporter, and vesicular monoamine transporter in chronic cocaine users. Ann Neurol 40:428–439, 1996.
195. GW Ashcroft, D Eccleston, JL Waddell. Recognition of amphetamine addicts [letter]. Br Med J 1:57, 1965.

196. HL Klawans, WJ Weiner. The effect of D-amphetamine on choreiform movement disorders. Neurology 24:312–318, 1974.
197. H Lundh, K Tunving. An extrapyramidal choreiform syndrome caused by amphetamine addiction. J Neurol Neurosurg Psychiatry 44:728–730, 1981.
198. LS Sperling, JL Horowitz. Methamphetamine-induced choreoathetosis and rhabdomyolysis [letter]. Ann Intern Med 121:986, 1994.
199. LS Seiden, KE Sabol. Methamphetamine and methylenedioxymethamphetamine neurotoxicity: possible mechanisms of cell destruction. In: Neurotoxicity and Neuropathology Associated with Cocaine Abuse. MD Majewska, ed. Rockville, MD: NIDA Research Monograph 163, 1996.
200. S Przedborski, V Jackson-Lewis. Mechanisms of MPTP toxicity. Mov Disord 13:35–38, 1998.

Index

Abuse, 242, 259
Acamprosate, 28
Acetylcholine (ACh) receptors, 43
Acquired immunodeficiency syndrome (AIDS), 204–239
ACTH, 44
Acting out, 174, 273
Addiction, 2, 259
Addiction psychiatry, 2
Addiction Severity Index (ASI), 22, 115
Adolescents, 133–167
Adolescent substance use disorder, 133–167
Adrenergic blocking agents, 27
Adrenocorticotropine hormone (ACTH), 83
Aerosol abuse, 45
Affective disorders, 6
African-Americans, 207
Aftercare, 28
Aggression, 125, 141

Agoraphobia, 17, 149
AIDS, 6
AIDS dementia complex, 211
AIDS Initial Assessment Questionnaire (AIA), 209
AIDS Risk Inventory (ARI-I), 209
AIDS-related illnesses, 205
Airplace crashes, 6
Akathesia, 28, 81
Alanine amino-transferase, 3
ALANON, 25
Alcohol, 18, 28, 65, 78, 85, 117, 146, 147, 180, 182, 221, 249, 256, 271, 278, 281, 284, 291
Alcohol abuse, 1, 7, 61, 62, 66, 146
Alcohol dependence, 146, 150, 153, 221
Alcohol heart-muscle disease (AHMD), 183
Alcohol-induced pseudo-Cushing's syndrome, 186
Alcohol intoxication, 7, 34, 35

307

Alcohol Urge Questionnaire (AUQ), 2
Alcohol Use Disorder and Associated Disability Interview Schedule (AUDADIS), 4
Alcohol use disorders, 5, 6, 34, 169, 174
Alcohol Use Disorders Identification Test (AUDIT), 2
Alcohol withdrawal syndrome (AWS), 36, 284
Alcoholic cardiomyopathy, 185
Alcoholics anonymous (AA), 25, 29, 118, 123, 171, 176, 222, 274
Alcoholism, 6, 34, 36, 59, 61, 64, 105, 106, 126, 134, 169, 174
Alcoholism in men, 36
Alcoholism in women, 36
Alcohol-related pancreatitis, 257
Alcohol-related seizures, 285
1-Alpha-acetylmethodol (LAAM), 28
Alpha$_2$-agonists, 27
Alpha$_2$-blocking agents, 27
Alpha-bungalotoxin, 88
Alprazolam, 26
Amotivational syndrome, 39, 40, 110
Amphetamine abuse, 78
Amphetamine challenge, 84
Amphetamine(s), 78, 84, 206, 258, 286, 287, 290, 292
Anemia, 13
Anger, 174
Anticonvulsants, 70, 247
Antidepressant medication, 23, 25, 27, 45, 46, 142, 242
Antihistamines, 23, 25
Antioxidants, 182
Antisocial behaviors, 119, 135, 137
Antisocial personality disorder (ASPD), 105, 134, 135
Antispasmodic agent, 247
Anxiety, 115, 135, 242
Anxiety disorders, 5, 11–32, 78, 149, 217, 242
Apomorphine, 83

Arachidonic acid, 281
Arterial embolization, 194
Aspartate amino transferase, 3
Ataxia, 291
Atrial fibrillation, 185, 186
Attention, 81
Attention deficit disorder, 141
Attention deficit hyperactivity disorder (ADHD), 134, 135, 139, 141
Atypical antipsychotic drugs, 89
Atypical depression, 41
AUDIT, 3
AUQ, 3
Avoidant personality disorder, 104, 121
Axis I disorders, 121
Axis I disorders in childhood, 111
Axis II diagnosis, 107, 114, 116
Axis II personality disorder(s), 106, 107, 119, 121
Axis II personality disorder (ASPD), 107
AZT, 194, 226

Barbiturate withdrawal syndrome, 285
Beck Depression Inventory (BDI), 38, 215
Behavioral disinhibition, 111
Behavioral sensitization, 82, 84, 89
Behavioral therapy, 24, 138
Benzodiazepine receptors, 40
Benzodiazepines, 25, 29, 46, 68, 217, 242, 248, 256, 285
Bereavement, 214
Beriberi, 184
Berkson's bias, 62
Beta-adrenergic blockers, 23, 25, 27
Beta-adrenergic receptor(s), 43, 185
Binge drinking, 180
Bipolar disorder, 6, 13, 59–75, 143
Bipolar disorder, type I, 6, 60
Bisexual men, 205
Blackouts, 39
Blood-brain barrier, 211

Index

Borderline personality disorder (BPD), 107, 213, 214
Bradycardia, 27
Brain infarcts, 290
Brain reward mechanisms, 45
Brain swelling, 280
Brain-mediated pathways, 218
Brief MAST, 2, 22
Brief psychiatric rating scale (BPRS), 80
Brief Symptom Inventory (BSI), 115
Buprenorphine, 28
Buspirone, 25
Butorphanol (Stadol), 251

CA1 hippocampal neurons, 286
Caffeine, 17, 21, 29, 105
CAGE questionnaire, 2, 21, 269, 270
Calcium channels, 281
Calcium-ion channels, 281
CALDATA Study, 19
California Psychological Inventory Socialization Scale, 117
cAMP-regulated phosphoproteins, 45
Cancer pain relief program of the world health organization, 251
Cancer, 243
Cannabinoid antagonist SR 141716A, 87
Cannabinoid withdrawal, 40
Cannabis abuse, 6, 78, 85, 86, 134, 179, 190, 258
Cannabis-induced dilated cardiomyopathy, 191
Cannaboid use disorders, 6
Carbamazepine, 70, 126, 226
Carbohydrate-deficient transferrin (CDT), 3
Carbon tetrachloride, 45
Carboyhemoglobin, 190
Cardiac antiarrhythmics, 23, 188
Cardiomyopathy, 183, 289
Cardioprotection, 182, 187
Cardiovascular disease, 179–202

Carpal tunnel syndrome, 245
Case management, 274
Casual models, 143, 150
Catecholamine reuptake, 42
Catecholamines, 44, 290
Categorical diagnoses, 119
Caucasians, 207
Causalgia, 245
CD4 cell count, 212
CD4+ cell counts, 210
CD4+ T-lymphocyte count, 205
Ceiling effect, 252
Center for Education and Drug Abuse Research (CEDAR), 136
Centers for Disease Control and Prevention (CDC), 205
Central dopaminergic effects, 188
Cerebrovascular disease, 188
Cervical cancers, 205
c-fos, 89
Childhood abuse, 147
Childhood anxiety disorders, 150
Childhood trauma questionnaire, 148
Chocolate, 29
Chronic pain, 241-263
Cirrhosis, 6
Cirrhotic cardiomyopathy, 185, 193
Citalopram, 27
Classical psychoanalytical treatment, 171
Clonazepam, 26, 248
Clonidine, 27
Clozapine, 89, 90
Cluster A personality disorders, 104, 126
Cluster B personality disorders, 104, 113, 126
Cluster C personality disorders, 104, 125
personality disorders, 104
Cocaine, 17, 65, 78, 81, 84, 179, 187, 188, 192, 206, 219, 220, 249, 258, 286, 289, 290, 292
Cocaine abuse, 7, 41, 62, 81, 188

Codeine, 44, 251, 254
Cognitive-behavior therapy (CBT), 24, 25, 117, 118, 120, 122, 123, 149
Cognitive impairments, 211, 212
Comorbidity, 2, 4, 34, 35, 77, 211
Conduct disorder (CD), 134, 135
Confusion, 43
Consolidation therapies, 24
Contact injuries, 279
Contaminated needles, 205
Convulsions, 284
Cookers, 209
Coping styles, 115, 116
Coping-skills therapy, 25
Coronary artery disease, 179, 180
Cortical system, 243
Corticotropin-releasing factor, 42
Cost-benefit ratio, 271
Countertransference, 175
CPK, 188
Crack, 220, 289
Crash, 42
Craving, 42, 82, 254
Criminality, 1
Cultural factors, 225
Cushing's disease, 13
Cyclothymia, 62
Cytochrome p450 3A3/4, 226
Cytochrome p450 3A4, 226
Cytomegalovirus, 218

D_1 receptors, 90
D_2 receptor, 89, 90
D_2-receptor agonist, 87
D_2-receptor binding, 84
D-amphetamine, 293
DAST, 3
Deep venous thromboses, 186
Delirium, 28, 191
Delta-9-tetrahydrocannabinol (THC), 40
Dementia, 212
Denial, 269
Dependence, 2, 104, 242, 259

Depression, 5, 33–58, 115, 118, 135, 214, 216, 242
Desipramine, 27
Detoxification, 22, 25, 46
Dexamethasone suppression test (DST), 37, 83
Dextroamphetamine, 216
Diabetes mellitus, 270
  diabetic neuropathy, 245
Diagnostic and Statistical Manual of Mental Disorders (DSM-IV), 12, 16, 104, 242, 265, 277
Diagnostic Interview Schedule (DIS), 39, 255
Dialectic behavioral treatment (DBT), 214
Diaphragmatic breathing, 24
Diazepam, 248, 256
Dihyrocodeine, 251
Dilated cardiomyopathy, 183, 186
Dimensional approach, 119
Disability, 179
Disinhibited behavior, 134
Disulfiram, 28, 226
Doctor-shopping, 253
Dopamine (DA), 27, 42, 188
Dopamine receptors, 39, 84, 87, 89, 90, 291
Dopamine system, 40
Dopamine-2 receptor antagonist, 26
Dorsal column, 243
Dorsal lateral tract, 243
Doxepine, 27
Drinking problem, 169
Drownings, 6
Drug abuse, 278
Drug Abuse Screening Test (DAST), 2, 22
Drug craving, 17
Drug interactions, 226
Drug traffickers, 206
Drug use disorders, 6
Drug Use Screening Inventory, 153
Drug-free periods, 112

Index

Drug-induced parkinsonism, 80
Drugs of abuse, 83
Dry beriberi (Peripheral neuropathy), 185
DSM-IV, 2, 16, 21, 40, 105, 278
Dual diagnoses, 5, 16, 59, 110
Dyskinesias, 291
Dysphoria, 34, 45
Dysthymia, 36, 41, 143, 245

ECA, 19
ECT, 38
EEG, 248, 284
Ejection fraction, 191
Elderly, 265–276
Emboli, 289, 291
Embolic stroke, 290
Emotional expression, 174
Emotional healing, 7
Endocarditis, 193, 290
Endocrine disorders, 13
Ephedrine, 290
Epidemiologic Catchment Area survey (ECA), 4, 60, 77, 105
Epilepsy, 13
Epstein-Barr virus, 218
Ethanol, 179, 180
Executive function, 81
Exposure techniques, 24
Extrapyramidal side effects, 79, 81

Face-recognition test, 81
False positives, 2
Familial risk, 86
Family history, 64
Female drug users, 63
Fentanyl (Sublimimaze), 252
Fetal transmission, 208
Fibromyalgia, 245
Fluoxetine, 27
Free radicals, 280
French paradox, 181

G proteins, 45

GABA, 291
GABA neurotransmitter system, 248
$GAGA_A$ chloride channels, 281
Gamma-glutamyl-transpeptidase (GGT), 3
Gastroesophogeal reflux, 270
Gay men, 205, 213
Gender, 63
Generalized anxiety disorder (GAD), 12, 25, 149, 217
Glucocorticoids, 84, 85, 281
Glutamate, 280
Glutamatergic excitatory neurotransmission, 280
Grandiosity, 110
Group psychotherapy, 28
Group sessions, 69
Growth hormone, 44
Guided imagery, 24

Halfway houses, 28
Hallucinogen use disorders, 7, 78, 134
Hallucinogens, 46
Haloperidol, 82, 89
Hamilton Anxiety Rating Scale, 150
Hamilton Depression Rating Scale (HDRS), 36
Harvard Anxiety Research Project (HARP), 18
Head injuries, 6, 277–305
Healthcare costs, 1, 19
Heart attack, 179
Heart failure, 6, 183
Heat/cold, 249
Hepatitis B, 218
Heroin, 192, 206, 219, 287
Heroin abuse, 7
Heroin addicts, 219
Heroin overdose, 193, 194
High average risk (HAR), 136
High-output state, 185
High-risk behaviors, 209
High-risk sexual activity, 209, 220
Histrionic personality disorders, 104

HIV, 194
HIV counseling, 210
HIV dementia complex, 212
HIV encephalopathy, 205
HIV risk in mothers, 208
HIV Risk-Taking Behavior Scale (HRBS), 209
HIV-1-associated cognitive/motor complex, 211
HIV-associated dementia, 211
HIV-positive patients, 213
Holiday heart dysrhythmias, 186
Holiday heart syndrome, 185
Homeostasis, 170
Homosexual activity, 204
Homosexual men, 213
Homovanillic acid (HVA), 83
5-HT levels, 187
5-HT$_{1A}$ receptor, 90
5-HT$_{2A}$ receptor, 89, 90
Human Immunodeficiency Virus (HIV), 203-239
Hydrocodone, 251
Hydromorphone (Dilaudid), 252
5-Hydroxyindoleacetic acid (5-HIAA), 38
Hyperactivity, 141
Hyperlipidemia, 185
Hyperphagia, 42
Hypersomnia, 42
Hypertension, 186, 270, 289
Hyperthyroidism, 13
Hyperventilation, 24
Hypoglycemia, 13
Hypotension, 27
Hypothalomic-pituitary-adrenal (HPA), 83
Hypothermia, 7

Illicit drug use, 7
Imipramine, 27
Immune system, 208
Immunosuppression, 218
Impulsive personality disorders, 112

Impulsiveness, 35
Impulsivity, 125, 141, 213
Inattention, 141
Inhalant abuse, 7, 45
Inhaled nitrate drugs, 223
Injection drug, 205, 220
Injection drug use, 204
Injection drug users (IDUs), 206
Insomina, 43
Interactive model, 112
Interpersonal therapy, 124
Intervention challenges, 267
Isolation, 214

J-shaped curve, 186
Juvenile offenders, 138

Karnofsky Scale of Physical Performance, 215
Kindling, 286
K-SADS, 150

LAAM, 126
Lateral spinothalamic tract, 243
Legal problems, 114
Lethargy, 42
Levorphenol (Levo-Dromoran), 252
Limbic system, 47, 243
Lithium, 68, 70, 126
Liver disease, 184
Liver transaminases, 70
Lorazepam, 26
Low average risk (LAR), 136
Low-density lipoprotein (LDL), 182
Lung disease, 191
Lymphadenopathy, 204
Lysergic acid diethylamide (LSD), 46

Major depression, 13, 33, 36, 45, 46, 60, 143, 145
Major depression (posttraumatic), 134
Major depressive disorder, 6, 245
Maladaptive behavior, 122
Male-to-male sexual behavior, 221

Index

Malnutrition, 281
Maltrexone, 226
Mania, 60, 61, 115, 216
MAOIs, 27
Marginalization, 214
Marijuana, 7, 39, 85, 86, 110, 146, 190, 249, 257, 258
Marijuana abuse, 7, 86
Marijuana withdrawal syndrome, 39
Meclofenamate, 247
Melancholia, 41
Menopause, 266
Mental Disorders in Adolescents, 133–167
Meperidine (Demerol), 255, 287
Mesenteric ischemia, 189
Mesolimbic DA system, 84
Mesolimbic dopamine (DA) neurons, 82
Methadone, 28, 44, 126, 226
Methadone (Dolophine), 252
Methadone maintenance, 219
Methamphetamine, 290
Methamphetamine, 293
3-Methoxy-4-hydroxyphenylglycol (MHPG), 38
3,4-Methylenedioxymethamphetamine (MDMA, Ecstasy), 46
Methylphenidate, 216
1-Methyl-4-phenylpyridinium (MPP+), 294
Methyl-phenyl-tetrahydropyridine (MPTP), 293
Methylxanthines, 29
MHPG, 42
Michigan Alcoholism Screening Test (MAST), 2, 3, 21, 270
Michigan Alcoholism Screening Test-Geriatric Version (MAST-G), 269
Microangiopathic hemolytic anemia, 194
Microemboli, 194
Migraine headaches, 13
Mini-mental state examinations, 81

Minor depression, 35
Misoprostol, 247
Misuse, 242, 259
Mitral valve prolapse, 13
Mixed Mania, 64
Mixed opiate agonist-antagonists, 251
Mixed states, 66
MMPI, 259
Moderate drinking, 180
Monoamine oxidase type B (MAOb), 294
Mood disorders, 135, 143
Mood stabilizer, 70
Mood stabilizers, 126
Mood-stabilizing medications, 243
Morphine, 84, 192, 252
Motivational enhancement therapy (MET), 118
Motor vehicle deaths, 6
Movement disorders, 291, 292
Motor vehicle injuries, 6
Multicenter AIDS Cohort Study, 212
Multidimensional treatment programs, 155
Multiple sexual partners, 208
Multisystemic treatment, 138
Muscle damage, 243
Muscle relaxants, 247
muscle-strain syndromes, 245
Mycotic aneurysms, 194
Myocardial infarction, 188
Myofascial pain, 244, 245, 247

NA, 29
Nalbuphine (Nugain), 251
Naltrexone, 28, 126, 219
Narcissistic personality disorder, 104, 107
Narcotics Anonymous (NA), 25
National AIDS Demonstration Research Projects, 222
National Comorbidity Survey (NCS), 4, 16, 60

Index

National Head Injury Foundation (NHIF) Task Force, 282
National Institute of Mental Health Epidemiologic Catchment Area Program (ECA), 16
National Longitudinal Alcohol Epidemiological Survey (NLAES), 4
Natural-killer-cell activity, 218
Necrotizing angitis, 194
Needle and syringe exchange programs (NSEPs), 223
Needle exchange, 223
Needles, 209
Negative emotional states, 135
Negative life events, 35
Negative symptoms, 79
Nerve damage, 243
Neurobiological mechanism, 23, 38
Neurohormonal systems, 125
Neuroimaging techniques, 284
Neuroleptic-induced dysphoria, 81
Neuroleptics, 28, 83, 91, 126
Neurological Disorders, 277–305
Neuropathic pain, 244, 245, 247
Neuropeptide Y, 42
Neuropsychological Impairment Scale (NIS), 212
Neurotoxicity, 293
Neurotransmitter receptors, 23
Neurotransmitter systems, 34, 38, 62
Neurotransmitters, 45, 286
Nicotine, 21, 29, 43, 78, 83, 87, 105
Nicotine dependence, 150
Nicotine withdrawal, 43, 44
Nicotinic receptors, 88
Nigrostriatal DA neurotransmission, 89
Nitric oxide, 281
N-methyl D aspartate (NMDA), 211, 280, 281
Nonaffective psychosis, 6
Noncompliance, 29
Nonsteroidal anti-inflammatory drugs (NSAIDs), 247
Nonverbal memory tests, 213

Noradrenergic systems, 17
Norepinephrine (NE), 27, 42, 188
Nortriptyline, 27
Nutritional deficiencies, 183

Obsessive-compulsive, 104
Obsessive-compulsive disorder (OCD), 12, 25, 119, 149
Odds ratio (OR), 5
Opiate abuse/dependence, 45, 252, 254
Opiates, 44, 179, 192, 218, 242, 248,
Opiate-withdrawal, 45
Opioids, 82, 192
Oppositional defiant disorder (ODD), 134, 135
Organic brain syndromes, 13
Oxycodone, 254, 255
Oxydodone (Roxicodone), 252

Pain disorder associated with both psychological factors and a general medical condition, 245
Pain disorder associated with psychological factors, 245
Pain medications, 29
Pain pathways, 243
Pancreatitis, 270
Panic attacks, 28
Panic disorder, 12, 17, 149
Panic reactions, 191
Paranoia, 86, 111, 114, 119, 125, 191
Paranoid personality disorder (PPD), 86, 104, 111, 119
Parent training, 142
Parkinsonism, 28, 80, 291
Paroxetine, 27
Passive-aggressive personality disorder, 104
Passivity-withdrawal, 110
Pathological personality processes, 105
Pathophysiology, 82
Peer pressure, 28
Pentazocine (Talwin), 251, 287
Pentozocine, 255

Index

Peptide systems, 42
Personality, 103
Personality characteristics, 170
Personality clusters, 103
Personality dimensions, 125
Personality disorders, 103–131
    phantom pain, 245
Pharmacotherapies, 25
Phencyclidine (PSP), 46
Phenelzine, 27
Phenylalanine, 38
Pheochromocytoma, 13
Phobias, 6, 12
Phobic avoidance, 177
Phospholipase A$_2$, 281
Physical disabilities, 6, 7
Physical therapy, 249
Pill popping, 250
Pittsburgh Adolescent Alcohol Research Center (PAAR), 136
Platelet activity, 182
Pneumonia, 205
Polysubstance dependence, 15
Positive re-enforcing effect, 81, 82
Positive symptoms, 79
Posterior thalamus, 243
    postherpetic neuralgia, 245
Postsynaptic alpha$_2$-adrenoceptor, 39
Posttraumatic stress disorder (PTSD), 6, 12, 25, 135, 145
Prefrontal cortex, 82
Presynaptic nicotinic receptors, 44
Prevention, 222
Primary brain injury, 279
Primary depression, 37
Primary-secondary depression dichotomy, 37
Profile of Mood States (POMS), 40
Progressive muscular relaxation, 24
Project Match, 118
Propoxphene, 255
Propoxyphene (Darvon), 251

Psychiatric Research Interview for Substance and Mental Disorders (PRISM), 3
Psychoanalysis, 170
Psychoanalytical approaches, 176
Psychoanalytical therapy, 177
Psychoanalytically informed treatment, 169–178
Psychoanalytical treatment, 169–178
Psychogenic pain, 245
Psychological treatments, 151
Psychopathology, 19, 34, 80, 154, 211
Psychosis, 28, 66
Psychosocial programs, 90
Psychosomatic, 245
Psychostimulants, 83, 216, 258
Psychotherapy, 24, 69, 142, 175, 177, 220
Psychotic mania, 66
Psychotic symptoms, 83
PTSD, 28, 147
Puerto Rican Americans, 207
Pulmonary hypertension, 186
Pulmonary tuberculosis, 205

QT interval, 189
Quinpirol, 87

Rage, 174
Rapid cycling, 64, 65, 66
Rational Recovery, 25
Receptor down-regulation, 27
Receptor-gated channels, 280
Receptor mechanisms, 89
Receptor sensitivity, 23
Red wine, 187
Reflex sympathetic dystrophy, 245
Regressions, 174
Rehabilitation, 7, 274
Rehabilitation patients, 6
Rehabilitation program, 90
Relapse prevention, 274
Relationship enhancement (RE), 117
Relationship-focused treatment, 124

Relationship problems, 242
REM sleep, 42
Research Diagnostic Criteria (RDC), 35
Rey Verbal Memory Task, 212
Rhabdomyolysis, 193
Rifampin, 226
Right-heart failure, 186
Risk assessment, 209
Risk factors, 63
RISK for AIDS Behavior Scale (RAB), 209
Risk-reduction counseling, 224
Rotator cuff injury, 245

Scale for the assessment of negative symptoms, 80
Scale for the assessment of positive symptoms, 80
Schedule for Affective Disorders and Schizophrenia (SADS), 35
Schedule for Affective Disorders and Schizophrenia for School-Age Children—Present and Lifetime Version (K-SADS-PL), 148
Schedule for Affective Disorders and Schizophrenia-Lifetime (SADS-L), 44
Schizoid personality disorder, 86, 104, 106
Schizotypal personality disorder, 86, 108
Schizophrenia, 6, 77-101, 115
Schizotypal personality disorder, 104, 121
Screening Tests, 2
Secondary anxiety, 18
Secondary brain injury, 280
Secondary depression, 37, 41
Secondary-gain issues, 246
Sedation, 28
Sedative abuse, 46
Sedative/hypnotic withdrawal, 283

Seizures, 283, 285, 286, 287
Selective serotonin-reuptake blockers (SSRIs), 25, 126, 217
Self-centeredness, 110
Self-esteem, 170
Self-help groups, 29
Self-medication, 62, 81, 141, 147, 242
Septic emboli, 194
Serotonin, 27, 38, 42, 47, 187
Serotonin deficiency, 38
Sertraline, 27
Sex for drugs, 220
Sexual abuse, 146, 147
Sexual behavior, 221
Sexual risk behaviors, 210
Sexuality, 220
Shooting galleries, 206
Sigma opiate receptors, 45
Sinus tachycardia, 190
Sleep apnea, 185
Smokers, 80, 190
Smoking, 29, 43, 78, 88, 266, 288, 289
Snake neurotoxin, 88
Social competence, 148
Social pathology, 175
Social phobia, 25, 121
Social Phobia and Anxiety Inventory, 150
Social support, 214
Sociopathy, 117, 118
Specific phobias, 149
Specificity, 2
Speedball, 207
Spinal cord injury, 6, 7
Splitting, 214
Standardized risk assessments, 209
Staphylococcus aureus, 193
State Trait Anxiety Inventory for Children, 150
12-step facilitation, 118
Stimulant-abstinence cycle, 42
Stimulant-associated paranoia, 111
Stimulants, 17, 40, 110, 285, 292

Index

Stress, 83, 85
Stress reduction, 182
Stressful life event, 83
Stressors, 65
Stroke index, 191
Stroke, 186, 187, 288, 289
Structured Clinical Interview for DSM-III (SCID), 41
Structured Clinical Interview for DSM-IV Disorders (SCID), 3
Subdural hematoma, 280
Substance abuse, 7, 14, 68, 77, 78, 169, 242, 259
Substance use disorders, 6, 13, 15, 33
Substance-abusing pregnant population, 208
Substance dependence, 14
Substance-induced anxiety disorder, 17
Substance-related disorders, 5
Suicidal attempts, 35, 89
Suicidal ideation, 214
Suicide, 32, 66, 79, 214
Suicide rate, 39
Supersensitivity, 43
Supraventricular tachydysrhythmias, 185
Symbol digit testing, 213
Sympathoadrenal discharge, 190
Symptom Checklist 90 (SCL-90), 45

Tardive dyskinesia, 28, 79, 80
Temporomandibular joint dysfunction syndrome (TMJ), 245
Tendinitis, 245
Tension headache, 245
Tetrahydrocannabinol (THC), 87
Theophylline, 29
Therapeutic communities, 28
Therapeutic community, 219
Therapeutic relationship, 172
Thiamine deficiency, 184
Thoracic outlet syndrome, 245
Thrombi, 186

Thyroid-releasing hormone (TRH), 37
Thyroid-stimulating hormone (TSH), 37
T-lymphocyte counts, 218
Toxin exposure, 293
Trail-making, 81, 213
Transcutaneous electrical nerve stimulation, 249
Transdermal fentanyl, 252
Tranylcypromine, 27
Trauma, 146, 187
Trauma history, 145
Traumatic brain injury, 278, 282
Traumatic experiences, 147
Traumatic injury, 6
Traumatic nest, 266
Trazodone, 27
Treatment Improvement Protocol (TIP), 19
Treatment-resistant depression, 47
Tricyclic antidepressants (TCAs), 27, 217, 247
Triggers, 115
Tripelennamine (pyribenzamine), 287
Tryptophan, 38
Tryptophan pyrrolase activity, 38
TSH, 41
12-Step facilitation (TSF), 118
Type B alcoholic, 114
Type II alcoholic, 114
Tyrosine, 38
Tyrosine hydroxylase, 45

U- or J-shaped curve, 180
Ulcers, 270
Unipolar depression, 38, 78
Urine drug screens (UDSs), 4, 22
Urine toxicological screens, 22
U-shaped curve, 180

Valproic acid (valproate), 68, 70, 126
Vascular disease, 183
Vasopressin, 44

Ventral tegmentum, 82
Verbal fluency, 81
Verbal recall, 81
Victimization, 147
Violent behavior, 1, 79
Viral hepatitis, 193
Vitamin E, 281

Weight gain, 28
Wernicke-Korsakoff, 185

Wet beriberi (congestive heart failure), 185
Wine drinking, 181
Withdrawal, 23
Withdrawal symptoms, 217
Withdrawn personality disorders, 113
Working memory, 81

Zidovudine (AZT), 208, 213